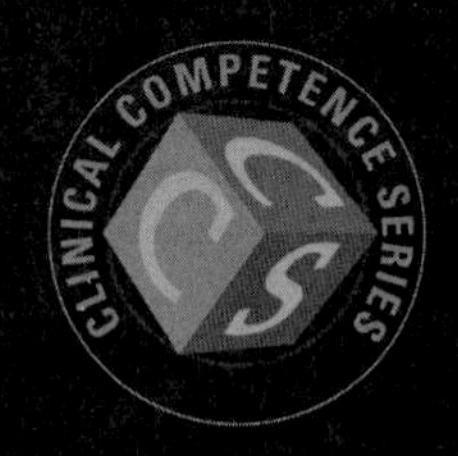

Medical Speech-Language Pathology

A Desk Reference

THIRD EDITION

Lee Ann C. Golper

Clinical Competence Series

Series Editor
Robert T. Wertz, PhD

Medical Speech-Language Pathology: A Desk Reference, 3rd ed.
Lee Ann C. Golper, Ph.D.

Approaches to the Treatment of Aphasia
Edited by Nancy Helm-Estabrooks, Sc.D., and Audrey C. Holland, Ph.D.

Assessment and Intervention Resource for Hispanic Children
Hortencia Kayser, Ph.D.

Clinical Manual for Laryngectomy and Head/Neck Cancer Rehabilitation, 2nd ed.
Janina K. Casper, Ph.D., and Raymond H. Colton, Ph.D. with contributions from Carla DeLassus Gress, Sc.D.

Developmental Reading Disabilities: A: Language Based Treatment Approach, 2nd ed.
Candace L. Goldsworthy, Ph.D.

Manual of Articulation and Phonological Disorders: Infancy Through Adulthood, 2nd ed.
Ken M. Bleile, Ph.D.

Manual of Stuttering Intervention
Patricia M. Zebrowski, Ph.D. and Ellen M. Kelly, Ph.D.

Manual of Voice Treatment: Pediatrics Through Geriatrics, 3rd ed.
Moya L. Andrews, Ed.D.

For more information on Delmar Cengage Learning's Clinical Competence Series, please log on to www.delmar/healthcare.com.

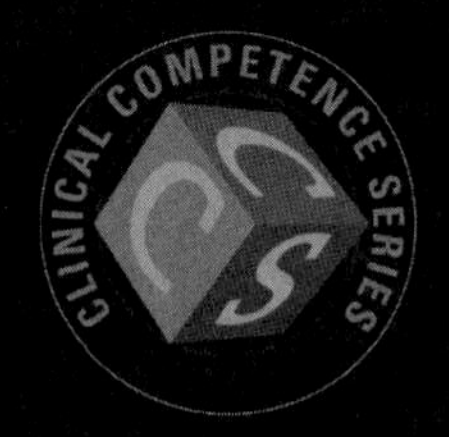

Medical Speech-Language Pathology

A Desk Reference

THIRD EDITION

Lee Ann C. Golper, PhD
Professor
Director, Speech-Language Pathology Clinical Division
Department of Hearing and Speech Sciences
School of Medicine
Vanderbilt University

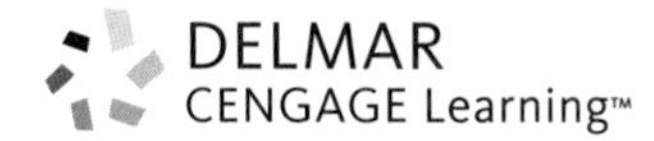

Australia • Brazil • Japan • Korea • Mexico • Singapore • Spain • United Kingdom • United States

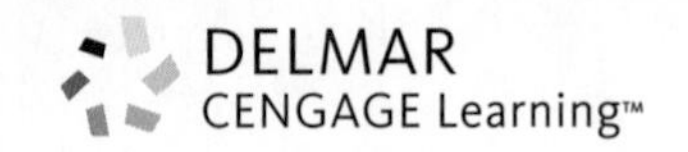

Medical Speech-Language Pathology: A Desk Reference, Third Edition
Lee Ann C. Golper, PhD

Vice President, Career and Professional Editorial: Dave Garza

Director of Learning Solutions: Matthew Kane

Senior Acquisitions Editor: Sherry Dickinson

Managing Editor: Marah Bellegarde

Product Manager: Laura J. Wood

Editorial Assistant: Anthony R. Souza

Vice President, Career and Professional Marketing: Jennifer McAvey

Executive Marketing Manager: Wendy E. Mapstone

Senior Marketing Manager: Kristin McNary

Marketing Coordinator: Scott A. Chrysler

Production Director: Carolyn Miller

Production Manager: Andrew Crouth

Senior Content Project Manager: Elizabeth C. Hough

Senior Art Director: David Arsenault

Library of Congress Control Number: 2009922775

ISBN-13: 978-1-4283-4057-2

ISBN-10: 1-4283-4057-2

Delmar
5 Maxwell Drive
Clifton Park, NY 12065-2919
USA

Cengage Learning is a leading provider of customized learning solutions with office locations around the globe, including Singapore, the United Kingdom, Australia, Mexico, Brazil, and Japan. Locate your local office at:
international.cengage.com/region

Cengage Learning products are represented in Canada by Nelson Education, Ltd.

To learn more about Delmar, visit **www.cengage.com/delmar**

Purchase any of our products at your local college store or at our preferred online store **www.ichapters.com**

Notice to the Reader

Printed in Canada
1 2 3 4 5 6 7 13 12 11 10 09

CONTENTS

FOREWORD

com•pe•tence (kom' pə təns) n. The state or quality of being properly or well qualified; capable.

Clinicians crave competence. They pursue it through education, experience, evidence, emulation, and innovation. Some are more successful than others in attaining what they seek. This book, titled ***Medical Speech-Language Pathology: A Desk Reference,*** is a third edition of the previously published texts titled ***Sourcebook for Medical Speech-Language Pathology***, by Lee Ann C. Golper. Like the first and second editions, the third edition's purposes are to keep speech-language pathologists current, competent, and afloat in the depths of medical environments. For over 30 years, Dr. Golper has mended speech and language deficits, administered clinical programs, taught generations of students, and conducted clinical research in a variety of medical settings. When she speaks, I listen. When she writes, I read. Herein is the information that makes speech-language pathologists in medical settings infinitely more knowledgeable about what their medical and allied health colleagues do than either knows about what speech-language pathologists do. Herein are the terminology, procedures, and practices that significantly increase the probability of the successful practice of Speech-Language Pathology in medical environments. Your attention to what Dr. Golper provides indicates your competence and your effort to improve it, because competent clinicians seek competence as much as for what it demands as for what it promises.

Robert T. Wertz, PhD

Co-Series Editor

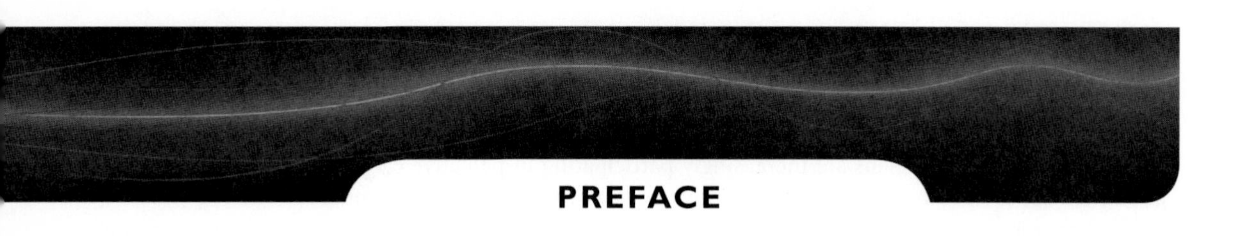

PREFACE

The practice of *medical* speech-language pathology includes the evaluation and treatment of communication, cognition, and swallowing within the context of medical conditions. In medical settings, the speech-language pathologist's (SLP's) treatment decisions may directly affect health and safety as well as communication; thus, clinicians who work in medical settings should have a basic understanding of the conditions that bring patients to the hospital or clinic and what is being done to manage them. This text is intended to provide that *basic* understanding with a handy reference for clinicians who are practicing or are in training to practice speech-language pathology in hospitals and in other health care-related facilities, such as rehabilitation programs, private practice, outpatient clinics, nursing homes, and home health agencies. It is also intended as a desk reference for clinicians who work in school and preschool settings, where children with medically related communication and swallowing disorders are a part of the caseload.

In my practice over the past 30 years as a clinician, teacher, supervisor, and administrator, I have often puzzled over medical chart notes, trying to decipher abbreviations, symbols, and terminology, and I have sat through conferences wondering, "What does that word mean?" "What does that finding reveal?" I have read, and undoubtedly written, reports containing incorrect uses of medical terminology. I have written background summaries containing abstracted medical histories that listed two names for the same disease. But, probably worst of all, I may have unwittingly made recommendations regarding communication or swallowing management that were contraindicated by the patient's medical status. Through a great deal of trial and an embarrassing amount of error, I gradually learned to communicate—to interpret and present information—in a credible manner in the hospitals where I have worked. I have had to ask a lot of questions and consult a lot of references through the years. In an attempt to become more comfortable with a medically oriented practice, I have acquired a substantial library of resource materials, textbooks, manuals, dictionaries, hospital memos, charts and illustrations, PowerPoint handouts, lecture notes, and so on, which were consulted in the preparation of this text. As a gauge for deciding what to include in each edition of this text, I have drawn on comments and observations of my coworkers and from student clinicians and included information that reflected their needs, problems, and confusions. One of the nice features of technological advances since preparing the last edition of this text 10 years ago is the ease of access to electronic libraries and reference articles. If I ran into an inconsistency, needed to check the spelling of a word, or wanted to find out about a new procedure, I could "Google it" and instantly find hundreds of links and articles on the topic. Increasingly, we literally have the information we need at our fingertips. For example, at my medical center the electronic patient record provides links to medical terminology and the current, recommended evidence-based, management of many diseases.

Reflected in this third edition is the vastly changed role of the SLP in the neonatal intensive care unit and inpatient services in children's hospitals. Information related specifically to newborns and young children has been added to nearly every chapter. Additionally, tremendous medical advances have occurred over the past decade, particularly in two areas of medicine—genetics and oncology. Accordingly, a new chapter has been added related to *Medical Genetics* (Chapter 6), and the chapter on *Oncology* (Chapter 12) has been expanded to include current therapies. The SLP affiliation with geriatric medicine has also expanded; thus, a chapter on *Rehabilitation Medicine and Geriatrics* (Chapter 14), specialties that share many principles and practices, was added. That chapter includes a discussion of biomedical ethics and end-of-life issues across the life span, because clinicians are increasingly participating in palliative care teams, particularly when patients choose to have their end-of-life hospice care in a hospital or nursing home.

New terminology, abbreviations, and medical tests and procedures have been added, and errors in previous editions that somehow escaped multiple sets of editing eyes in the earlier editions have been corrected. My hope is that this version is flawless, but no textbook is perfect and this type of text is particularly challenging to edit given all of the lists of terminology, abbreviations, glossaries, and details. Experts disagree as to how to define medical terms. In those cases, we have looked at multiple resources (listed at the end of each text) for a general consensus agreement. Ultimately, when there were questions about spelling, usage, or definitions, we opted to let *Taber's Cyclopedic Medical Dictionary* (19th edition) serve as the final arbiter.

Due to the comprehensive and broad brush scope of this text, the definitions and descriptions contained in it are, by necessity, terse, and superficial. Be cautioned that this book was written by a medical *speech-language pathologist.* Nearly every definition or brief description contained in this text should be read with the caveat, "Of course, it is a lot more complicated than that!" When a complex medical condition, for example, *leukemia*, is reduced to a one-sentence quick reference definition, the result will be incomplete and sorely in need of further elaboration. Additional reference texts and medical authorities should be consulted. Each chapter and Appendix A were initially read by at least one subject matter expert and then reviewed by the Series Editor (Robert T. Wertz, PhD), a medical content editor, and copy editors. Any queries that emerged from those reviews were checked against other references and my "in house" medical expert (Thomas A. Golper, MD), who read all of the chapters in this edition. It was he who made the observation found in Chapter 1 that most physicians know far less about the practices of speech-language pathology than SLPs know about medicine.

Finally, we should recall that this text is a general desk reference *about medical practices.* It is *not about how to practice* medical SLP. Presumably, knowledge and principles and practices about medical SLP have been acquired in graduate classes and clinical practica, during Clinical Fellowships, and in postgraduate courses. Comprehensive texts covering medical SLP practices with children and adults are available. Most are cited in this text. Other texts, including some in the Clinical Competence Series, focus on SLP practices with particular clinical problems and disorder populations, such as pediatric dysphagia, voice disorders, laryngectomy, videoendoscopy, and others. This book is intended to complement texts on clinical-medical practices in SLP. The information included here and the terminology reviewed cover topics and facts about medical care delivery and procedures that seemed important, or at least potentially useful, for clinicians to know or have readily available. The content of some of the chapters includes a review of related "fundamental principles" to add some background and context across the disorders or practices and terminology found in those chapters or to better prepare clinicians to understand that medical specialty better. Some of the information in this text is intended for reference only, and some could be viewed as rarely needed but "nice to know." Most of the information contained in this text applies directly to the day-to-day work life of a medical SLP.

This text has been given an updated title, *Medical Speech-Language Pathology: A Desk Reference*, but as with the previous editions, the overriding purpose of this text is to advance the practices of SLP clinicians and help them to become comfortable with the principles and practices found in hospitals and related settings so they can practice their profession and take their place among other health care providers with confidence and competence.

ACKNOWLEDGMENTS

This third edition has built upon the material contained in the first and second editions with new sections added where needed and deletions, corrections, updates, expansions, and clarifications made on the original text. This text contains previously published and new material, data, and figures adapted from other sources or reproduced with permission for this edition. The attributions for these sources are cited and any prepublished material is used with the author's gratitude. The array of reference texts that were consulted in preparing this desk reference are listed following each chapter (References and Resources Consulted). I am most grateful to the Delmar Cengage Learning reviewers whose comments were addressed in this edition and to all of the support I received from the Delmar Cengage editors in its preparation. I am especially grateful to the medical artists who revised several of my hand-drawn figures from previous texts.

I remain indebted to my longtime friend and mentor, Robert T. (Terry) Wertz, PhD, for all of his support and help in this project and in so many other areas of my career. I was offered the opportunity to write the first edition of this text in 1987 at his invitation. I doubt if he expected his obligation as editor to carry well into his retirement! I also remain grateful to those people who helped with the expert reviews of the first and second editions of this text: Marvin N. Golper, MD (deceased); Lillian O. Seligman, MS, CCC-SLP; Suzanne Boone, RD; Nancy Owen, RD; Bernie McIntyre, RD; Lisa Green, RD; Janice Sargent, RN, NP; Pamela Hagen, RN; Ann Teaford, OTR; Jane Salat, PT; Kara Carr, MD; Todd Kirchoff, MD; and Dennis Briley, MD. For her guidance with the Medical Genetics chapter of this text, sincere thanks are extended to my colleague in the Vanderbilt University Department of Hearing and Speech Sciences, Linda Hood, PhD. And I am eternally grateful to my husband, Thomas A. Golper, MD, for his careful reading and editing of this edition and for bringing its content into the twenty-first century.

Reviewers

Delmar Cengage Learning would like to extend appreciation to the following reviewers for their valuable feedback during the revision process:

Alice P. Armbruster, MA, CCC-SLP
Lead Hospital SLP and Student Intern Supervisor
Mayo Clinic Arizona Hospital
Phoenix, Arizona

Patti Bailey, MS, CCC-SLP
Speech Pathology Coordinator
Greater Baltimore Medical Center
Baltimore, Maryland

Stephanie M. Bednar, MA, CCC-SLP
Speech and Language Program Specialist
Osceola District Schools
Kissimmee, Florida

Jane Clem, MA, CCC-SLP
Instructor and Clinical Director of USD Scottish Rite Children's Clinic
University of South Dakota
Vermillion, South Dakota

Melinda Corwin, PhD, CCC-SLP
Assistant Professor, Department of Speech, Language, and Hearing Sciences
Texas Tech University Health Sciences Center
Lubbock, Texas

Cheryl Gunter, PhD, CCC-SLP
Professor of Communicative Disorders, Department of Communicative Disorders
West Chester University
West Chester, Pennsylvania

Melissa Rose, MEd, CCC-SLP
Clinical Instructor, Communication Disorders
Georgia State University
Atlanta, Georgia

DEDICATION

To the memory of my mother, Georgia Lee,
and with love always to my husband and children,
Tom, Stefanie, and Zach

ABOUT THE AUTHOR

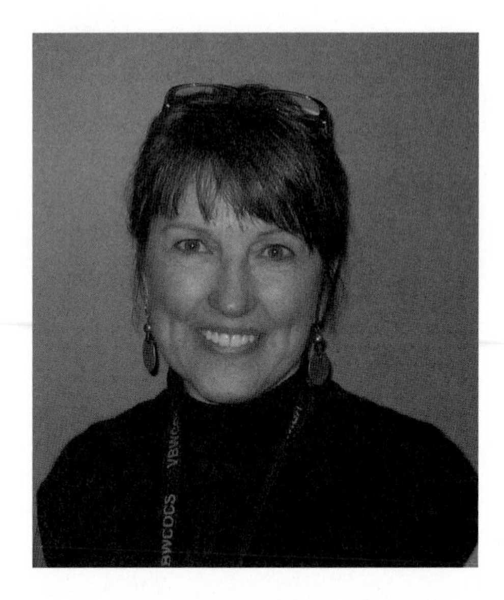

Lee Ann C. Golper, PhD, CCC-SLP, BC-ANCDS

lee.ann.golper@vanderbilt.edu

Lee Ann C. Golper is a professor in the Department of Hearing and Speech Sciences (DHSS), Vanderbilt University, School of Medicine, and the Administrative Director of SLP Clinical Programs at the Vanderbilt Bill Wilkerson Center. She received her academic training from Indiana University (BA, 1971), Portland State University (MS, 1976), and University of Oregon (PhD, 1982) and completed clinical fellowships in the Portland VA Medical Center (1976) and the University of Oregon for Health and Sciences, Child Development and Rehabilitation Center (1977). She has worked as a clinician, an administrator, and a member of the faculty for over 30 years in academic medical center settings and has published and presented in the areas of neurologic communication disorders, medical speech-language pathology, evidence-based practices, professional issues, and health services delivery. Dr. Golper is Board Certified by the Academy of Neurologic Communication Disorders and Sciences; she is a Fellow of the American Speech-Language-Hearing Association, a Scientific Fellow of the American Academy of Otolaryngology/Head and Neck Surgery, and a Fellow of the American Heart Association-American Stroke Association.

CHAPTER 1

Speech-Language Pathology in Medical Settings

In medical settings, **speech-language pathologists (SLPs)** do essentially what they do in any of their other professional work settings. They assess communication and swallowing status; provide information to confirm or establish a diagnosis; and select, plan, and, when appropriate, implement treatment to improve communication, cognitive, or swallowing functions. **Medical SLPs** work with individuals who have communication, cognitive, and swallowing disorders resulting from diseases and other medical conditions. They work mainly in acute, subacute, or postacute care medical settings such as **hospitals, rehabilitation facilities, home health agencies, outpatient clinics, long-term care** and **skilled nursing facilities**, and **private practice**. Medical SLPs also provide services to clients with medically related conditions in settings that are not strictly "medical," such as day care centers, preschools, public and private schools, and early intervention programs.

I. CHAPTER FOCUS

This chapter describes the medical work environment, including the range of professionals who treat the different types and severities of illnesses. The terminology and abbreviations related to professional preparation and credentialing, the financial and administrative aspects of health service delivery, and the descriptions of the range and rankings for the levels of care are provided.

II. SPEECH-LANGUAGE PATHOLOGY IN MEDICAL SETTINGS

A. Concurrence, Cooperation, and Coordination

In the majority of medical settings, SLPs see patients only by referral. SLPs are required to work on the "order" and explicit concurrence of physicians, even though the physicians may know less about the practices of speech-language pathology than the SLPs know about medicine.

Diagnostic, treatment, and even screening services provided by SLPs in medical settings usually require a written order from the patient's physician. In some settings, a **physician's assistant (PA)**, a **nurse practitioner (NP)**, or an **advanced practice nurse (APN)** may also have privileges to write orders.

In hospitals, physicians are the only health care professionals with **admitting privileges** (allowed to admit patients under their care to the facility). The levels of privileging in hospitals are discussed later in this chapter, but by virtue of their licenses, staff appointment, credentialing, and privileging rank, physicians have the ultimate say about what transpires during the course of their patients' hospital stays. They also carry the ultimate **risk management** burden for any problems that may arise during the hospitalization. Physicians and nurses appreciate that cognitive-communicative processes and swallowing abilities are important to the health and well-being of their patients. SLP services are particularly valued when those services contribute to reducing the length of stay (LOS), facilitate discharge planning, reduce the occurrence of medical complications such as pneumonia, and enhance the outcome of medical management.

Medical SLPs collaborate closely with other members of the health care team. Collaboration with the nursing staff is essential to ensure that the SLP recommendations are followed. During hospitalizations, nurses have ongoing and frequent contact with patients and are in direct communication with families and physicians throughout the day. Although physicians and nurses are the central members of the care team, medical SLPs spend a considerable amount of time obtaining concurrence, cooperation, and coordination with many other disciplines.

Collaboration with staff in providing nutrition services is necessary in order to have food prepared and presented in the manner that may be managed best by the patient. Collaboration with case managers and staff providing social work services helps to ensure that the patient has access to continued speech-language rehabilitation after discharge. Scheduling visits for assessment and therapy when the patient is least fatigued and maximally alert often requires working cooperatively with nursing and staff from other rehabilitation therapy services. Treatment of the ventilator-dependent patient in an intensive care unit may require coordinating visits with the pulmonologist or the respiratory therapist. Diagnostic evaluations of persons with dysphagia often require coordination with their physicians, nursing staff, radiology staff, and dietitians.

B. Scope of Practice and Responsibilities

The following outline lists the areas of concern and types of referrals made to the SLP who works in a medical facility. The publication *Scope of Practice in Speech-Language Pathology* (American Speech-Language-Hearing Association [ASHA], 2001) as well as ASHA position papers and policies on the roles, knowledge, skills, and competencies that are required in order to work with specific conditions or perform specific procedures may be obtained from the ASHA's Web site (http://www.asha.org/). A comprehensive discussion of the scope of practice in speech-language pathology and a wide range of professional issues can be found in *Professional Issues in Speech-Language Pathology and Audiology* (Lubinski, Golper, & Frattali, 2007).

1. Mental Status Assessment

Brief bedside screenings or more formal standardized assessments of attention, memory, orientation, and communication are frequently required to determine the patient's mental status as it relates to his or her level of cognitive recovery from acquired brain injuries, readiness for rehabilitation efforts, amount of assistance required for feeding, and discharge planning.

2. *Swallowing and Feeding Evaluation and Treatment*

SLPs are frequently asked to evaluate a patient's swallowing ability, identify the presence of dysphagia, or "rule out" (RO) the presence or risks of aspiration. Evaluation usually begins with a review of the patient's medical record; interviews with the ward staff, patient, and family; and a noninstrumental or **clinical (bedside) assessment**. Although a noninstrumental evaluation may be viewed as preliminary, it is a comprehensive assessment and should not be described as "screening." The clinical assessment includes evaluating the patient's oral motor and sensory functions and the structures of the mouth, pharynx, and larynx. Any evidence of factors that are likely to compromise safe oral intake, including respiratory or laryngeal compromise such as labored breathing, coughing, "wet-sounding" phonation and the inability to phonate a vowel for at least 10 seconds, are identified. The characteristics of the gag reflex response and observations of the patient's level of alertness, mental vigilance, orientation, verbal (auditory and written) comprehension, and fatigue level are noted. As mentioned earlier, the swallowing evaluation includes a review of the patient's medical record to determine the current diet orders, nutritional status and needs, and any medical concerns or precautions related to nutrition and hydration. All of these factors are considered to determine the next steps and recommendations, including the instrumental studies of swallowing status such as a **videofluoroscopic swallow study (VFSS)** and a **fiberoptic endoscopic evaluation of swallow (FEES)**.

The management of dysphagia, or swallowing status, requires the ability to recognize the indicators for a good or poor prognosis of a patient to regain functional swallowing and the potential to benefit from treatment designed to improve swallowing and reduce the risks of aspiration. Treatment may include recommending dietary adjustments and teaching the patient or caregivers how to use facilitative feeding procedures or adaptive devices. Treatment may also include training in swallow safety precautions and procedures; behavioral programs and sensory therapies for problem eaters; oral, pharyngeal, or laryngeal neuromotor and sensory stimulation therapies; and consideration of alternative methods of nutrition and hydration support, such as nonoral feeding tubes or **enteral feeding**. In **neonatal intensive care units (NICUs)** or **pediatric intensive care units (PICUs)** SLPs may select the preferred methods, nipples, and timing and duration of feedings, or supervise the infants' feedings and work with other specialists such as a **lactation nurse specialist**.

3. *Neurogenic Language Disorders*

Diagnostic assessment of neurogenic language disorders involves a brief nonstandardized bedside assessment and a more comprehensive standardized language testing. Neurogenic language disorders include **aphasia** and other language impairments associated with the cognitive-communicative deficits frequently found with **right hemisphere brain damage, traumatic brain injury (TBI), dementias**, and other acquired conditions. SLPs may, for example, differentiate frank language impairment typical of acute focal neurologic damage from delirium and confused language caused by metabolic disorders. Diagnosing the type of communication disorder, determining candidacy for treatment, selecting and implementing the appropriate treatment for neurogenic language disorders, and providing education and counseling for family members about the communication disorders and the expected improvement are provided by SLPs.

4. *Neurogenic Speech Disorders*

Like neurogenic language disorders, neurogenic speech disorders, or **motor speech disorders**, require skilled assessment, differential diagnosis, and, when appropriate, treatment by an SLP. Assessment involves a standard oral motor examination and speech intelligibility assessment, which may be performed at bedside. Assessment may also require instrumental evaluation of phonation, resonance, velopharyngeal sufficiency, respiration function, and perceptual or acoustic analysis of speech. Treatment may require highly skilled procedures that should be performed only by trained providers (e.g., the application of *Lee Silverman Voice Therapy [LSVT]®* techniques with parkinsonism). When speech intelligibility is severely impaired, treatment may require selecting, programming, and training the patient to use an **augmentative or alternative communication (AAC)** device or nonoral method of communication. These AAC speech aids range from simple picture, symbol, and alphabet boards to computerized systems capable of communicating complex ideas and language structures. The selection depends on the patient's functional communication needs and visual, motor, and cognitive abilities.

5. *Assessment and Treatment of Cognitive Status*

In acute care settings, referrals to the SLP for an evaluation of speech, language, and cognitive status may be a routine part of the "care pathways" for certain diagnoses (see Chapter 2). SLPs are usually involved in the standard care pathway assessments or screenings made with patients who have had cerebrovascular accidents (CVAs) and head injuries, or SLP services may be ordered when there has been an acute change in communication or cognitive status. In some settings, there may be "standing orders" for SLPs to see all patients admitted with a given diagnosis, such as TBI, or once a patient reaches a certain level on the **Rancho Levels of Cognitive Functioning** (see Chapter 4). Assessment and treatment of cognitive-communicative disorders is a part of the scope of care provided by the SLP. Services range from procedures explicitly aimed at improving orientation, attention, vigilance, and other cognitive functions or to providing education and counseling to family members about the nature of the disorder and the expected course of recovery.

6. *Voice and Resonance Disorders*

SLPs in medical settings work closely with otolaryngologists when evaluating and determining treatment options for voice and resonance disorders. Evaluation requires specialized knowledge of articulatory, phonatory, and respiratory anatomy and physiology as well as skill in instrumental assessments (such as computerized "speech lab" *acoustical analysis*, and the use of *nasometry, nasendoscopy*, and *laryngostroboscopy*). The physician uses many of the same instrumental assessments to make a medical diagnosis of the voice and resonance disorder that the SLP uses to evaluate the behavioral side of the disorder and any structural and functional abnormalities that affect phonation and resonance to determine the appropriate treatment and evaluate treatment outcomes. The SLP's assessment includes listing the *perceptual characteristics* of phonation and resonance, deciding whether they deviate significantly from normal, and determining the adequacy of phonation and resonance for an individual's everyday communication or other voice use (public speaking, singing) needs. The SLP also assists in differentiating a nonorganic functional disorder (e.g., hyperfunctional misuse of the voice) from an organic (e.g., neurologic) condition.

Speech treatment for individuals with voice and resonance disorders requires specialized knowledge and familiarity with various forms of medical and surgical procedures employed by otolaryngologists and other surgeons to improve velopharyngeal and laryngeal adequacy. Palatal surgery may be required to correct velopharyngeal insufficiency, and phonosurgery may be performed to improve vocal fold functions. Clinicians should also have knowledge of pharmacologic and other nonsurgical medical therapies for disorders of the vocal folds and pharynx, for example, treatment for **gastroesophageal reflux disorder (GERD)**. The SLP brings to the team unique skills in the *behavioral management* of voice and resonance disorders secondary to functional or organic causes that may bring about more normal sounding phonation and resonance; reduce the habitual, behavioral factors contributing to the voice disorder; eliminate or reduce the need for surgery in certain conditions; and, if surgery is required, produce an optimal postsurgical outcome.

7. *Pre- and Post-Head and Neck Surgery Speech Assessment*

Any patient who is about to undergo surgery of the structures of the head and neck that are involved in speech or swallowing should be seen by an SLP for **presurgical counseling** and **postsurgical speech rehabilitation**. Individuals who require laryngectomies, for example, are especially in need of pre- and postsurgical attention from the SLP.

Postlaryngectomy treatment includes determining the most efficacious method for alaryngeal communication (**electrolarynx, esophageal speech, tracheoesophageal puncture [TEP] voice prosthesis**) and helping the patient achieve a functional level of intelligibility with the selected method. Treatment also includes instruction in safety concerns and lifestyle changes when the patient becomes a "neck breather" following a total laryngectomy. SLPs assist patients with purchasing adaptive equipment (e.g., "shower shields" for showering) and encourage participation in community support groups. In cases where the patient with a laryngectomy is a candidate for a TEP voice prosthesis, SLPs assist with or conduct **air insufflation tests** to determine upper esophageal adequacy for a good alaryngeal speech result following the TEP prosthesis fitting. In some settings, the SLP is the professional who fits the patient with the appropriate type and size of TEP prosthesis; instructs the patient or family member to insert, clean, and care for the prosthesis; and trains the patient in procedures to achieve maximal TEP speech skills.

8. *Patients with a Tracheostomy*

It is increasingly common for SLPs to be consulted about patients in intensive care units (ICUs), such as to see children and adults who are unable to speak (phonate) due to the presence of a **tracheostomy** or **endotracheal tube**. These patients often have cognitive and motor deficits, which complicate management. The ICU staff is usually anxious to assist these patients to communicate. Medical SLPs must be familiar with how respiratory status is managed in patients of all ages who have a tracheostomy and who are ventilator dependent. They may need to examine a patient's language and mental status and oral motor abilities to determine options for communication. In concert with the respiratory therapist, primary nurse, or physician, the SLP may determine the patient's potential for using a speaking valve, such as the **Passy-Muir Valve™** or a mode of augmentative communication that does not require phonation (e.g., writing, hand gestures, pointing to letters on an alphabet board, using an electrolarynx).

9. *Pharmacologic, Surgical, or Rehabilitation Therapy Outcomes*

In some medical settings, the SLP may be asked to make baseline and follow-up assessments of speech, language, or swallowing status to evaluate the outcome of drug therapies, surgeries, rehabilitation, or other medical therapies. This request is more frequent in settings where **clinical trials** are being conducted, for example, in university-affiliated **teaching hospitals** (see Chapter 2).

10. *Interdisciplinary and Multidisciplinary Teams*

The SLP is often a key member of a number of interdisciplinary and multidisciplinary teams in a medical setting. These teams may include rehabilitation medicine and intermediate care teams; geriatric unit teams; extended care rehabilitation teams; feeding and swallowing, or dysphagia, management teams; and special treatment protocol consultation teams, such as the velopharyngeal insufficiency (VPI) team, tumor board, and otolaryngology/head and neck surgery indications team (see Chapters 2 and 14).

11. *Staff Education*

The medical center setting provides frequent opportunities for **teaching conferences, rounds**, and **in-services**. SLPs are often asked to provide lectures and staff education on various topics that are related to communication, cognition, and swallowing. Topics may vary across a variety of disorders and procedures, such as indicators for aspiration risks, optimal feeding procedures following acute strokes, enhancing communication with the person with severe aphasia, the use of augmentative communication devices, the management of primary progressive aphasia, communication with dementia, methods for managing food aversions in children with autism spectrum disorder (ASD), determining candidacy for speaking valves in the ICU, alaryngeal speech options following a total laryngectomy, cognitive-communicative disorders in mild TBI, reducing communication barriers in long-term care facilities, and evidence-based practices in voice therapy.

12. *Data Collection and Research*

Although practicing clinicians are not typically engaged in formal research projects, data collection is a necessary part of any plan of treatment as a means to assess the effectiveness of the clinical services. Clinicians are increasingly participating in the **National Outcomes Measurements System (NOMS)** of the ASHA. The NOMS applies functional rating scales that are applicable to clients with certain diagnoses in certain settings who are undergoing treatment of a defined duration. These rating scale data taken at intake and discharge are submitted to the ASHA and aggregated into a large database to provide an examination of treatment outcomes within both health care and education settings. Clinicians also routinely collect outcomes data as a part of **quality assurance** (QA) monitors.

Any data collecting or other research activity, including retrospective reviews of clinical records, currently requires a number of steps and assurances to protect the rights and privacy of the patient (even if the patient is deceased). Many of these protections are the result of the implementation of the **Health Insurance Portability and Accountability Act (HIPAA)**, which is directed at ensuring privacy of an individual's medical data and the internal and external communication of **protected health information (PHI)**. As a consequence, institutions have strict regulations regarding confidentiality of medical information, and research activities are closely scrutinized by **Institutional Review Board (IRBs)**, which review and approve a number of aspects of a proposed study, including the research rationale, design, methods of obtaining informed consent, subject selection, data collection and maintenance of records, risks to and protection of human subjects, and statistical analysis. The department's data collection methods for its QA monitors may require IRB approval, depending mainly on how the data are gathered, stored, and reported.

13. *Continuing Education*

In most states, SLPs who work in medical settings are required to have licensure. The majority of licensure laws mandate continuing education for renewals. Additionally, the ASHA now requires evidence of continuing education for certified members to maintain their **Certificate of Clinical Competence**. Certification maintenance reports are now required to be filed with the ASHA triennially.

14. *Ensuring Reimbursements*

The **Centers on Medicare and Medicaid Services (CMS)** and other third-party payers, such as insurance payers, require documentation to support any claim for reimbursement. The documentation should support the need for therapy and allow the claims reviewers to determine if the therapy was necessary, appropriate, and effective. To obtain reimbursement for services, clinicians must know what the payer requires with claims submissions and how to use any terminology, abbreviations, and documentation protocols required on medical reimbursement forms.

15. *Risk Management*

Risk management includes a systematic process for identifying, reducing, and eliminating the occurrence of anything that puts the patient, care provider, or provider organization at some legal or financial risk. Preventing or reducing risk should improve the quality of services provided and reduce the costs to provide care.

16. *External and Internal Reviews and Audits*

Like all staff in a medical facility, SLPs participate in *internal reviews* (performed within the facility) and *external reviews* (performed by an accrediting agency or commission) to ensure that standards of appropriate care are met. These audits may be conducted on medical record documentation or with site visits and interviews, as described in Chapter 2.

17. *Cost Containment*

All SLPs contribute data to the facility's cost-containment studies, or **utilization reviews**, which ultimately determine the most cost-effective way to provide services. In large facilities, various metrics, such as the **cost per unit of service**, or cost per visit, may be "benchmarked" and compared to the averages and percentile performances for similar facilities or programs across the country. Managers of programs with costs that exceed the comparison groups or productivity that is less than the comparison standard may be asked to find ways to reduce costs and increase productivity.

18. Quality Assurance and Performance Improvement

All health care organizations are expected to conduct ongoing program evaluation for QA and performance improvement to identify problems in patient care, plan and implement corrective actions, and monitor the results. These activities may be formalized within the organization and may be overseen by a *QA program coordinator* within the facility's administration. Typically, QA programs are concerned with maintaining a safe **environment of care (EOC)** and monitoring any procedures that are performed frequently, at a **high volume**, or pose a **high risk** for morbidity or mortality (e.g., heparin therapy).

19. Professional Involvement

Involvement in professional issues and advocacy is a special concern for SLPs in medical settings. Legislation and public policies influence access to SLP services and funding for reimbursements or payment for services. Working within professional peer groups can help clinicians have a greater influence on a variety of issues related to the "what, when, who, where, how, and how much" of clinical services in medical settings. Participation in professional affairs and advocacy helps to ensure that patients who might benefit from speech-language pathology services will have access to them. Providing leadership and participating in local, state, and national professional organizations also allow clinicians to influence the priorities of their professional associations concerning the training, education, research, knowledge, skills, and practice needs of clinicians.

III. HEALTH CARE PERSONNEL

A. Professional, Technical, and Clerical Support Staff

There are over 200 different professions or work titles related to the health care and medical professions. The following list introduces the clinician to medical personnel and their specialties and some of the clinical staff. This list applies to medical personnel typically affiliated with hospitals, training programs, rehabilitation programs, home health, and long-term care facilities in the United States. Career preparation, certification requirements, licensures, and registration are administered in a variety of ways across professional disciplines in the United States, and there are variations among states. Most health care careers, however, are subject to the training and practice guidelines established by the regulatory, licensing bodies (usually the State Boards of Health) within the state in which the health care providers practice. In addition, some health care professions in the United States have independent national certifying bodies. **Occupational therapists (OTRs)**, for example, are "registered" by a national examining body, but in most work settings therapists are also required to have state licensure in the state where they practice (OTR/L). National association certification may be required for **physical therapists (PTs)**, but in most states they also must take state qualifying examinations and meet that state's licensure standards. Presently, graduates of accredited occupational therapy and physical therapy programs are required to complete graduate-level classroom and field experience training leading to a clinical doctorate. These degrees are clinical in their focus and nature and are not research degrees, they are not "PhDs." Although therapists may have earned a PhD, the correct designations for the *clinical degrees* are **Doctor of Physical Therapy (DPT)** and **Doctor of Occupational Therapy (OTD)**.

In the United States physicians are always required to be licensed and usually, but not always, are board certified in their specialty of practice. Some professionals, for example, **physician assistants-certified (PA-Cs)** or **advanced practice nurses (APNs)** are recognized and licensed (or certified) in some states but not in others. For certain types of Medicare reimbursement, providers are required to have a **National Provider Identification (NPI)** number and be designated as a **licensed individual provider (LIP)**. In some states, nurses' aides are not required to have completed a formal academic degree (BS, BA, AA) program and may have received training in a certification program within the hospital or institution in which they work. Other states, however, may require a minimum training (anywhere from 5 weeks to 6 months) in an accredited program. Usually, therapy providers, such as SLPs, OTs, and PTs, are not required to have formal hospital privileging credentials because they work under a physician's direction. SLPs and rehabilitation therapists are often referred to as **ancillary service providers** or **technical providers**.

In addition to national and state credentialing, the health care facility or organization itself has policies regulating the **credentialing** and **privileges** that are extended to certain members of its professional staff (discussed later in this chapter). Physicians must receive approval by the hospital's medical director, chief of staff, or credentialing board to have the *privilege* of admitting patients to and making use of the services in that facility. This is referred to as *admitting privileges*. Health care facilities are required by their credentialing bodies to list the privileges afforded to various members of the professional staff, including physicians and nonphysicians. Facilities are also required to have policies related to how the competency of *all* clinical staff is determined when hired and how competency is assessed and monitored thereafter.

The following list provides a review of the personnel and consultants encountered in medical settings. This list does not include all health care careers, and the list of nursing subspecialties is only partially elaborated.

B. Health Care Personnel

Anesthesiologist. A physician who specializes in the use of various forms of sedation and anesthesia.

Attending. The senior staff physician working in a teaching hospital who is a member of the faculty in a medical-surgical training program and who is designated to be legally responsible for the care of all patients being cared for within his or her "service." (See *Bed service*.)

Audiologist. Professionals with graduate degrees in audiology; the ASHA and the American Academy of Audiology (AAA) currently require completion of the Doctor of Audiology, or AuD, degree. Audiologists diagnose and treat disorders of hearing, balance, and auditory related conditions in individuals of all ages.

Biomedical Engineer, Biomedical Equipment Technician (BET). An individual who provides technical assistance with the selection, ordering, use, and repair of the adaptive devices, equipment, and instruments found in medical facilities.

Cardiologist. A physician who specializes in the diagnosis and treatment of the heart and circulatory diseases.

Cardiovascular Disease Specialist. A physician who specializes in the diagnosis and management of diseases of the heart and blood vessels.

Cardiovascular Surgeon. A physician who specializes in the surgical treatment of the heart and circulatory vessels.

Case Manager. An individual who coordinates and oversees the referrals for services and continuity of care for a patient assigned to him or her or assesses the patient's eligibility for services and authorizes and monitors funding for services.

Certified Occupational Therapy Aide (COTA). An individual who has technical training in occupational therapy and who works under the supervision of a registered and licensed occupational therapist (OTR/L).

Certified Medical/Nurse's Aide. An individual who has completed an accredited certification training program in basic nursing skills who works under the supervision of a licensed practical nurse, registered nurse, or physician.

Certified Registered Nurse Anesthetist. A registered nurse (RN) who has completed advanced training and is certified to assist with anesthesia under the supervision of a physician-anesthesiologist.

Chaplain. A member of the clergy from any religious denomination or community who performs religious rites and services and provides spiritual counseling for patients, their families, and friends, or the facility's personnel.

Chief Resident. A resident (individual who has completed medical school and is engaged in postgraduate medical training) who is in his or her final year of residency, or has taken an additional year of residency, and was chosen or elected to administer certain aspects of the medical or surgical training program and to participate in teaching more junior residents and students.

Circulating Nurse. Operating room nurse who assists with tasks outside of the sterile field that are necessary during a surgery (obtaining additional instruments and supplies, transferring specimens, clearing contaminated materials, etc.).

Clinical Nurse Specialist. A registered nurse with advanced training in a specialty of medical care (e.g., clinical nurse specialist in oncology).

Clinical Pathologist, Pathologist. A physician who specializes in pathology, the study of the essential nature of disease especially of the structural and functional changes in tissues and organs that cause disease, and the use of clinical laboratory methods in diagnosis. Pathologists may have subspecialties (e.g., renal pathologist).

Colon-Rectal Surgeon. A physician who specializes in surgeries of the colon and rectum, which are the lower portions of the large intestine.

Community Care Coordinator, Discharge Coordinator. An individual, usually a nurse or social worker, who serves as a liaison between the staff in a hospital or rehabilitation program and community health care programs or services.

Compliance Officer. An individual, usually with a law degree, Master's of Health Services Administration degree, or Master's of Business Administration (MBA) degree, who oversees the Compliance Office of the organization. The Compliance Office ensures that the mandates and statutes of the Centers on Medicare and Medicaid Services (CMS) are followed within the organization as well as other legal obligations and standards, such as adherence to the confidentiality and conflict of interest policies, and ensures the security of protected health information and the patient's right to privacy.

Critical Care Registered Nurse (CCRN). A registered nurse with training and experience in the nursing management of critically ill patients in intensive care units.

Critical Care Specialist, Intensivist. A physician, usually an internist or critical care surgeon, who has had subspecialty training in pulmonary, cardiac, or renal disease with additional advanced training in critical care surgical or medical management, specializing in the care of patients in intensive care units.

Deglutition Therapist. An individual, usually a nurse, who specializes in the management of disorders of deglutition, including dysphagia and nutritional problems.

Dental Hygienist. An individual with a professional degree in dental hygiene who specializes in the prevention of dental and periodontal diseases.

Dentist. An individual with a professional (doctoral) degree in dental surgery (DDS) or dental medicine (DMD) who diagnoses and treats disorders and diseases of dentition and the oral structures.

Dermatologist. A physician, usually an internist, with subspecialty training and certification in the diagnosis and treatment of the diseases of the skin.

Diagnostic Radiologist. A physician who specializes in diagnostic imaging (e.g., x-ray or computed radiology) procedures.

Diener. A laboratory worker who assists the pathologist with laboratory tasks, such as autopsies.

Dietitian, Dietician, Nutritionist. An individual with academic training (usually a bachelor's or master's degree) in nutrition who is responsible for managing food services and determining and managing the nutritional needs of patients in hospitals.

Dietary or Nutrition Technician. An individual with technical skills in dietary management who works under the supervision of a dietitian.

Dosimetrist. An individual with technical training in dosages for radiation oncology therapies.

Dysphagia Therapist. An individual, usually an SLP or nurse, who specializes in the diagnosis and management of swallowing disorders.

Electrocardiography Technician (EKG Tech). An individual with the technical skills necessary to make recordings of the electrical activity of the heart through the use of electrocardiography (EKG, ECG).

Electroencephalography Technician (EEG Tech). An individual with the technical skills necessary to make recordings of the electrical activity of the brain.

Electromyography Technician (EMG Tech). An individual with the technical skills necessary to make recordings of the electrical activity within the muscles through the use of electromyography (EMG).

Emergency Medical Technician (EMT). An individual who has completed a course of training in emergency medical procedures and, in most cases, has passed a state certifying examination.

Emergency Medicine, Trauma Physician (ER/ED Doctor, Trauma Doc). A physician who specializes in the emergency medical management of acute diseases or injuries, including life-threatening traumatic injuries.

Endocrinologist, Metabolism Specialist, Diabetologist. A physician, usually an internist, who has specialized training and certification in the diagnosis and treatment of diseases of metabolism or the endocrine system and who may subspecialize in the management of specific endocrine diseases or disorders, such as diabetes, growth disorders, and endocrine-related osteopathies.

Environmental Safety Engineer. An individual who ensures that health care facilities and their staff maintain a healthy, safe environment and that the facilities comply with the *environment of care (EOC)* standards of their accrediting and regulatory agencies.

Epidemiologist. An individual who specializes in the study of the relationship between environmental and behavioral factors and the frequency and distribution of infection or diseases in a given population or community. Epidemiologists are often a part of the faculty in medical training programs. In addition to the study of the incidence and prevalence of medical conditions in populations, the origins of **evidence-based medicine (EBM)**, or **evidence-based practice (EBP)**, evolved from the observations, statistical analyses, assessment of outcomes, and algorithms that were developed by researchers in the field of epidemiology.

Exercise Physiologist. An individual, usually with at least an undergraduate degree in physiology, who has expertise in the use of exercise to promote health, wellness, and fitness.

Extern. A fourth-year medical student who works outside of his or her typical clinical training rotations, usually in private hospitals, as a physician's assistant.

Family Practitioner, General Practitioner (GP). A physician who typically is board-certified in Family Practice, and who provides general medical care and minor surgical treatment for patients from birth through adulthood.

Fellow. A physician who has completed a postgraduate residency training program and is selected for 2 to 3 years of additional training and research in a medical or surgical specialty or subspecialty. Nonphysician *fellows* are also found in medical training facilities (e.g., psychology "post-docs," and Clinical Fellows (CFs) in speech-language pathology).

Forensic Pathologist. A physician who specializes in pathology with emphasis on medical-legal issues and the adjudication of the cause of death due to criminal and other unnatural causes.

Gastroenterologist (GI), Hepatologist. A physician who specializes in the diagnosis and treatment of diseases of the gastrointestinal tract and its primary organs, such as the stomach, pancreas, and liver.

General Surgeon. A physician who specializes and usually has board certification in general surgery.

Geneticist. An individual, usually an MD or PhD, who specializes in the study of genetics and inherited conditions and diseases.

Genetics Counselor. Any medical professional who is qualified to provide genetics counseling. There are professional master's and doctoral degree programs in genetics counseling with professional certification requirements. A certified genetics counselor in the United States has passed the qualifying standards and a national examination administered by the American Board of Medical Genetics or the American Board of Genetics Counseling.

Geriatrician. A physician who specializes in internal medicine of the elderly. A geriatrician may or may not be a **gerontologist**. A *gerontologist* specializes in the psychosocial and physical (including medical) conditions associated with aging and usually holds a graduate degree in one of the social or behavioral sciences, such as psychology or sociology.

Gynecologist/Obstetrician. A physician who specializes in uterogenital and reproductive diseases and conditions in women and the science of contraception, conception, fetal and maternal care, and birth.

Hand Surgeon. A physician, usually an orthopedist, who subspecializes in the plastic, neurologic, orthopedic, and vascular reconstructive and corrective surgeries of the hand.

Hand Therapist. An occupational therapist or physical therapist who specializes in the rehabilitation of the structures and functions of the hand, arm, and shoulder.

Head and Neck Surgeon. A physician who specializes in surgeries to the oral, nasal, pharyngeal, laryngeal, and esophageal structures.

Hematologist. A physician who specializes in the diseases of the blood and blood-forming processes.

Home Health Nurse. A registered nurse or licensed practical nurse who practices nursing in the patient's home.

House Staff, House Officers. The residents, interns, and fellows in a teaching hospital.

Immunologist. A physician who specializes in the diagnosis and treatment of diseases of the immune system.

Infection Control Nurse. A registered nurse or advanced practice nurse with special training in infectious disease and hospital infection prevention and control who assists the infectious disease officer (usually an infection disease physician) in preventing and controlling the occurrence of infections and the spread of contagious diseases within the medical facility.

Infectious Disease Specialist (ID Doctor). A physician, usually an internist, with specialty training and board certification in the diagnosis and treatment of infectious and communicable diseases.

Information Technology (IT) Specialist. In medical settings, an individual with wide knowledge of computerized systems and programming and has specialized training in secure electronic clinical documentation and financial records management and communications.

Intern. A physician who is in the first year of training after graduation from medical school; interns are also referred to as first-year residents, or more commonly; **PGY 1, referring to postgraduate year one**.

Internist. A physician who specializes in the diagnosis and treatment of diseases of the organs of the body.

Interventional Radiologist. A board-certified physician who specializes in minimally invasive, targeted treatments using radiologic therapies and procedures.

Kinesiotherapist (KT). An individual who specializes in the treatment of disease with movement or exercise.

Licensed Practical Nurse (LPN), Licensed Vocational Nurse (LVN). An individual who typically has completed at least a 1-year course in nursing techniques and skills and works under the supervision of a registered nurse.

Locum Tenens. A Latin phrase referring to a physician who temporarily fills in for or takes over the practice of another physician.

Maternal and Fetal Medicine Specialist. A physician who specializes in the prenatal gestational care of the mother and fetus, particularly in cases of at-risk pregnancies and deliveries.

Medical Librarian. An individual, usually with a master's degree in Library Science, who has had advanced training in the use and access to medical publications, education, and research resources.

Medical Media Technician. An individual with skills in the preparation of graphic and audiovisual materials for medical displays, presentations, and publications.

Medical Records Clerk, Medical Records Librarian. An individual who manages the facility's medical (paper and electronic) records, including controlling access to and release of records, and ensuring that the records of hospitalizations contain the appropriate documents and signatures.

Medical Student. An individual who is in postgraduate (usually postbaccalaureate) academic and clinical training in preparation for clinical practice in medicine or surgery. During their clinical rotations (sometimes called "clerkships") medical students may be referred to as "subinterns," indicating that they work under the supervision of house staff (interns and residents).

Medical Technician. An individual who has completed a training program in laboratory techniques and performs laboratory procedures and studies under the supervision of a medical technologist.

Medical Technologist. An individual who has completed a professional training program and certification in laboratory sciences and interpretation of laboratory studies.

Medical Supply Clerk. An individual who is responsible for maintaining an appropriate inventory and ordering and distributing medical-surgical supplies.

Microbiologist. An individual, usually with a doctoral degree (PhD) in Microbiology or Bacteriology, who specializes in laboratory sciences and studies dealing with microorganisms.

Neonatologist. A physician, usually a pediatrician, with specialty training and board certification in the critical care management of neonates and infants.

Nephrologist, Renal Physician. A physician who specializes in the diagnosis and treatment of kidney diseases and related conditions (e.g., hypertension).

Neurologist. A physician who specializes in the diagnosis and treatment of diseases of the nervous system.

Neuroradiologist. A radiologist who specializes in neurologic imaging procedures and their interpretation.

Neurosurgeon. A physician who specializes in surgeries involving the structures of the nervous system. Subspecialties may include back (or spine) surgeons, skull base surgeons, neck surgeons, and neurooncologic (brain and spinal cord tumor) surgeons.

Nuclear Medicine Specialist. A physician who specializes in the therapeutic uses radioisotopes and diagnostic interpretation of radioisotopes studies.

Nurse Practitioner (NP). A registered nurse with a bachelor's or master's degree in a specialty of nursing whose practice is limited to that specialty (e.g., pediatric nurse practitioner, geriatric nurse practitioner). NPs are usually permitted (credentialed) to write some orders and in consultation with the patient's physician may perform certain duties or procedures normally conducted by a physician (see *Clinical Nurse Specialist*).

Nurses' Aide (NA). An individual with training in basic nursing skills who assists and works under the supervision of licensed practical nurses (LPNs) and registered nurses (RNs).

Occupational Therapist (Registered/Licensed) (OTR/L). An individual with a minimum of a bachelor's degree in Occupational Therapy (increasingly graduates hold a Doctor of Occupational Therapy, or OTD, degree) who specializes in the occupational, functional, or adaptive restoration of physical disabilities and rehabilitation.

Officer of the Day (OD). The most senior house officer (resident) or fellow.

Oncologist. A physician who specializes in the diagnosis and treatment of cancer, including neoplasms (tumors) and systemic malignancies (e.g., leukemia).

Operating Room Technician (OR Tech). An individual who has completed a training program in operating room skills and who assists during surgeries.

Ophthalmologist. A physician who specializes in the diagnosis and treatment, including surgeries, of the diseases of the eye.

Oral Surgeon. An individual who has a professional (doctoral) degree in Dental Surgery and specializes in surgery limited to the oral cavity and its structures.

Orderly. An individual who performs duties assigned by physicians, nurses, and other hospital staff.

Orthopedist, Orthopaedist, Orthopod. A physician who specializes in surgeries to the bony and connective structures of the body. Orthopedists may specialize in surgeries involving a particular body area or joint (e.g., spine, knee, hip, shoulder) or certain types of injuries (e.g., sports injuries or spinal cord injuries and diseases).

Osteopathic Physician (OD). A physician who has received medical school training in a professional, degree-granting, osteopathic medicine training program and utilizes accepted medical, physical, and surgical methods of diagnosis and therapy with emphasis on normal body mechanics and manipulative methods.

Otolaryngologist. A surgeon who specializes in the medical and surgical treatment of ear, nose, and throat diseases; depending on the areas of specialty, these physicians may be referred to as ear, nose, and throat (ENT) doctors or eye, ear, nose, and throat (EENT) doctor, or rhinologist).

Pediatric Neurologist. A physician who specializes in the diagnosis and treatment of neurologic disorders and diseases in children.

Pediatrician. A physician who specializes in the medical diseases and developmental disorders in children (usually from birth to young adulthood).

Pharmacist. An individual who has completed a professional training program in the study of pharmacology and who is registered (RPh) and licensed to dispense drugs. In most settings, the pharmacy service is directed by a pharmacologist, who has postgraduate education (usually a doctoral degree) in pharmacology (PharmD, DPh).

Phlebotomist. An individual with skilled training in vascular invasive (incision, aspiration, or puncture) techniques for the treatment of blood and circulatory diseases who works under the supervision of a physician.

Physiatrist/Physical Medicine and Rehabilitation (PM & R) Specialist. A physician who specializes in rehabilitation medicine.

Physical Therapist (PT), Physiotherapist. An individual with a minimum of a bachelor's degree in Physical Therapy (increasingly, graduates hold a Doctor of Physical Therapy [DPT] degree) who specializes in physical rehabilitation methods to achieve functional and adaptive restoration of movement in individuals who are physically disabled by disease, injury, or developmental disabilities.

Physical Therapist Assistant (PTA). An individual who holds an associate of arts degree as a PTA, with technical training in physical therapy procedures who works under the supervision and implements the treatment plans of the physical therapist.

Physician Assistant (PA), Physician Assistant–Certified (PA–C), Advanced Practice Nurse (APN). A registered nurse with advanced professional training in clinical procedures who may have privileges to write orders and perform the medical procedures that are normally conducted by physicians.

Plastic and Reconstructive Surgeon. A physician who specializes in cosmetic or reconstructive surgeries.

Podiatrist. An individual with a professional (doctoral) degree (DPM) who specializes in podiatry, which is the treatment of disorders of the feet, including orthotic therapies.

Postanesthesia Nurse. A registered nurse with advanced training in postsurgical recovery nursing management who works in the surgical recovery room.

Primary Care Physician (PCP). The patient's primary physician (usually a general practitioner, internist, or pediatrician) who orders and coordinates specialty or subspecialty consultations and has "gatekeeping" control for referrals within managed care plans.

Proctologist. A physician who specializes in the diagnosis and management of diseases of the rectum.

Prosthestist. An individual with board certification and technical training in the fabrication and fitting of prosthetic body parts and devices (e.g., breast prostheses, artificial limbs, eye and nose prostheses, etc.).

Prosthodontist. A dentist who specializes in the fabrication and fitting of oral prosthetic devices (e.g., palatal obturators and palatal lifts).

Psychiatrist. A physician who specializes in the diagnosis and treatment (medical and behavioral) of cognitive, emotional, and mental disorders.

Psychologist, Child Psychologist, Clinical Psychologist, Medical Psychologist, Neuropsychologist, Geropsychologist. An individual with a master's or doctoral degree (PhD, PsyD), or equivalent, and professional training in Clinical Psychology. Psychology includes the the study of practices dealing with emotional and mental operations, especially as they relate to behavior. Psychologists provide assessment, diagnosis, and (nonmedical) treatment of cognitive, emotional, and mental disorders and are required to be licensed within the states in which they practice. *Neuropsychologists* and *geropsychologists* usually have completed "post-docs" in these specialty areas and may also have obtained board certification from the American Psychological Association (APA) in their specialty area.

Psychometrist. An individual with training in psychological test administration.

Psychology Assistant. An individual with technical skills in testing and clinical-clerical procedures used in psychology who assists and works under the supervision of a psychologist.

Public Health Specialist. An individual who has completed a master's or doctoral degree (MPH, DPH, ScD, MS, PhD) in the study of environmental/public health principles, epidemiology, and the behavioral and biological basis of diseases.

Pulmonary Disease (PD) Specialist. A physician who specializes in pulmonology, which is the diagnosis and treatment of diseases of the respiratory system.

Radiation Safety Specialist, Radiation Safety Officer. An individual with training in nuclear science who oversees the hospital's program for the radiation protection of its employees and patients.

Radiologist. A physician who specializes in the methods of body structure imaging and the use of radiotherapies.

Radiology Technologist. An individual who has completed a training program (typically a 2-year associate of arts degree) in radiology techniques and procedures and who assists the radiologist by preparing the patient, equipment, and instruments, as well as processing the films, DVDs, or tapes from radiology studies.

Registered Nurse (RN). An individual who has completed a comprehensive professional training program leading to a degree, usually a Bachelor of Science in Nursing (BSN) and who is trained to serve a variety of roles in patient care, including dispensing medication, monitoring vital signs, performing procedures, educating patients and families, and implementing the physician's orders.

Resident. A physician who is completing a 3- to 6-year clinical training program in a specialty area (e.g., medicine, surgery, pediatrics, psychiatry, neurology, radiology, etc.). In the United States, medical and surgical residents have completed a postgraduate medical degree (MD) and after completing their first year of residency/internship, they usually are licensed medical practitioners within the state in which they are training. In academic training programs, these "junior" physicians, or *house staff*, are responsible for providing direct care for patients in the teaching hospitals and their clinics under the supervision of senior physicians (fellows and attending physicians). The residency year is designated as *postgraduate year (PGY)*; thus PGY 1 refers to first-year residents, PGY 2 refers to second-year residents, and so forth.

Respiratory Therapist (RT). An individual with professional training in the ventilator (respirator) management and respiratory therapies for the prevention and management of pulmonary disease.

Rheumatologist. A physician who specializes in the diagnosis and treatment of diseases affecting the joints and connective tissues.

Scrub Nurse. A nurse, usually a registered nurse, who assists surgeons in the operating room.

Social Worker. An individual who has at least a bachelor's degree and is licensed in clinical social work (LCSW) who assists the patient and health care team with financial arrangements, serves as a liaison to other community agencies and services, and provides counseling therapies to patients and families.

Speech-Language Pathologist (SLP). An individual with a minimum of a master's degree, or equivalent, in speech-language pathology who provides diagnostic and rehabilitation services for speech, language, voice, and cognitive disorders and dysphagia across all ages.

Stoma Therapist, Enterostomal Therapist. An individual, usually a nurse, with an expertise in patient and family training for stoma management.

Surgical Assistant, First Assistant. A physician or an individual trained in particular surgical techniques who provides surgical assistance to the primary surgeon during an operation.

Teratologist. An individual who specializes in the study of the relationship between the environment and disorders of embryologic development.

Therapeutic Radiologist. A radiologist who specializes in the therapeutic uses of radiologic agents (e.g., radioisotopes).

Thoracic Surgeon, Cardiothoracic Surgeon, Chest Surgeon. A physician who specializes in heart and lung surgeries.

Transplant Surgeon. A physician who specializes in organ transplantation surgery and the pre- and postsurgical medical management of patients with transplanted tissues and organs.

Transportation Aide, Escort Aide. An individual who transports patients among various locations within the facility.

Ultrasound Technician. An individual (usually a radiology technician) with training in conducting ultrasound studies for interpretation by the radiologist.

Urologist. A physician who specializes in surgeries of the urinary tract.

Vascular Surgeon. A physician who specializes in repairs, reconstructions, and anastomoses of blood vessels.

Volunteers. Individuals who provide volunteer (nonpaid) service in various capacities within the facility to assist patients and the professional, technical, and clerical staff.

Ward Secretary, Clinic Secretary, Medical Secretary. An individual with training in medical terminology and medical administrative-clerical skills who is typically responsible for relaying doctors' orders, scheduling special procedures and therapies, preparing and maintaining charts and files, filing reports, and answering telephone inquiries.

C. Personnel Preparation for Health Care Careers

Most physicians, nurses, dentists, and specialty technologists in health care professions who are trained in the United States receive their training in academic medical centers; "Health Sciences Universities;" or university-affiliated Schools of Medicine, Dentistry, Pharmacy, Nursing, Osteopathy, and Allied Health. These institutions offer professional degrees, such as **Doctor of Medicine** (MD), **Doctor of Dental Surgery/Medicine** (DDS/DMD), **Medical**

Technologist (Med. Tech.), **Doctor of Osteopathy** (DO), **Registered Nurse** (RN), and **Doctor of Pharmacy** (PharmD) degrees. Other health care personnel, such as PTs, OTs, dietitians, audiologists, and SLPs usually receive their training in colleges or universities that have schools or departments with professional programs leading to bachelor's, master's, doctoral, or professional doctorate degrees (e.g., **Doctor of Optometry**, [DO]; **Doctor of Public Health**, [PHD]) in their disciplines. Some health care professionals, such as microbiologists, may have received their career preparation either from a basic science department within a medical school or from the Biologic Science Department in the College or Arts and Sciences (CAS) within a university with no administrative affiliation with a medical school. Hospitals, both private and teaching hospitals (discussed later), may have in-house training programs for assistants, aides, or technicians such as operating room technicians nurses, practical nurses, and nurses' aides.

Physicians trained in the United States normally have completed 4 years of medical school, a postbaccalaureate academic and clinical training program in medicine leading to the MD degree, and a minimum of 1 year of postgraduate (medical, surgical, family practice) residency, or internship, prior to obtaining their license to practice in their state. The physician who is planning to enter a nonspecialized, general medical practice might take additional residency training in **family medicine** or could enter practice as a **general practitioner (GP)** after completing a degree in medicine, completing a year of internship and obtaining state licensure, and usually obtaining **board certification** in family medicine. **Internists** are physicians who, following medical school, have completed at least a 3-year residency training program leading toward a specialty in diseases of the internal organs and their systems and structures. Physicians who practice any one of the dozen or more subspecialties of **internal medicine** usually have had a minimum of 3 years of residency in internal medicine and a national board-certifying examination in internal medicine before entering a 2- or 3-year fellowship program in their subspecialty areas. Surgeon subspecialists are usually required to have taken one or more years of **general surgery** before they begin their subspecialty training. Some general surgeons obtain board certification in general surgery. Some subspecialties require more than one residency; for example, a pediatric urologist usually has had both general surgery and urology residencies and then completed a pediatric urology clinical fellowship followed by, in some settings, an additional 1- to 2-year research fellowship. A physician who has become board certified in a particular specialty or subspecialty is said to be a **diplomate** of the accrediting body.

D. Aides, Assistants, and Technicians

Among health care professions, a wide variety of job titles that reflect specialized technical skills are designated as "aides," "assistants," and " 'technicians." These are individuals who usually have completed a relatively brief training course ranging, for example, from a few months for nurses aides to 2-year "associate of arts degree" (AA) programs, for example, **physical therapist assistants (PTAs)**. Aides, assistants, and technicians may or may not be required to have a license or registration, depending on the state licensure laws, but will invariably be required to work under the supervision of a member of the licensed staff. One exception is the **first assistant** surgeon, who is typically another surgeon who assists the principal surgeon with a complicated surgery.

Aides and assistants help the professional staff with routine tasks. In some professions, there are notable differences between a *technician* and a *technologist*. Technologists, such as **medical technologists**, usually have completed longer and more specialized degree training and certification programs than medical technicians. Consequently, medical technologists have more responsibilities and greater independence. Similarly, one sometimes finds aides and assistants designated to have a hierarchical relationship. For example, PTAs and **certified occupational therapy assistants (COTAs)** have completed an accredited training program and certifying examinations but, depending on the state, are not usually permitted to conduct evaluations independently or prepare a plan of treatment and they provide treatment only under the supervision of a licensed therapist. Similarly, speech-language pathology assistants (SLP-As), where allowable by state licensure/registration laws, practice under the direct supervision of a licensed practitioner.

E. Health Services Administration

Hospitals and most other health care facilities are generally organized under two administrative structures: One branch is responsible for operations and the staff (Human Resources) involved in direct patient care services (i.e., clinical staff administration and clinical operations) and the other is responsible for operations and the staff involved in indirect patient services (i.e., support staff administration and support operations). Although there are overlapping areas of concern, *direct* patient care services, or clinical services, include the medical, surgical, dental, laboratory, pharmacy, rehabilitation therapy, and nursing services that the hospital provides directly to the patient. The *indirect* patient services, or support services, include services such as patient accounting, facilities and plant management, records management, food services, parking, transportation, laundry, clerical, engineering, housekeeping, safety, security, volunteers, and medical supply services.

Direct patient care staff and services are usually administered by a physician who is selected to serve either permanently, or for a designated tenure, as the **medical director**, or **chief of staff**. Reporting to the chief of staff are the **department chairs** who may have several **division chiefs** and **directors** reporting to them. For example, there will be division chiefs in pulmonology, rheumatology, nephrology, infectious disease, cardiology, internal medicine, and so forth reporting to the chair of the Department of Medicine. In medical center training programs, where there is a School of Medicine and School of Nursing, there are **deans** over those schools. The overall academic administrator in a university typically is the **chancellor**, who may have some number of vice chancellors, including a **vice chancellor for health sciences/health-related affairs**. In the **Department of Veterans Affairs (DVA) Medical Centers**, there are **service chiefs** for specialties and subspecialties and **associate chiefs of staff (ACOS)** for education, research and development, and the like, who report to the chief of staff (COS).

The facility's indirect, or support, services are usually administered by individuals with degrees in business administration, management, law, or health services administration, but these individuals may be administrators who have a background in a health-related profession (e.g., physical therapy), who move up the administrative ladder to leadership roles in the organization. Typically, the **hospital administration** is directed by the **chief executive officer (CEO)**, or **hospital director**, who oversees the **chief operating officer (COO)** and the **chief financial officer (CFO)**. Each of these administrative officers, correspondingly, has a number of **associate hospital administrators** reporting to them who, correspondingly, have a number of **department heads** or **program directors** reporting to them.

There is, of course, variation among institutions and facilities. The extent to which a system of elaborated tiers and subordinations exists within the facility's administration depends mainly on the nature and size of the facility and its programs and whether or not it is a part of a large health care organization or is an independent entity. In most settings, the CEO, or hospital director, is responsible to a **board of governors** or **trustees**. The board of governors or trustees is ultimately responsible for monitoring the organization's services, programs, and operations and the integrity of all fiduciary concerns.

IV. HEALTH SERVICES ORGANIZATIONS

As suggested previously, health services facilities and organizations in the United States are highly varied and provide services to patients in a number of ways and under a variety of delivery schemes. **Primary care provider** organizations, for example, may include group practices, multispecialty groups, government health services, or single specialty groups and providers. **Acute care provider** organizations typically are hospitals but may also be "urgent care" centers or ambulatory surgery centers. **Rehabilitation care provider** organizations include home health agencies, therapy and nursing contractors, and inpatient or outpatient rehabilitation facilities. **Disease-specific care** refers to services aligned with a particular medical condition, such as *end-stage renal disease (ESRD)*. **Maintenance and palliative care provider** organizations include entities such as nursing homes and hospice programs. **Supplier organizations and vendors** include pharmaceutical companies, biotechnology companies, durable medical equipment providers, and multipurpose medical and laboratory supply providers. Other important entities involved with the provision of health services in this country include third-party payers; professional and trade organizations; educational and research organizations; employers; and federal and state government supported programs, for example, the DVA; Social Security Disability (SSD); the CMS, and accrediting bodies such as state departments of health or The Joint Commission. Increasingly, many aspects of these health service organizations are linked into an integrated delivery system of health care. In such settings, acute care, recuperative care, rehabilitation, and home health programs are all a part of one health system, or **provider network**. Separate facilities or health services organizations also may be networked financially through the facilities' **managed care** contracts. Even though a facility or health care network is not formally incorporated as a **managed care organization (MCO)** per se, the same principles—referrals restricted to only certain providers and copayments or restrictions on services "outside of network"—will be applied.

V. HEALTH CARE SERVICES SETTINGS AND LOCATIONS

The following is a list of the locations, settings, facilities, and the abbreviations employed to refer to the location where health care services are provided or the administrative personnel.

A. Locations and Settings

Admitting Office/Area. The administrative intake location where payment status and authorization and eligibility for services at that facility are determined and admission forms (e.g., insurance forms, Right to Privacy, Advanced Medical Directives) are completed prior to or at the time of admission.

Ambulatory Care Clinic, Outpatient Clinic. Any area where outpatients are seen, which may be attached to or within the main facility or off site.

Bed Service, Ward Service. The hospital beds or wards designated for inpatient admissions to a particular specialty (e.g., neurology bed service, cardiology bed service).

Blood Bank. The area in the hospital's laboratory service where blood and blood products are kept and blood chemistry panels and blood typing take place. Often hospitals share blood and blood products, and a central laboratory facility serves several hospitals.

Burn Care Unit (BCU). An intensive care unit devoted to patients with burns; these units are found only in specially designated hospitals.

Cardiac Care Unit (CCU). An intensive care unit devoted to patients with acute or critical cardiac disease.

Cardiac Rehabilitation Unit/Center/Program. An inpatient or outpatient rehabilitation program devoted to patients who have undergone heart surgery or have chronic cardiac disease.

Comprehensive Outpatient Rehabilitation Facility (CORF). An outpatient facility that provides, at a minimum, physician services, physical therapy, and social work or psychology services. Typically, CORFs also have speech-language pathology services and occupational therapy services for patients who require comprehensive rehabilitation.

Day Surgery Center. A freestanding facility or part of a hospital facility where relatively minor elective surgeries are performed.

Day Treatment Center (DTC), Day Treatment Facility (DTF). A medical program or facility that provides comprehensive therapies for patients who do not require hospital or nursing facility admissions. DTCs and DTFs include programs that provide comprehensive outpatient treatment for targeted groups (e.g., alcohol and drug abuse, Alzheimer's disease day care programs, etc.).

Dialysis Unit. The area of the hospital or an outpatient clinic devoted to hemodialysis. Some hospitals have an inpatient unit ("acute unit") for patients admitted to the hospital who require dialysis either due to acute renal dysfunction or chronic kidney disease, and a "chronic unit" for outpatient hemodialysis for chronic renal insufficiency.

Emergency Department (ED), Emergency Room (ER). The location and department of the hospital where patients with emergent, acute, or life-threatening illness or injuries are seen for treatment.

Endoscopy Unit/Endo Lab. Usually the location for GI endoscopy and bronchoscopy studies.

Episodic Care, Urgent Care Centers. Facilities or programs that provide limited emergency and on-call physician services. These centers are sometimes referred to condescendingly as "doc-in-the-box."

Extended Care Facility. A nursing home or residential center for individuals who require nursing care or supervision.

File Room/Record Room. The area in the facility where paper medical records are kept. Access is usually restricted. Incomplete files (files that are missing signatures or documents) are usually kept separately in a "signature room" or medical records room. Increasingly, medical facilities are moving to "paperless," or electronic, medical records, which are kept on secure servers, and electronic signatures (using personal identification numbers) are the norm (see Chapter 2).

Geriatric Medicine Unit, or Bed Service. A bed service (see previously) or ward devoted to admissions and transfers of elderly patients who require specialized care. These units are common in hospitals with a geriatric program or geriatricians on its staff.

Home Health Agency/Program. A program and an agency that provides nursing, social, and rehabilitation services to patients in their homes.

Hospice Program. A program that provides brief inpatient treatment, day treatment, or home health nursing; and counseling, social, and other support services to patients with known terminal illnesses usually for an anticipated time period of up to 6 months.

Hospital-Based Outpatient Rehabilitation. Rehabilitation services extended to patients seen in the hospital outpatient clinic facilities.

Inpatient Rehabilitation Unit. A hospital bed service (see previously) or ward devoted to patients who require physical and other rehabilitation therapies. These units are found in facilities where there are rehabilitation therapists and physical medicine and rehabilitation physicians (physiatrists) on staff.

Intensive Care Unit (ICU). A ward equipped with special monitoring capability and staffed with specially trained nurses and support staff for the purpose of managing life-threatening, acute, and critical illness.

Isolation Bed / Ward. A room or ward designated for admission or transfer of patients with contagious diseases, especially when the infectious process is airborne, or when the patient has a susceptibility for infections from others, for example, due to immune suppression therapies.

Laboratory. The area in a medical facility where laboratory studies, such as blood, urine, and tissue analyses, are conducted on the request of a physician or individuals with clinical privileges for ordering laboratory studies.

Medical Intensive Care Unit (MICU). An intensive care unit devoted to the management of patients with acute or critical medical problems involving the internal organs, for example, hepatic coma.

Medical and Surgical Hospital (Med-Surg Hospital). A hospital with personnel and facilities to provide basic medical and surgical services.

Morgue. The area in the hospital where postmortem anatomical examinations are made by the pathologist. *Postmortem* pathologic studies (autopsies) are sometimes required to determine the cause of death or factors that potentially contributed to a patient's demise.

Neonatal Intensive Care Unit (NICU). An intensive care unit devoted to critically ill neonates and infants.

Nurses' Station. The area in an intensive care unit, hospital ward, or clinic where medical records and the nurses' "Kardex" are kept. This is the area where nurses conduct their "charting," write progress notes, complete other documentation, access computerized records and data, and monitor a patient's status with central monitors.

Operating Room (OR). The area or suite of rooms devoted to surgical procedures.

Pain Center. The bed service or outpatient program devoted to the interdisciplinary management of chronic, debilitating pain syndromes.

Pediatric Intensive Care Unit (PICU). The intensive care unit for children.

Postanesthesia Care Unit (PACU). The recovery room.

Private Office. The clinical facility where health care professionals with private practices treat outpatients.

Pulmonary Function Laboratory (PFL). The area of the hospital equipped with instruments and staffed with personnel trained to evaluate pulmonary status and functions. Invasive pulmonary studies, such as a lung biopsy, are performed in the operating room, outpatient surgical suite, or specially designed area within the PFL.

Radiology Department/Unit/Clinic. An area in a hospital or freestanding clinic specially equipped with instruments and staffed with personnel trained in the use of various imaging techniques to diagnose disease.

Recuperative Care Unit. A ward or bed service for patients who require a less acute level of care but are not quite ready for transfer to a home, rehabilitation, home health care, or other program; includes "step down" units, intermediate care units, and the like.

Respite Care. A brief inpatient or day treatment program that provides time-limited nursing and rehabilitation services mainly for the purpose of providing caregiver respite.

Skilled Nursing Facility (SNF). An extended care facility, or nursing home, for patients whose medical status requires continuous monitoring and skilled nursing services.

Surgical Intensive Care Unit (SICU). An intensive care unit for patients who remain critically ill following surgery or who need to have their vital signs closely monitored and require intensive nursing care before transferring to a room or ward.

Surgical Recovery. The area adjacent to the operating room or day surgery suite where patients' vital signs are monitored following surgery and during recovery from anesthesia.

Tertiary Care Facility. A facility capable of providing care to the critically ill patient or patient with complex medical conditions who requires specialized personnel and equipment.

Transitional Care Unit (TCU), Subacute Care Unit (SACU), "Step Down Unit." In some hospitals a unit that is available for patients who no longer require the degree of continuous monitoring and nursing supervision found in an intensive care unit but who are not yet sufficiently stable to be transferred to a standard ward.

Ward/Unit. A single large room with multiple patient beds, or a designated wing or sections of a hospital floor with several adjacent patient rooms attached to a particular service or specialty (e.g., neurology ward, burn unit).

Ward Administration Desk. The ward secretary's desk.

B. Abbreviations for Health Care Settings, Locations, and Personnel

ACOS. Associate Chief of Staff

AuD. Doctor of Audiology

BCU. Burn Care Unit

CCU. Cardiac Care Unit

CMHC. Community Mental Health Clinic

CNH. Community Nursing Home

CORF. Comprehensive Outpatient Rehabilitation Facility

COTA. Certified Occupational Therapy Assistant

DO, OD. Doctor of Optometry, Doctor of Osteopathy

DON. Director of Nursing

DPT. Doctor of Physical Therapy

EMT. Emergency Medical Technician

ED/ER. Emergency Department, Emergency Room

HH. Home Health

ICU. Intensive Care Unit

LIP. Licensed Individual Provider

LPN. Licensed Practical Nurse

MICU. Medical Intensive Care Unit

MD. Doctor of Medicine

MS.I, II, III, IV. First-year, second-year, third-year, and fourth-year medical students, respectively

NICU. Neonatal Intensive Care Unit; Neurologic Intensive Care Unit

OD. Officer of the Day

OR. Operating Room

OT. Occupational Therapist/Therapy

OTD. Doctor of Occupational Therapy

PA-C. Physician's Assistant-Certified

PGY 1, PGY 2, PGY 3. Postgraduate year one, two, three, etc.

PhD. Doctor of Philosophy

PMD. Private MD

PM & R. Physical Medicine and Rehabilitation

PsyD. Doctor of Psychology

PT. Physical Therapist/Therapy

PTA. Physical Therapist Assistant

RN. Registered Nurse

RR. Recovery Room

RT. Respiratory Therapist/Therapy, Recreation Therapist/Therapy

SACU. Subacute Care Unit

SICU. Surgical Intensive Care Unit

SLP. Speech-Language Pathologist

SNF. Skilled Nursing Facility

SW, MSW, LCSW. Social Worker, Master of Social Work, Licensed Clinical Social Worker

TCU. Transitional Care Unit

C. Levels of Care Rankings in Special Settings

In medical settings special programs, or units, may have been awarded national or state rankings related to their **levels of care**. For example, trauma centers are ranked as: *Level I Trauma Center*—provides the highest level of surgical and anesthesiology at all times; *Level II Trauma Center*—provides emergency medicine and comprehensive trauma care in collaboration with a Level I center; *Level III Trauma Center*—provides emergency care to trauma patients who do not require Level I or II care; or *Level IV Trauma Center*—provides stabilization and treatment to trauma patients when no other alternative is available.

Postnatal care services and NICUs within hospitals in the United States may also have levels of care certification rankings. Facilities that are equipped and staffed to provide only minimally complex postnatal care are designated as *Level I* care. Most university medical center affiliated children's hospitals have highly skilled and neonatal nursing and physician staff in units equipped to provide **tertiary care**. In the NICU ranking system, the highest level of certification is a **Level III NICU**.

VI. ROUNDS AND CONFERENCES

In training program hospitals, conferences for the purpose of discussing the care of patients are called **rounds** and, sometimes, **care conferences**. The types of rounds and conferences typically found in these settings are listed next.

A. Morning Rounds

Sometimes called "work rounds," **morning rounds** are usually conducted by fellows and attended by residents, interns, and medical students and take place on the hospital wards in the early morning. During morning rounds, the residents who were assigned care of patients the previous night inform the rest of the team of the status of their patients.

B. Attending Rounds

Attending rounds are scheduled and administered by the staff physician who is overseeing the care of patients on a given service. For newly admitted patients, the **history and physical (H & P) examination**, admitting problem, laboratory findings, current vital signs, and indications and plans are presented to the attending physician.

C. Evening Rounds

Evening rounds take place in the early evening during which time the plans for any procedures, concerns, or special monitoring orders are discussed and conveyed to the house staff on call for that evening.

D. Morning Report, M & M, and CPC Conferences

In most training programs, the entire house staff and attending physicians meet daily for a "**morning report**" and weekly for a **morbidity and mortality (M & M)** conference during which any deaths, iatrogenic problems, and medical or surgical complications are discussed. In training facilities, **clinicopathologic conferences (CPCs)** are formal teaching conferences during which the clinical data from an interesting "teaching case" are presented to an expert or panel of experts for discussion of the management options.

E. Grand Rounds

Ground rounds are teaching conferences held in virtually all hospitals, not just in teaching hospitals, in which clinical or research topics, management challenges, or interesting teaching cases are presented for **continuing medical education (CME)** credits. Most hospitals have surgery grand rounds, medicine grand rounds, neurology grand rounds, pediatric grand rounds, renal grand rounds, and so forth.

F. Change of Shift Conferences

Change of shift conferences occur at each nursing shift change (day, evening, and night). The primary care nurses either dictate or discuss face to face in conference with incoming nurses what has transpired during the previous shift and what needs to occur during the next shift. It is *highly advisable* to avoid interrupting nurses during this conference, because it causes the nurses going off shift to be delayed. It may be helpful to discuss with the day shift nurse any special requests or plans that need to be communicated to the evening and night nurses so that he or she may convey these requests during the shift change conferences.

G. Discharge Planning Conferences

Nurses or social workers usually conduct **discharge planning conferences** and welcome input from any discipline that has been involved in a patient's care.

H. Team Conferences and Clinical Care/Case Conferences

For special purposes **team conferences** and **clinical care/case conferences** are often scheduled on a regular basis, depending on the needs of the facility. These multidisciplinary conferences may include neuropathology rounds, pathology rounds, tumor board or cancer team rounds, rehabilitation team rounds, cardiac care rounds, dysphagia management team conference, and the like.

VII. MEDICAL STAFF PRIVILEGES, CREDENTIALS, AND HIERARCHIES

In most hospitals, staff members are categorized according to the extent of their clinical and administrative privileges. **Clinical privileges** refer to the extent or level to which an individual is permitted to perform particular procedures without prior authorization. Clinical privileges may be general; for example, a surgeon may have privileges to admit patients, order tests, prescribe drugs, and perform surgeries. Privileges may also be "limited" or specific; for example, a PA, clinical nurse specialist, or APN may be permitted to write most orders except for certain medications. **Administrative privileges** refer to participation on hospital boards and voting in medical staff elections. The following illustrates the levels and types of privileges found in health care settings.

A. Medical Staff

Physicians who are fully eligible for all medical privileges and administrative privileges. Certain other nonphysician staff (dentists, psychologists, and other doctoral level professional staff) are sometimes elected to the medical staff, but they do not receive full medical privileges; for example, psychologists are not privileged to admit patients to the hospital.

B. Associate Staff

Physicians and certain other nonphysician staff who have not met all the requirements for full staff privileges and have limited administrative privileges.

C. Provisional Staff

Physicians and certain other nonphysician staff who are newly appointed to the staff and are still under review. *Provisional* staff typically do not have full clinical or administrative privileges.

D. Courtesy Staff

Physicians and certain other nonphysician staff who are given privileges for occasional admissions but do not have administrative privileges.

E. Temporary Staff

Physicians and certain other nonphysician staff who are given specific clinical privileges for a specified period.

VIII. STATES OF ILLNESS

States, or levels, of patient illness categories are defined relative to the acuity or severity of the illness or the level of care required.

A. Acute Illness

Acute illness refers to conditions characterized by an abrupt or life-threatening change in vital signs or mental status. Examples of these conditions are pneumonia, acute psychosis, stroke, sudden fever, or appendicitis. Acute illness can be designated as **life threatening** (cardiac arrhythmia), and described in the medical record as an **acute life-threatening event (ALTE)**, or as **non-life threatening** (broken pelvis). The term **subacute** is sometimes used to refer to a condition that is not fully obvious or has not reached a critical or life-threatening state. **Postacute** references the point at which the acute episode has subsided.

B. Critical Illness

Critical illness includes conditions that are potentially life threatening and require treatment in intensive care or critical care units. Critically ill patients require urgent medical care; special monitoring; highly skilled nursing; and specialized therapies, for example, respiratory care. Patients with a critical illness may have conditions that are reversible, such as pneumonia, or irreversible. The term *gravely ill* is used to refer to patients who are critically ill and potentially near death.

C. Serious Illness

Patients described as seriously ill are those whose acute conditions have stabilized but continue to *require close monitoring* of cardiac and respiratory status; support therapies, such as oxygen support; intravenous (IV) drug therapies; and nonoral nutrition and hydration.

D. Chronic Illness

Patients with chronic illness, or chronic disease, are those who have largely irreversible minor or major conditions that in some way affect their physical or mental well-being. For example, patients with stroke residual may require daily medications, rehabilitation maintenance programs, and periodic checkups by their physician, and generally live with at least some persistent functional limitations secondary to their chronic condition.

E. Subclinical Illness

Medical conditions that have not yet been revealed to be significant or in need of treatment, conditions with signs and symptoms too mild to be found on examination, or conditions that the patient is not aware of having may be referred to as subclinical conditions.

F. Clinically Significant Illness

Medical conditions sufficiently severe to be of concern to the patient or health care provider and require treatment or monitoring are referred to as clinically significant illnesses.

G. Factitious Illness, Functional Disorders

These are conscientiously faked, nonorganic, conditions (see Chapter 10, Neurologic and Psychiatric Disorders) and may include conditions that are self-induced or falsely reported. Various terminology may be encountered with this category of disorders, including **Munchausen syndrome, Munchausen syndrome-by-proxy**, factitious illness, *pseudologia fantastica*, Ganser syndrome, narcissism, sociopathy, somatoform illnesses, malingering, somatization disorder, hypochondriasis, pseudocyesis, pain disorder, body dysmorphic disorder, delusional disorder, and somatic delusions. Psychogenic communication and swallowing disorders are of particular interest to SLPs. These disorders include a variety of nonorganic, psychologically based speech, language, and swallowing behaviors; for example, hyperfunctional, muscle tension (voice) disorders; elective mutism; mutational falsetto; psychogenic stuttering; childlike speech, and *globus hystericus*, food aversions, and other functional feeding and swallowing disorders (see Chapter 5) (Mahr, Yost, & Jacobson, 2007). Although there may be no frank evidence of a physical medical cause, these disorders often have a psychiatric comorbidity. In addition some functional disorders, for example, **muscle tension voice disorders** and mutational falsetto, can eventually cause physical abnormalities and lesions to the vocal folds owing to the inappropriate use of the vocal mechanism.

Feigned "neurogenic" speech or language disorders often vary from the typical behavioral pattern for the condition that is being mimicked. For example, individuals who consciously fake "aphasia" might display an implausible pattern or severity of language symptoms across modalities not typical for any neurogenic aphasia syndrome.

H. Conversion Disorders

Conversion disorders include a broad range of conditions that cannot be explained by a medical disease or condition and thus appear to be functional, nonorganic disorders, but these disorders are *not consciously faked*. The origin for these conditions is thought to lie with a psychological conflict that is "converted" to a physical disorder (Mahr et al., 2007). Certain voice disorders may have a physical or psychological origin; for example, spasmodic dysphonia may be caused by neurologically based dysphonia, or may ultimately be diagnosed as a conversion disorder, or **conversion-type spasmodic dysphonia**. Knowledge of the expected performance differences typical for an organic versus nonorganic condition aids in the differential diagnosis. A conversion disorder is diagnosed after consideration of factors such as the onset and history; comorbid psychiatric disorders; the speech characteristics compared to the typical pattern for organic disorders; and the individual's response to treatment.

IX. CLINICAL COMPETENCIES

The learner outcomes, skills, and competencies gained from information contained in this chapter include the ability to:

- List the roles and responsibilities of professional, technical, clerical support, and administrative personnel encountered in medical settings.

- Read, interpret, and use terminology and abbreviations that refer to health care settings and personnel.
- Describe the variations in how professions train to work in health services delivery.
- List reasons why physicians and nurses have a primary role in decision making in medical care settings.
- List the roles and responsibilities of SLPs who work in medical settings.
- Describe the types of conferences and rounds conducted in hospitals.
- Discuss how health services administration is typically organized.
- Discuss the difference between *credentialing* and *privileging* for professionals who work in medical settings.
- List and define levels of care rankings that are awarded to NICUs and trauma centers in the United States.
- Define the medical and administrative hierarchies of health services administration in medical facilities/organizations in the United States.
- List the primary work settings for health services delivery in the United States.
- Discuss the differences and provide examples of acute, critical, and chronic illness.
- Describe and give an example of how knowledge of the expected performance for individuals with truly organic speech, language, cognitive, and swallowing disorders can aid in the identification of functional (nonorganic), psychogenic, and faked conditions.

X. REFERENCES AND RESOURCES CONSULTED

American Speech-Language-Hearing Association (ASHA). (2001). *Scope of practice in speech-language pathology*. Rockville, MD: Author.

Avery, M., & Imdieke, B. (1984). *Medical records in ambulatory care*. Rockville, MD: Aspen.

(The) Belmont Report (1979, April). Retrieved July 2008, from http://www.hhs.gov/ohrp/humansubjects/ guidance/belmont.htm

Davies, J. J. (2008). *Essentials of medical terminology* (3rd ed.). Clifton Park, NY: Delmar Cengage Learning.

Gray, B. H., & Field, M. J. (Eds.). (1989). *Controlling costs and changing patient care*? Washington, DC: National Academy Press.

Haller, R. M., & Sheldon, N. (1976). *Speech pathology and audiology in medical settings*. New York: Stratten International Medical Book.

Jabonski, S. (2005). *Dictionary of medical acronyms and abbreviations* (5th ed.). Philadelphia: Elsevier Saunders.

Johnson, A. H., & Jacobson, B. H. (Eds.). (2007). *Medical speech-language pathology: A practitioner's guide* (2nd ed). New York: Thieme.

Lubinski, R., Golper, L. A. C., & Frattali, C. M. (Eds.). (2007). *Professional issues in speech-language pathology and audiology* (3rd ed.). Clifton Park, NY: Delmar Cengage Learning.

Mahr, G., Yost, W. B., & Jacobson, B. H. (2007). Psychogenic communication disorders. In A. F. Johnson & B. H. Jacobson (Eds.), *Medical speech-language pathology: A guide for practitioners* (2nd ed.). New York: Thieme.

Miller, R. M., & Groher, M. E. (1990). *Medical speech pathology*. Rockville, MD: Aspen.

Nicolosi, L., Harryman, E., & Kresheck, J. (1983). *Terminology in communication disorders* (2nd ed.). Baltimore: Williams & Wilkins.

Strand, E. A., Yorkston, K. M., & Miller, R. M. (2007). Medical ethics and the speech-language pathologist. In A. F. Johnson & B. H. Jacobson (Eds.), *Medical speech-language pathology: A guide for practitioners* (2nd ed.). New York: Thieme.

The Joint Commission (2008). *Accreditation and certification manuals*. Naperville, IL: Author.

Wolper, L. F., & Pena, J. J. (Eds.). (1987). *Health care administration*. Rockville, MD: Aspen.

CHAPTER 2

Communicating Information and Record Keeping

Efficient and accurate communication in health care settings requires knowledge of the medical terminology routinely encountered in written documentation and verbal reports. To be able to record and report findings and plans within the health care team, clinicians should have a basic knowledge of terminology, abbreviations, pronunciations, and usage. The patient's medical record is the primary vehicle for communication within medical facilities. Notes in the medical record that document the completion of procedures often need to be copied or sent electronically to the patient's insurance carrier to support reimbursement. The methods for ensuring accreditation standards set by the Joint Commission on Accreditation of Healthcare Organizations (JCAHO), more commonly, "The Joint Commission," are evaluated by site visitors who use an audit system called Tracer Methodology. The site visitors "trace" the documented records of care and the sequence of each procedure, medication, professional service provider, and others involved in an individual's medical care (assessments and treatment) to ensure compliance with standards across all areas throughout the admission, or incident of care. Thus, the medical record allows the organization and its providers to demonstrate that they have met all standards of care by verifying that appropriate care decisions, protocols, and sequences were followed by qualified and competent providers across the continuum of care from admission through discharge. There is a saying in health service delivery that goes, "If it wasn't documented, it wasn't done." That is, if a record of the service cannot be traced there is no way to verify that it was performed and therefore should not be billed.

Because documentation is both crucial and time consuming, the use of approved **abbreviations**, **acronyms**, and **eponyms** is common in handwritten and electronic medical records. The use of appropriate abbreviations also is encouraged when completing reimbursement forms and insurance claims. *Abbreviations* are shortened words or letters that stand for a word or phrase, such as "PT" for "physical therapy." *Acronyms* are words formed from the initial letters of a compound term; for example, the word *l*aser is an acronym for light *a*mplification *s*timulated *e*mission of *r*adiation, and the word *rads* refers to *r*adiation *a*bsorbed *d*oses. *Eponyms* are words or phrases derived from the name of a person, as in the *Babinski* sign.

I. CHAPTER FOCUS

This chapter reviews medical communication and what to consider when gathering and recording information in medical charts. All personnel should be comfortable with the conventional language and format encountered in medical settings. This chapter introduces basic concepts in medical terminology and discusses the purposes and types of medical notations, including prescriptions and other notations. Abbreviations and symbols that are commonly found in progress notes, laboratory findings, and doctors' orders are included. Issues, such as confidentiality protections and informed consent, as well as guidelines for appropriate entries in medical records and other methods of communicating in medical settings are also discussed.

II. SOURCES FOR MEDICAL TERMINOLOGY

Speech-language pathology (SLP) clinicians who practice in medical settings should have at least one comprehensive textbook on medical terminology and a medical dictionary in their professional libraries. These texts provide definitions and explanations on word origin, spelling, and pronunciation of medical terms. It is helpful to define the suffixes and prefixes and the meanings of the root words to understand the polysyllabic language of medicine. The majority of medical terms are derived from Greek or Latin; thus, knowing etymologic features of medical terms will help to determine both their meaning and pronunciation.

Throughout this book are lists of terminology and abbreviations likely to appear in medical records, reports, and progress notes. In cases where a word is entirely unfamiliar to the clinician, a medical dictionary should be consulted to determine pronunciation and meaning. Medical terminology can be misused and mispronounced in the popular media, so the best source for the preferred pronunciation is experience listening to how terms are pronounced and used in the context of descriptions and verbal reports made by physicians and nurses.

The preparation of this text required consulting and comparing several comprehensive books on medical terminology as well as medical dictionaries, textbooks in pediatric and adult critical care, medical manuals, physicians' pocket guides, nursing care handbooks, and the like. The sources consulted in preparation of this edition and previous editions are listed at the end of each chapter. These references and similar texts would be useful additions to the SLP's departmental or personal libraries. Most facilities have a medical library with comparable terminology resource texts. In addition to published texts on medical terminology, medical centers are required to have a list of "acceptable abbreviations" and legends for their facility. That list is periodically updated and can usually be obtained from the Compliance Office, Transcription Office, Medical Records Department, Medical Administration Office, Hospital Administration Office, or the facility library. In large health care facilities, the **Compliance Office** is charged with overseeing adherence with various federal and state mandates and statutes as well as the facility's accreditation standards. The Compliance Office requires the use of only the facility's **approved abbreviations**. Many abbreviations are easily confused, causing medical errors and putting the patient and the organization at risk. Consequently, it is mandatory that SLPs and other service providers use only the accepted and appropriate terminology and abbreviations for their facility. For example, the abbreviation "DC" might refer to "discharge," "discontinue," "diagnostic code," "dilation and curettage," "death certificate," "day care," "decrease," "critical dilution rate," "distal colon," and other terms. As a part of the **Risk Management** program, the Compliance Office will publish and enforce the use of approved abbreviations. Steps to ensure consistently accurate communication and create a "safety culture" in hospitals are key to the **prevention of medical errors**. Medical errors include actions, or failures to perform actions, that cause unintended, and often catastrophic, harm to the patient. These errors include, for example, administering the wrong medications or the wrong dosages, treating the wrong patient or the wrong body part, and causing the development of decubitus ulcers (bed sores) or pneumonia due to inadequate care. Nearly 100,000 people die each year in hospitals as a result of medical errors; increasingly, Medicare and other payers are refusing to cover costs for the consequences of these events.

III. COMMON MEDICAL TERMINOLOGY

A. Terms for Direction

Afferent. Going toward a body or center

Anterior. Toward the front or before

Cephalad. Toward the head

Deep. Away from the surface

Distal. Away from the body or point of attachment

Dorsal. In back of or posterior

Efferent. Going away from a body or center

Inferior. Below or in a downward direction

Intermediate. Between the medial and lateral parts

Lateral. Toward the side

Medial. Toward the midline

Posterior. Toward the back or behind

Proximal. Toward the body or nearest point of attachment

Superficial. Near the surface

Superior. Above or in an upward direction

Ventral. In front or anterior

B. Terms for Spatial Orientation or Planes

Apex, apical. Referring to the top or tip of a body organ or part

Base, basal. Referring to the foundation or lowest part

Frontal, or coronal. Vertical plane parallel to the coronal suture of the cranium, dividing the body's front from the back at right angles to the midsagittal plane

Longitudinal. Any plane parallel to the long axis of a structure

Midsagittal. Vertical division of the body through the midline to make a left and a right half

Sagittal. Parallel to midline

Transverse, or horizontal. Dividing superior (upper) from inferior (lower) portions of the body

C. Terms Used to Indicate Regions of the Body

Figure 3–1 illustrates some of these regions.

Axillary. In the armpit

Cervical. Area involving the neck

Clavicular. Near the clavicle

Epigastric. Lower midchest; above the stomach

Flank. Part of the body extending below the ribs to the ileum, the distal portion of the small intestine

Hypogastric. Abdominal; below the stomach

Inguinal. Lower pelvic regions; groin area

Lumbar. Midlateral regions of the back

Perianal. Around the anus

Perineal. Between the anus and the genitalia

Peritoneal. Pertaining to the membranous sac lining the abdominopelvic cavity containing the viscera (internal organs)

Sternal. Near the sternum

Umbilical. Near the navel

IV. ROOTS, PREFIXES, SUFFIXES, PLURALS, AND PRONUNCIATION

A. Roots

Aden– Gland, lymphatic, lymph nodal

Adip– Fat

Aer– Pertaining to air

Angio– Vessel

Arterio– Artery

Arth– Joint

Athero– Fatty substance

Blephar– Eyelid

Cardi– Heart

Cerebro– Brain

Cephal– Head

Cerv– Neck

Cheil–, chil– Lip

Chol– Bile

Chondr– Cartilage

Cost– Rib

Crani– Skull

Cysto– Bladder, biliary, urinary

Cyt– Cell

Dactyl– Finger, toe

Enter– Intestine

Gastr– Stomach

Gloss– Tongue

Glyco– Sweet

Hem– Blood
Hepa– Liver
Histo– Pertaining to tissue
Hyster– Uterus
Ile–, elie– Ileum (distal part of the small intestine)
Ili– Ilium (pelvis, hip bone)
Inguino– Groin
Leuk– White
Lipo– Fat
Lith– Stone
Mening– Membrane
Metr– Uterus
Morph– Form, shape
Myel– Marrow
Myo– Muscle
Nephr– Kidney
Ophthalm– Eye
Oro– Mouth
Ortho– Straight
Osteo– Bone
Parentr– Not directly into the intestine
Pneum– Lung
Proct– Rectum
Psych– Mind
Pyel– Pelvis
Pyo– Pus
Radi– Ray, radiation
Spondyl– Vertebral
Trache– Neck
Viscer– Organ

B. Prefixes

a–, an– without
ab– from, away from
ad– increase, near, toward
ana– up, increase
ante– before
anti– against
bi– two, both
cata– down, decrease
con– together
contra– opposite, against
cost– rib
cysto– sac, bladder
dia– through, between
dys–bad, poor
ecto– outside
ed– out of or from
em–, en– in
endo– within
epi– upon, in addition
ex– out
eu– good, normal
hemi– half
hyper– above, excessive
hypo– beneath, deficient
iatro– related to medicine or a physician
intra– within
leuko– white
mega– large
meta– beyond, change
micro– small size
neutr– neutral
pan– all, total, wide
para– beside, near, abnormal
per– through, by
peri– around
poly– much, excessive
pre– before
pro– in front of, forward

pseudo– false
retro– backward, behind
semi– half
sub– below, under
super–, supra– above, beyond, superior
sym–, syn– with, together, beside
trans– across

C. Suffixes

–algia. Pain
–cele. Herniation, tumor, protrusion
–centesis. Puncture
–cyte. Cell
–dynia. Pain
–ectomy. Excision, removal
–edasis. Expansion, dilatation
–emesis. Vomiting
–emia. Blood
–genic. Origin, caused by
–iasis. Condition, formation of
–itis. Inflammation
–lysis. Breaking down, destruction
–malacia. Softening
–megaly. Enlargement
–oma. Tumor
–osis. Condition, disease
–pathy. Disease
–penia. Deficiency
–pexy. Suspension, fixation
–plasty. Surgical correction or repair
–plexy. Fixation
–ptosis. Falling, drooping
–ptysis. Spitting, coughing (e.g., hemoptysis—coughing blood)
–rrhage. Gushing, flowing
–rrhaphy. Suture
–rrhea. Discharge, flow
–rrhexis. Rupture
–scopy. Inspection
–stalsis. Contraction
–stasis. Stopped
–staxia. Dripping
–stomy. Creation of a new opening
–tomy. Incision into
–tripsy. Crushing
–trophy. Development, nourishment

D. Plurals

Singular		Plural
a as in bursa	to	**ae** as in bursae
us as in incus	to	**udes** as in incudes
us as in alveolus	to	**i** as in alveoli
um as in datum, or ovum	to	**a** as in data, or ova
ex as in apex	to	**ices** as in apices
ix as in appendix	to	**ices** as in appendices
ax as in thorax	to	**axes** as in thoraxes
nx as in larynx	to	**nges** as in larynges[1]
or phalanx	to	phalanges
oma as in adenoma	to	**omata** as in adenomata

or stoma	to	stomata[1]
u as in cornu	to	**ua** as in cornua
ur as in femur	to	**ura** as in femura
us as in nucleus	to	**i** as in nuclei
is as in crisis	to	**es** as in crises
is as in iris	to	**ides** as in irides
er as in tuber	to	**era** as in tubera
en as in foramen	to	**ina** as in foramina
on as in criterion	to	**a** as in criteria

1 "Larynxes" and "stomas" are also conventional and acceptable.

E. Pronunciation

ae– When the *ae* ending is a plural of a Latin word, it is pronounced like the diphthong "i," for example, the plural word "petechiae," referring to small hemorrhages, is pronounced as /pe–ti-ki-a•I/. Words beginning with the letters *aer* are derivatives from Greek or combined forms using Greek and Latin. These letters are pronounced "air" (e.g., "aerosol").

cn–, gn–, kn–, mn–, pn– Words beginning with *cn*, *gn*, *kn*, *mn*, and *pn*, as in cnemical, gnathic, knot, mnemic, and pneumonia, are pronounced as though they begin with "n."

ps– Words beginning with *ps*, as in psychology, are pronounced as though they begin with "s."

phth– Words beginning with *phthir* are pronounced as though they begin with "thir"; words beginning with *phthis* are pronounced as though they begin with "tiz."

pt– Words beginning with *pt*, as in ptosis, are pronounced as though they begin with "t."

–gm. Words ending in *gm*, as in diaphragm, are pronounced as though they end with "m" (the "g" is silent).

V. PURPOSES, TYPES, AND FORMATS OF MEDICAL RECORDS

A. Purposes

The primary purpose of the medical chart is to provide a permanent record of the patient's health status and laboratory and vital sign data as they relate to the sequence of diagnostic studies, procedural interventions, observation of responses to treatment, and medications that have been administered. As an ongoing log of every incident and procedure in the health care continuum, the medical record is:

- A documentation procedure to *protect the patient's safety*
- A means to *communicate the observations and plans* among members of the care team
- A *verification* of services provided to support billing
- A *legal record* of events

B. Types and Formats of Medical Records

A hospital maintains both paper and electronic types of medical records that pertain to its patients' current admissions and an integrated file of any previous care at that facility. Although the use of electronic technologies in medical records is rapidly growing, very few medical facilities are entirely "paperless." Inpatient units, intensive care units (ICUs), and some outpatient clinics often maintain some kind of paper record. The paper documents amassed during a hospital admission are sorted, and much of the paper record information is ultimately scanned into the electronic medical record following discharge. As facilities gradually transfer their records to electronic files, computerized records will become the primary, or *official*, medical record, and paper records, or "shadow charts," will be discouraged. Issues related to computerized medical records are discussed in more detail later in this chapter. The most common types of organizational formats for medical records include:

- *Flow Sheets* and *Clinical (Critical) Pathway* Documentation
- *Source-Oriented* (SO) or *Source-Indexed (SI)* medical records
- *Problem-Oriented Medical Records (POMRs)*
- *Standards-Based Documentation* or *Documentation by Exception*
- *Problem-Intervention-Evaluation (P.I.E.) Format*
- *Chronologic Records of Episodes of Care*

1. Flow Sheets and Clinical Pathway Documentation

The type of paper documentation most commonly found at a patient's bedside is the **flow sheet**. Flow sheets typically span a 24-hour time frame and contain spaces, or "cells," for the pertinent parameters to be recorded, for example, vital signs, ins and outs, nutrition, mental status, respiratory therapy treatments, and rehabilitation therapy treatments. Similar to the flow sheet documentation are the **clinical (or critical) care pathway** documents. Care pathways, or **care paths**, are "maps" of best practices protocols and standards of care for particular diagnoses or conditions. These care paths span the entire admission from the Emergency Department (ED) through the projected day of discharge. In some cases, preadmission data are included. For example, a routine labor and delivery (L and D) care path covers the preadmission onset of labor instructions and the postadmission sequence of procedures and interventions. Care paths stipulate the anticipated time frame from admission to discharge and the discharge plans and follow-up instructions. The care pathways are sometimes documented in individual booklets, or flow sheets, that contain cells to check whether the elements in the plan have been completed and signed by the responsible person. For example, the clinical care pathway for the patient undergoing a total hip replacement might include a space to document any presurgical teaching and training, any admitting x-ray and laboratory studies, the physical examination at admission, and the surgeon's and anesthesiologist's presurgical visits prior to or during the first hours or day of admission. The pathway maps out the course, schedule, and expected duration of each of the critical elements of care based on "best practices" standards for management of the condition.

2. *Source-Oriented Medical Records*

Source-oriented (SO), or **source-indexed (SI)**, **records** contain separate sections for physicians' orders, progress notes, nurses' notes, x-ray reports, laboratory findings, and so forth. SO electronic records have tabs for the various types of notes, such as "Rehab Therapies." Entries may include templates or may be written or typed in a narrative format that documents the problem or reason for the visit, the duration of the problem, physical findings, laboratory and other study findings, diagnosis and secondary conditions, therapeutic and preventive services or medications prescribed, and the follow-up plan. Entries may also be made in a "SOAP" format, which is described in the next section.

3. *Problem-Oriented Medical Records*

Problem-oriented medical records (POMRs) are organized relative to the patient's "Problem List," including both the reason for the admission or visit and any preexisting or other active diseases. The patient's medical problems are listed and numbered and the list might include medical, surgical and previous surgeries, and psychiatric and social problems. Previously treated problems or surgeries are sometimes listed with the word "resolved" next to them. The problem list can also include the need to "R/O," or rule out, a questionable diagnosis. In general, POMRs are organized with the following sections:

- Introductory section, or the *Data Base*
- *Problem List*
- *Initial Plan*
- *Progress Notes*

Progress notes are itemized, or headed, relative to each problem. For example, the SLP's notes might be headed "Problem #1: Aphasia, secondary to left CVA" followed by "Speech-Language Pathology Initial Plan." Progress notes may be organized in a format termed "SOAP," or notes may be briefly written narratives.

SOAP Format

S *Subjective observations* (behavioral observations about the patient, comments, observations related to the patient's mental status, or the patient's complaints), for example,

"S — Pt. said, 'I'm feeling sick all over.' "

"Pt. c/o (complains of) fatigue."

"Pt. was inattentive during this visit."

O *Objective observations or findings* (data and facts), for example,

"O — Pt. reliably indicated yes and no to 10 orientation questions."

A *Assessment* (your analysis and formulation), for example,

"A — Mental status has improved from yesterday."

P *Plan* (steps and measures to be taken or recommended), for example,

"P — Standardized testing is scheduled to begin tomorrow."

4. Standards-Based Documentation or Documentation by Exception

Standards-based documentation, or *documentation by exception*, is a method of documentation of care that references predefined norms, protocols, and standards of care. If care is provided in accordance to these prestated standards and the response to care does not vary from the expected response, then only symbols, such as check marks, or notations, such as "P" for *progressing* or "E" for *evaluation*, are required in the notes. If there are variations in the typical plan or in the patient's response, then a *focused note* will be written. Focused notes are one- or two-phrase narrative notes. Usually, the standards-based or documentation by exception format uses a 24-hour flow sheet that refers to predetermined standards. For example, if the facility has established a standard care pre- and postsurgical protocol for "Total Laryngectomy," the SLP's Laryngectomy Communication Protocol will be referenced. The flow sheet contains a place for the clinician to note that the standard protocol is being followed, and daily, long narrative notes will not be needed unless there is some variation from the protocol due to a complication or abnormal response.

5. Problem-Intervention-Evaluation (P.I.E.) Format

A documentation format used occasionally in nursing notes is referred to as *problem-intervention-evaluation*, or P.I.E., format. This system consists of a running list of nursing diagnoses that is subdivided into three components: "**P**," statements of the problems; "**I**," interventions made; and "**E**," evaluation of the outcomes of the interventions.

6. Chronologic Records of Episodes of Care

Chronologic records place all notes, laboratory findings, procedures, consultation reports, and so forth in the file *sequentially in time* as they are written or received. This sort of file might be found in some outpatient clinic records, such as a voice clinic, where there is a single problem or condition that is followed longitudinally and involves relatively few visits. Electronic medical records allow for automatic documentation of the date and the exact time episodes of care were recorded. A facility may have a policy that all notes and reports be filed within a given time frame (e.g., on the date of service or within 24 hours), and auditors will look at the filing date for notes to ensure that the policy has been followed.

VI. COMPUTERIZED RECORDS AND COMMUNICATIONS

A. Electronic Records

Bedside computer stations and portable notebook computers are becoming increasingly available for clinicians. These small, handheld, or wall-mounted devices use either a touch sensitive screen or a keyboard. Computerized record keeping has some disadvantages inherent in the technologies (e.g., "ye ole' server problems") and it requires technical support to maintain and upgrade. Consequently, many settings and clinics maintain paper forms of documentation as either a backup or the preferred method of record keeping. The advantages to computerized systems for documentation are: *increased legibility; standardization of information*; *outcomes data measurement*; *off-site access* to medical records; and most importantly, *confidentiality* of the records.

B. Confidentiality of Electronic Records

Confidentiality of protected health information is mandatory in medical settings. Access to any patient record or private data is limited to a "need to know" basis. As a rule, communication with e-mail regarding patient appointments and health-related communication is discouraged, unless these communications take place in a secure, encrypted format. Some facilities offer certain staff members the opportunity to access medical records from their home computers through what is sometimes called a "virtual private network" (VPN). This access is restricted and measures are taken to ensure that transmissions are encrypted and secure. Individuals who access an electronic medical record from their home or office leave their "electronic fingerprints" on that record. Medical record audits will generate a list of all the individuals who have accessed a given record. Anyone who has accessed **protected health information** (PHI) should have authorization *and* a defensible reason to access that confidential information or risk dismissal.

C. Efficiency and Completeness

Computerized records and orders increase accuracy, completeness, and efficiency of noting. For example, when multiple disciplines are needed for an evaluation, such as the dysphagia team, the computer can generate several orders simultaneously. Reports and progress notes can be seen by multiple disciplines at the same time. Additionally, the development of standardized forms and templates reduces typing time and ensures that every concern that payers (e.g., Blue Cross-Blue Shield or Centers on Medicare and Medicaid Services [CMS]) and accrediting bodies (e.g., The Joint Commission, State Health Department) require be addressed in the record is noted and documented by the providers. For example, The Joint Commission requires providers to assess any "barriers to learning" in patient education. Templates help to make sure that providers remember to address these questions. Most payers require evidence of measurable, functional progress toward the stated rehabilitation goals. Templates can be designed to provide therapists with a record of progress that is clearly linked to each of the short- and long-term goals.

VII. GUIDELINES FOR ENTRIES IN PROGRESS NOTES

Medical chart notes and reports should always be signed by the actual provider via an electronic *personal identification number* (PIN) or in writing. The name and title or degree of the provider should always be stated along with his or her discipline. Physician assistants (PAs) and nurse practitioners (NPs) acting on behalf of a physician should indicate their credentials. It is standard practice for therapy staff to put "PT," "OT," "RT," or "SLP" after their name, if that is not obvious. The designation "MS, CCC-SLP" may not translate as "speech-language pathologist" to some readers, and the referent "Speech Path" may be preferred. Medical record departments require that the nature of the note and the author's discipline also be designated in the note headings. For example, progress notes might be headed as "Speech-Language Pathology Consultation," "Speech Path (or SLP)-Admitting Note," "Speech Path-Progress Note," "Speech Path-Treatment Note," "Speech Path-Transfer Note," or "Speech Path- Discharge Plan." Because the styles and procedures for medical charting vary among institutions, SLPs should follow the local format and policies.

A. Handwritten Entries in Medical Records

When making handwritten medical chart entries, you should:

- Use a pen, preferably with *black ink.*
- Write (or print) *legibly.*
- Enter the *date and time* of the note and *duration of the visit.* Some facilities require entering the time of the note and may prefer a 24-hour clock or "military time," where 6:00 p.m. equals 1800 hours. Payers are increasingly requiring rehabilitation therapy notes to include the actual duration of the visit in time units, usually in minutes or "units" of 15 minutes.
- Record only information related or significant to *your* assessment or plan.
- *Correct all mistakes.* If you make an error or information is omitted do not erase or "white out" the error; draw a line through your mistake or insert the missing information with a caret (^). Put your initials next to any corrections and write "error" above the mistake.
- Avoid phrases such as "seems to," "appears to," or "apparently."
- Avoid *personal comments* or assigning blame for a problem.
- Avoid *excessive spacing* within and between notes.
- If notes exceed one page, write *"continued on pg 2"* at the bottom of the first page and then *"Speech Path Note continued from pg 1"* at the top of the second page.
- Use *descriptions in place of labels.*
- Use the facility's published or conventionally *accepted abbreviations* and omit words such as "an," "a," and "the" whenever possible.
- Be *brief.*
- Sign all notes with your *name and professional title.*

B. Verbal Communication

Verbal communication with physicians and other health care providers in telephone calls or oral reports should get directly to the point and include only the pertinent information. One communication method that was developed to meet that objective is referred to as **SBAR**, an acronym that stands for: **S**ituation, **B**ackground, **A**ssessment, and **R**ecommendation, to delineate how the verbal reporting format is structured. Increasingly, SBAR is becoming the preferred, standardized way of communicating among health care providers, particularly nurse and physician communications. The intention of SBAR is to improve patient safety and communication efficiency by applying a standardized format. SBAR communication helps caregivers communicate about patients in a predictable, concise, and complete way.

VIII. PATIENT AND FAMILY EDUCATION

An essential area that must be addressed in health service delivery is **patient and family education.** All of the accrediting standards for health care facilities require an assessment of the patient's and caregiver's needs for education, which includes a determination of any barriers to learning.

This assessment addresses any difficulties with understanding or using English and any cultural or religious issues that could affect patient or caregiver education and compliance with instructions. Sensory losses (hearing, vision); speech, language, or cognitive barriers to learning; the preferred learning method (demonstration versus spoken, or written versus videotaped or oral instruction); and the motivation level of the learner are also taken into account. Every member of the care team who provides patient or family education is expected to document the *topic of the instruction*, the *teaching method*, the *materials used*, and the *recipient's response* to the instruction (i.e., how the patient or family member demonstrated the knowledge gained from the instruction). In acute care settings, a standard patient education flow sheet, patient education form, or chronological notebook for patient education documentation is maintained throughout the admission.

IX. ORGANIZATION OF INFORMATION

A. Medical Chart Organization

Medical charts are generally organized to contain the following information:

- **Admitting History and Physical (H & P) Examination**. An outline of the **chief complaint (CC)**, admitting diagnosis, pertinent medical history, vital signs, and findings of the physical examination of the patient.
- **Doctors' Orders.** Section containing every lab study, test, procedure, therapy, consultation, or medication ordered by the physician(s).
- **Progress Notes.** Narrative or problem-oriented notes of observations, data, and plans for treatment. Occasionally, charts will contain separate sections for Physicians' Progress Notes and the progress notes made by other staff.
- **Nurses' Care Plan and Progress Notes.** A separate section of notes made by the patient's primary nurse(s) at the end of each shift or whenever a notable change has occurred or a problem arises.
- **Nutrition Care Plans.** Diet histories, nutritional status notes, and nutrition plans prepared and implemented by the dietitians, dietary technicians, or unit nurses.
- **Consultation Reports.** Written responses to requests for consultation from various disciplines.
- **Lab Findings.** Data summaries of laboratory studies, or lab "panels" ordered by the physician (lists or graphs of laboratory findings and special notations for abnormal findings).
- **ECG.** Section containing selected electrocardiograph strips.
- **Imaging Studies.** Reports from any radiology studies.
- **Procedure Notes.** The narrative summary describing details of specific procedures, for example, surgeries.
- **Miscellaneous Data and Notes.** Special administrative forms, medical coverage information.
- **Discharge Summaries.** The physician's narrative summary of the hospital course and discharge plan.

- **Subspecialty Discharge Summaries.** Discharge summaries from various subspecialists who have provided treatment and who are participating in the discharge plan.
- **Patient Data.** Patient's address, phone number, next-of-kin contact, insurance plan, and employer.
- **Consents and Directives.** Research releases, special protocol forms, informed consents, and **advance medical directives** or a copy of the patient's **living will**.

B. Consent Forms

The paper copies, containing original signatures, of any special consent forms or waivers are filed with the patient's medical record and/or scanned into the electronic record. The format for these forms will have been reviewed and approved by several entities, such as the individuals responsible for *Risk Management*; the *Compliance Office*; the **Medical Records Committee**; the **Human Subjects Committee**; and in some cases, an **Institutional Review Board**.

Consent forms must adhere to rigorous guidelines as to who is giving consent and assurances that the patient is fully informed of the risks and benefits of any procedures or studies and to protect the rights of the patient (discussed further later and in Chapter 14). In some cases it may be necessary to use alternative communication methods, assistive devices, or interpreters to ensure that all parties (patient and family) understand the informed consent. In cases when the SLP, translator, family member, or another member of the hospital staff has assisted with an explanation of the consent form, the method used to obtain consent should be stated.

C. Advance Medical Directives

Increasingly, some type of *advance medical directives*, or a copy of the patient's *living will*, is required prior to admission. These documents specify the patient's preferred emergency contacts, who, if any, are legally authorized to make medical care decisions on behalf of the patient, and directives if the patient does or does not wish to be resuscitated (*do not resuscitate*, or *DNR*) in the event of a catastrophic cardiopulmonary emergency. Advance medical directives is discussed further in Chapter 14.

D. Admitting Orders

The conventional format used for the physician's admitting medical notes and orders varies according to the preferences of the facility's medical staff. Admitting notes usually include "notifications," which is a list of individuals who need to be notified of the admission (such as the senior resident, the private physician, etc.) and the medication and admitting orders. The admitting orders may follow a format referenced by the mnemonic "**ADC VAAN DISCL**," which refers to:

- **Admit** (to a stated ward, team, doctor, or service)
- **Diagnosis** (admitting medical diagnoses)
- **Condition** (indicating whether the patient is critical or stable)
- **Vitals** (listing temperature, heart rate, respiration rate, blood pressure, height, and weight)

- **Activity** (indicating degree of allowable activity)
- **Allergies** (drug, food, environmental agents, and any known sensitivities or reactions)
- **Nursing** (stating bed positioning, preps, wound care, etc.)
- **Diet** (stating the method for nutritional support)
- **Ins and outs** (listing the tubes and drains that are to be inserted)
- **Special** (listing special risks, observations, studies needed)
- **Consults** (SLP, occupational therapist [OT], physical therapist [PT], etc.)
- **Labs** (indicating which studies and special tests need to be made and the times they should be done)

E. Laboratory Findings

Further discussion of the history and physical examination and typical methods used to record findings is found in Chapter 3 and elsewhere in this text. It should be noted that along with conventional formats for the organization and method for making notes in medical records, there are also prescribed "shorthand" methods for recording specific data. For example, the format for recording the standard laboratory values that are part of the physician's chart work is provided in Figure 2–1. The top diagram shows how the "blood work," or hematologic analysis, is noted. **CBC** refers to **complete blood count** (WBC, *white blood count*; Hgb, *hemoglogin*; and HCT, *hematocrit*). The other two diagrams indicate how electrolyte and renal function parameters are recorded. Chapter 3 discusses the significance of fluid and electrolyte findings, and Chapter 9 describes the significance of certain hematologic parameters. The values for a normal range in these laboratory analyses are provided in Appendix A.

F. Nurses' Kardex

In acute care and subacute care facilities, a nurses' Kardex may be kept on the ward to provide a "hard" (not computerized), quick reference of the current orders and key parameters of the patients' care. The Kardex typically has plastic covered index cards with pertinent information for each patient affixed to a Rolodex-type holder, or in an index card file, in a sequence according to the room and bed numbers for that ward. The Kardex sometimes contains information that is not retrievable from a patient's medical chart, for example, an unlisted telephone number for the patient's closest relative, or the real identification of patients admitted under an alias. The most current diet and medication orders are also noted in the Kardex. In some facilities, there is one Kardex for medications and another Kardex for procedures.

G. Incident, Occurrence, and Variance Report Forms

A system for the reporting and facility's oversight of patient and employee accidents (incident or occurrence reports) or any variances in the care of patients will be in place as part of the facility's safety program and risk monitoring processes. Usually, there is a requirement that a formal report of any accident, incident, or variance in care be completed, be signed by a

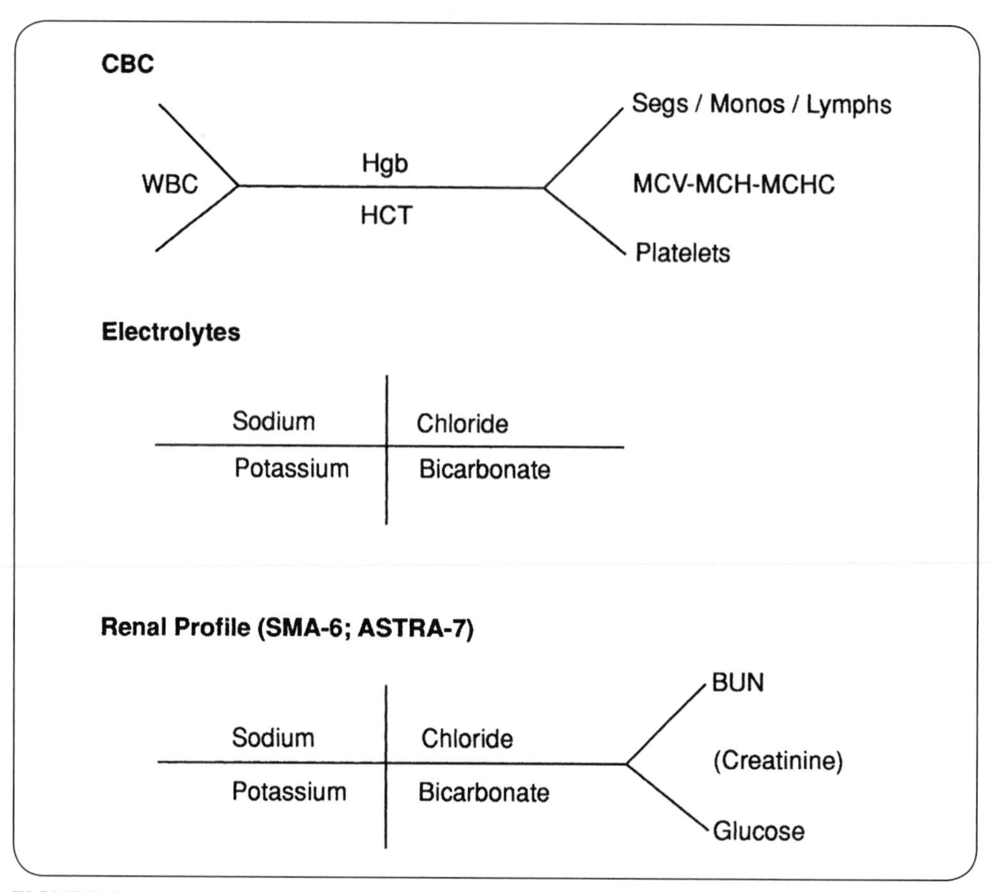

FIGURE 2–1 Common methods for noting laboratory values in medical charts. Source: Delmar/Cengage Learning

supervisor, and be filed with the Safety Office within 24 hours of the event. Occasionally an investigation by Risk Management personnel may be needed. The facility has policies and procedures for reporting these events. If the incident or variance involves a medical device, then the reporting guidelines for compliance with the **Safe Medical Devices Act** is followed.

X. NOTES IN MEDICAL CENTER TRAINING PROGRAMS

Hospitals that are affiliated with physician training programs, or teaching hospitals, have restrictions regarding what can and cannot be written by **medical students** and other students (SLP practicum students) in medical records. **House staff** (interns and residents), **fellows** (junior physicians involved in postresidency clinical or research fellowships), and **attending physicians** (staff physicians) and other licensed practitioners enter notes that are headed and signed to designate the author's status. Notes written by students are cosigned by the supervising staff members with an addendum declaring that they were present during and participated in the examination and that they fully concur with the plans. The medical students' notes, if allowed, may be headed "MS III AN," meaning the note was written by a third-year medical student and the note is his or her "Admitting

Note." The notation "RAN" denotes a "Resident Admitting Note," and "IPN" denotes an "Intern Progress Note," and so forth. Consultation requests to specialists and subspecialists for their opinions will usually receive a response from either the attending staff physician in a particular subspecialty or a "fellow" from that specialty (see Chapter 1). Thus, one might find consultation reports and notes headed, for example, as "Cardiology Fellow Consult."

XI. SYMBOLS, PRESCRIPTIONS, AND ADMINISTRATION OF DRUGS

A. Symbols and Abbreviations

Medical abbreviations, acronyms, eponyms, symbols, and prescription notations can be difficult to interpret, although one can frequently surmise the meaning from the context. Some abbreviations are idiosyncratic to the user or a given facility, and some notations are used inappropriately or mistakenly, even by medically trained personnel, especially medical students. Chapter 3, Vital Signs and the Physical Examination, contains a list of terminology and abbreviations commonly encountered in progress notes and reports.

Table 2–1 provides a summary of prescription order notations and their meanings. Table 2–2 lists common medical chart symbols. Additional symbols and discussions of the effects of drugs on communicative abilities and disorders can be found in the *Dictionary of Medical Acronyms and Abbreviations* (Jablonski, 2005) and in *The Effects of Drugs on Communication Disorders* (Vogel & Carter, 1995).

TABLE 2–1 Abbreviations used in prescriptions

ABBREVIATION	DERIVATION	MEANING
aa	*ana*	of each
a.c.	*ante cibum*	before meals
ad	*ad*	to, up to
ad lib	*ad libitum*	as desired
alt. dieb.	*alternis diebus*	every other day
alt. hor.	*alternis horis*	every other hour
aq.	*aqua*	water
b.i.d.	*bis in die*	two times a day
b.i.n.	*bis in nocte*	twice at night
c.	*cum*	with
Cap.	*capiat*	let him take
cf	*conferre*	compare to
Det.	*detur*	let it be given
e.g.	*exempli gratia*	for example, for instance
et al.	*et alii*	and others

continues

TABLE 2–1 Abbreviations used in prescriptions

ABBREVIATION	DERIVATION	MEANING
Ft.	*fiat*	make
id.	*idem*	the same
i.a.	*inter alia*	among others
i.e.	*id est*	that is
NB	*nota bene*	note well
o.d.	*omni die*	every day
O.D.	*oculus dexter*	right eye
o.h.	*omni hora*	every hour
o.m.	*omni mane*	every morning
o.n.	*omni nocte*	every night
o., os	*os*	mouth
O.S.	*oculus sinister*	left eye
p.c.	*post cibum*	after meals
per	*per*	through or by
p.o.	*per os*	by mouth
p.r.n.	*pro re nata*	when needed
QED	*quod erat demonstrandum*	that which was to have been shown
q.h.	*quaque hora*	every hour
q. 2h		every 2 hours
q. 4h		every 4 hours
q. 6h[a]		every 6 hours
q.i.d.[a]	*quarter in die*	four times a day
q.l.	*quantum libet*	as much as desired
q.n.	*quaque nocte*	every night
q.p.	*quantum placeat*	as much as desired
q.v.	*quantum vis*	as much as you please
q.s.	*quantum sufficit*	as much as required
q/s	*quaque*/shift	each shift
Rx	recipe	prescription

TABLE 2–1 Abbreviations used in prescriptions

ABBREVIATION	DERIVATION	MEANING
s̄	*sine*	without
Sig. or *S*	*signa*	write on label
s.o.s.	*si opus si*	if necessary
ss	*semis*	a half
stat.	*statim*	immediately
t.d.s.	*ter die sumendum*	to be taken three times daily
t.i.d.	*ter in die*	three times a day
t.i.n.	*ter in nocte*	three times at night
ut dict	*ut dictum*	as directed
v.i.	*vide infra*	see below
via	*via*	by way of
viz	*viz*	namely
v.s.	*vide supra*	see above

[a] **Note:** q.i.d. and q. 6 h are not the same orders. Q.i.d. means the medication will be administered 4 times a day; q. 6 h means it will be administered by designated clock intervals (12 noon, 6 p.m., 12 midnight, 6 a.m.).

TABLE 2–2 Common medical symbols*

SYMBOL	MEANING
a	Before
i̇, ii̇, iii̇	one, two, three (drops)
#	Number, pounds, size, fracture
+	Plus, excess, positive, acid reaction
–	Minus, deficiency; negative; alkaline reaction
↑	Increase; increasing
↓	Decrease; decreasing
⇄	Reversible reaction
□, ♂	Male
○, ♀	Female

continues

TABLE 2–2 Common medical symbols*

SYMBOL	MEANING
>	Greater than
<	Less than
≥	Equal to or greater than
≤	Equal to or less than
Δ	Change
°	Degree, secondary to
=	Equals
≠	Does not equal
::	As; equal ratios of
2°	Secondary to
∴	Therefore
$\bar{c}$.	With
$\bar{s}$	Without
→	Yields, causes, leads to, leading to
:	Ratio
n, N—	Negative
O	Normal
$\bar{p}$	Post, after
Λ	Systolic blood pressure
V	Diastolic blood pressure

* Although symbols continue to be commonly found in paper medical records and doctors' orders and prescriptions, The Joint Commissions strongly recommends against their use to prevent medical errors.

B. Prescriptions

In the United States, drugs and other pharmacologic therapies are regulated in that they are only prescribed by physicians who are licensed by the Medical Licensure Boards in the states where they practice and "registered" with the **Drug Enforcement Agency (DEA).** Prescriptions are not required for "over-the-counter" medications. The federal **Food and Drug Administration (FDA)** determines whether a drug may be distributed and sold and if a physician's prescription is required for its use. The **United States Pharmacopeia (USP)** sets standards for purity and determines if the drug is indeed a useful therapy based on an analysis of clinical trial evidence. Licensed pharmacists dispense drugs in accordance with the physician's verbal (by telephone) order, faxed order, or handwritten order either on a signed prescription form or by written request in the "Doctor's Orders" section of the medical chart. In medical progress notes, telephone orders are noted as T/O, or t/o, and verbal orders are noted as V/O, or v/o.

C. Drug Names

A drug can have three different names:

- The **chemical formula,** or chemical name
- The **brand name, proprietary,** or trade name, which will usually be followed by a superscript® notation to indicate it is registered
- The **generic,** or official name, of the drug that is its legal and scientific name

For example: *Alpha-aminobenzyl P* is the chemical formula; *Amcap, Amcill, D-Amp, Omnipen, Pfizerpen A, Polycillin, Principen, SK-Ampicillin, Supen, Totacillin* are the brand names; and *ampicillin* is the generic chemical name. Most facilities have reference links for drugs within the electronic medical record, or written publications by the hospital pharmacy, to access the **Hospital Formulary** and the ***Physicians' Desk Reference (PDR)***. The latter is published privately and updated yearly. Facilities with electronic medical records provide links to other electronic tools, such as ***Hippocrates***®.

D. Administration of Drugs

The method of drug administration varies depending on how the medicine is best absorbed. Drugs given *orally* are absorbed in the bloodstream through the gastrointestinal walls. Drugs administered *sublingually* are dissolved by the saliva and absorbed rapidly through the mucous membranes of the mouth. Drugs administered *transdermally* utilize adhesive patches placed on the skin. Some drugs are applied *topically* as pastes or creams on the skin, and some are *inhaled* as vaporous gases or aerosols. *Rectal administration,* through suppositories or enemas, is usually done when the patient is too ill or too nauseated to tolerate oral intake. Direct injection of a drug may be done through a syringe (needle) into the muscle tissue (*intramuscular*, or IM); under the skin, *subcutaneously* ("sub Q"); into the skin, *intradermally*; directly into a vein, *intravenously* (IV); or, as with some forms of chemotherapy, *intra-arterially*, directly into an artery.

XII. ADMINSTRATIVE TERMINOLOGY AND ABBREVIATIONS

In addition to the medical vocabulary and abbreviations encountered in medical settings, the health care system in the United States employs considerable health care administrative terminology, principally generated by third-party payers, CMS, and accrediting bodies. The following provides a short list of the more commonly found terms.

A. Administrative Terminology

Access. The ability to obtain medical care.

Advance medical directives. Living will.

Ambulatory patient classifications (APCs). In Medicare's prospective payment systems, the outpatient equivalent of inpatient "diagnosis-related groups, or DRGs."

Ancillary services. Hospital services provided in conjunction with medical care (e.g., physical therapy, radiology, laboratory services).

Appropriate. Medically justified and necessary.

Beneficiary. Insured person.

Capitation. A fixed rate of payment to cover specifically designated services.

Centers for Medicare and Medicaid Services (CMS). The federal agency charged with overseeing Medicare and Medicaid programs, formerly the *Health Care Financing Administration (HCFA).*

Claim. A reimbursement application or bill submitted to a payer, either a private or public health benefits plan.

Coinsurance. The percent of medical costs that the beneficiary (insured person) must pay after the deductible is satisfied.

Consolidated Omnibus Budget Reconciliation Act (COBRA). Federal legislation enacted in 1985 containing amendments to the Medicare and Medicaid entitlements.

Cost center. The facility's program or department budgeted for particular costs (e.g., an SLP salary may be budgeted in and paid from the rehab department's "cost center").

Coverage exclusions and limitations. Conditions (diagnoses) explicitly excluded from insurance coverage, or coverage limitations allowing a set number of visits and/or duration of treatment.

Covered service. Service or procedure that is covered in the patient's health care plan.

Criteria. Stated guidelines for determining the necessity and appropriateness of a health care service.

Current Procedural Terminology® (CPT). Referring to five-digit codes with modifiers as a standard for identifying the procedures performed for billing purposes; previously CPT referred to *Common* Procedural Terminology.

Deductible. The amount of a medical expense that must be incurred and paid by the beneficiary before the third-party payer becomes liable for payment.

Diagnosis-related groups (DRGs). Under Medicare payment procedures for hospitals, DRGs refer to categories of reimbursement for care based on the patient's diagnosis(es) and related cost factors. This payment system assumes that patients with certain diagnoses will require an estimated amount of cost that is determined by aggregated, actuarial data.

Edits. Medicare electronic coding audits that identify conflicts in procedure codes (e.g., codes that cannot be billed together on the same day for the same patient).

Effectiveness. Probability of benefit.

Encounter. Patient visit.

Enrollee. Insured person; person covered by a health benefit plan.

Evidence-based medicine. The application of the best available research evidence, and prevailing expert opinion, in addition to the provider's and the patient's preferences to guide diagnostic or management decisions.

Fee-for-service. Method of payment for treatment with reimbursement based on individual fees for each procedure or visit.

International Classification of Diseases, ICD-9-CM, ICD-10-CM. The official diagnostic coding system developed and published by the U.S. Department of Public Health Service's National Center for Health Statistics that is used in health care to identify by standard codes the diagnosed diseases, or conditions, the patient has. For psychiatric conditions, the ***Diagnostic and Statistical Manual for Mental Disorders*-4th Edition, DSM-IV,** coding system is applied. This "multiaxial" coding system for mental conditions is published by the American Psychiatric Association (APA).

Managed care. Various cost containment systems put in place with the goal of delivering cost-effective care without compromising the quality. Managed care plans include limits on inpatient hospitalization coverage by prospective payments (see DRGs, encourage the hospital to reduce the **lengths of stays (LOS)** as much as possible, and limit the services to only those essential for quality care. Outpatient services are usually provided through a "gatekeeper" mechanism, which requires that certain steps are followed in the referral processes and may place limits on the number of visits, the types of procedures that can be preformed in a given day, and the diagnoses covered. Managed care policies may have a pharmacy benefit, but usually medications also have restrictions so that less expensive, generic drugs are encouraged and accumulations of stockpiles of several months' supplies of medications are disallowed and discouraged.

Medicare Advantage. Extended insurance coverage in addition to the basic Medicare benefits. These programs typically place "gatekeeper" limits on coverage benefits, including access to only the hospitals and physicians that are associated with a given plan.

Medicare Part A. Referring to the schedule of payment in Medicare benefits covering nonspecific institutional expenses incurred by inpatients in hospitals and postdischarge for a fixed time frame (up to the first 100 days of treatment) and for certain conditions in skilled nursing facilities, home health care, and hospice care settings. Eligibility for Part A is automatic for U.S. citizens over 65 years of age and for certain medical conditions, such as end-stage renal disease (ESRD).

Medicare Part B. The optional medical insurance for people over 65 years of age that covers services rendered by physicians and other practitioners in outpatient hospitals and clinics, nonskilled nursing settings, rehabilitation agencies, and similar settings.

Medicare Part D. Medicare's prescription drug ("D") coverage.

Medicare Title XVIII of Social Security Act. A federal health insurance program for people age 65 or older and for individuals with certain chronic medical diseases or disabilities.

Outcome. A result.

Outliers. Patient outcome or laboratory data that vary widely from normal expectations.

Pay for performance. A Medicare initiative intended to differentiate among providers and provide incentives for quality outcomes.

Performance Improvement. The organization's quality assurance program that provides continuous monitoring, identification, correction, and study of corrective outcomes to improve the quality of health care services.

Practice guidelines. Standard recommendations for patient care.

Practice pattern. Data illustrating the characteristics of a given practitioner's use of medical resources (admissions of certain diagnoses, tests ordered, procedures performed, etc.).

Preadmission review. An administrative review of the justification for procedures prior to admission, usually a feature of managed care.

Precertification. A requirement made by certain forms of medical coverage, such as Medicare, whereby the **plans of treatment (POTs)** must be periodically reviewed, approved, and "certified" by the patient's referring physician.

Premium. The cost (to the employer or individual, or both) to purchase health insurance.

Prior authorization. A review by a third-party payer of the justification of a given service and permission to proceed with a procedure before it is provided to a beneficiary.

Product line. In health service administration, a product line refers either to a revenue center or a cost center for a particular "line" of service. For example, rehabilitation can be a line of service and all aspects of care required to provide that health service "product" would fall under that cost center. Thus, the SLP costs attached to the rehabilitation team or unit would be included in calculating the costs for that program or product line. There are a couple of advantages to having product line revenue and cost centers: One is the ease of determining costs for particular programs, and the other is the organization of multiple providers into a unit, or team, whose members are responsible for its costs, revenues, and outcomes.

Provider. The individual providing health care services. Licensed physicians, psychologists, and dentists are designated as **licensed individual providers (LIPs)** and are required to have a **National Provider Identification (NPI)** number from Medicare.

Reasonable cost basis. A method that determines the Medicare reimbursement amount based on the operational expenses of the provider.

Resource-Based Relative Value Scale (RBRVS). Refers to a valuation, or rating, of Medicare Part B services on the basis of the *relative resource inputs* (work and other practice costs) that is required to provide services. RBRVSs have been used by managed care groups, in addition to Medicare, and have replaced the previous physician fee schedules that were historically based on the "customary, prevailing, and reasonable" charges.

Relative value units (RVUs). RVUs are applied by Medicare to determine reimbursement rates. These values are derived by committees of the American Medical Association, which include all medical specialties and representatives from nursing and other health professions. RVUs are reviewed annually and studied in depth every five years. These AMA committees consider how many hours or minutes it takes to perform a given procedure (referenced by its CPT®); the level of skill, education, and training required; and the practice expense (including malpractice costs) associated with a procedure.

Retrospective utilization review. An examination of the appropriateness, cost, and outcome of medical services in an audit of medical charts.

State Children's Health Insurance Program (S-CHIP). A federally mandated system for providing health insurance to children based on eligibility criteria supported by both state and federal funds.

Surgical Care Improvement Project (SCIP). A national quality improvement project endorsed by CMS designed to improve surgical care in hospitals.

The Joint Commission. An autonomous, national (and now international) private sector, not-for-profit accrediting agency for hospitals and other health services organizations. The Joint Commission's mission is to elevate and maintain quality and performance standards for health care delivery. The Joint Commission is sometimes referred to as "J-Co" in oral communication or as "JCAHO" in written documents.

Third-party payer. An entity providing health care coverage on behalf of the patient (first party) to the health care provider (second party).

Total quality improvement (TQI), Continuous Quality Improvement (CQI). Refers to Quality Assurance, or Performance Improvement, programs that are explicitly directed toward continually monitoring and improving services to ensure consistent quality and prevent variations, defects, and deficiencies in the provision of services (see Performance Improvement).

Tricare. The managed care health services system for active duty and retired military personnel, previously referred to as CHAMPAS.

Unbundle. A charging practice where individual procedures are billed separately rather than under one inclusive procedure code.

Upcode. Refers to an illegal practice whereby a patient is billed for a procedure that reflects a higher level of care than was provided.

Utilization review. A method to manage health care costs through a case-by-case evaluation of the justification for clinical services.

B. Administrative Abbreviations

AEP. Appropriateness evaluation protocol

A & H. Accident and health (insurance)

AMA. American Medical Association; Against Medical Advice

ANSI. American National Standards Institute

BBA, BBRA, BIPA. Balanced Budget Act, Balanced Budget Refinement Act, Benefits Improvement and Protection Act

BCBSA. Blue Cross and Blue Shield Association

C.A.R.F. The Commission on Accreditation of Rehabilitation Facilities

CDM. Charge Description Master (the facility's published list of its procedures, codes, and fees)

CHAMPAS. Civilian Health and Medical Program for Armed Services, recently revamped into a managed care system called Tricare

CHAMPVA. Civilian Health and Medical Program for Veterans Affairs

CME. Continuing medical education

CMGs. Case mix groups

CMS. Centers for Medicare and Medicaid Services

COBRA. Consolidated Omnibus Budget Reconciliation Act

CORF. Comprehensive Outpatient Rehabilitation Facility

CPR. Customary, prevailing, and reasonable; **UCR** - usual, customary, and reasonable

CPT®. Current Procedural Terminology

DHHS. (U.S.) Department of Health and Human Services

DME. Durable medical equipment

DMERC. Durable Medical Equipment Regional Carrier

DRG. Diagnosis-related group

DSM-IV. *Diagnostic and Statistical Manual for Mental Disorders*, 4th Edition

DVA. Department of Veterans Affairs

FDA. Food and Drug Administration (United States)

FFS. Fee for service

FMG. Foreign medical graduate

FY. Fiscal year

GAO. General Accounting Office (federal government)

HCPCS. Healthcare Common Procedural Coding System

HICN. Health insurance claim number

HIPAA. Health Insurance Portability and Accountability Act (note the correct abbreviation is, ***HIPAA***, not HIPPA).

HMO. Health maintenance organization

HRGs. Health resources groups (home health)

ICD-9 (CM); ICD-10. International Classification of Disease - 9th Edition (Clinical Modification); International Classification of Disease—10th Version

IRF PPS. Inpatient Rehabilitation Facilities Prospective Payment System

IG. Inspector general

IPA. Individual practice association

IRB. Institutional Review Board

ISD-A. Intensity of service, severity of illness, discharge, and appropriateness (screenings)

JCAHO. The Joint Commission, formerly the Joint Commission on Accreditation of Healthcare Organizations. Even though The Joint Commission has shortened its name, references to JCAHO may still appear in written communications, such as memos and meeting announcements.

LOS. Length of (hospital) stay

MAC. Maximal allowable charge

MedPAC. Medicare Payment Advisory Committee

MDS. Minimum Data Set

MFS. Medicare fee schedule

MHB. Maximum hospital benefits

NIH. National Institutes of Health

NPI - National Provider Identification number (CMS)

OASIS. Outcome and Assessment Information Set (in Home Health)

OPPS. Outpatient Prospective Payment System

PAI. Payment Assessment Instrument

PCP. Primary care physician

PLOF. Previous (or prior) level of functioning

PN. Provider number

POC. Plan of care, point of care

POS. Point of service

POT. Plan of treatment

PPRC. Physician Payment Review Commission

PPS. Prospective payment system

PRO. Peer review organization

RACs. Recovery audit contractors

RBRVS. Resource-based relative value scale

RICs. Rehabilitation impairment categories

RUG. Resource utilization group (in skilled nursing facilities)

RVU. Relative value unit

SNF. Skilled nursing facility

SOC. Start of care

SS. Social Security

SSI. Supplemental Security Income

SSN. Social security number

TPO. Treatment, payment, and operations; or time post onset

TQI. Total quality improvement

WHO. World Health Organization

XIII. RIGHT TO PRIVACY, CONFIDENTIALITY, AND INFORMED CONSENT

A. Right to Privacy

As discussed earlier, there are strict and closely monitored policies in force in all health care facilities to ensure that patients' **rights to privacy** are protected and that they have given their "informed consent" for any procedures posing a risk or of an experimental (research) nature. Surgeries or special invasive x-ray studies require prior written permission. Patients or their authorized representatives will be requested to sign a consent form that describes, in the language they speak and with terminology the average person can understand, the procedures that are planned and delineating all of the risks associated with those procedures. Any patient who is to be included in a research project or whose clinical data might be included in a research study is required, with rare exceptions, to have agreed to that participation by signing a *consent to participate* form. Academic medical centers and other facilities have Human Studies Committees or Institutional Review Boards (IRBs) that must review and approve proposed research projects, including retrospective studies of clinical records. The IRB ensures that the wording of consent forms meets all of the regulatory and legal criteria and ethical care guidelines (see Chapter 14 for further discussion). The IRB also considers other factors, including the appropriateness of the research design; privacy protections in the research data, record storage, and disposal methods; and any access to PHI.

B. Protected Health Information

PHI is medical as well as other data that could allow an individual to be identified, for example, name, social security number, address, medical record number, and the like. With the possible exception of a concern for patient safety, there is probably no area more strictly monitored in health care facilities than the confidentiality of the medical record. Safeguarding protected information was a primary facet of the **Health Insurance Portability and Accountability Act**, or **HIPAA**. The implementation of the privacy protections contained in that statute have overshadowed the initial intent of the statute, which was to allow greater access to insurance and to facilitate transfers of health care coverage from one job to the next (i.e., "portability") by preventing denials of coverage due to a preexisting condition when employees changed jobs. Today, everyone working in a medical setting must receive annual training in the adherence to the privacy protections and confidentiality requirements related to HIPAA. These policies apply to all forms of health information communications by researchers, service providers, and any other person or entity in the facility, including any business associates (another organization or individual not employed by the facility).

C. Releasing Medical Information

Generally, legal guidelines maintain that, although the medical record belongs to the facility, patients have the right to access the information contained in the record. The patient's physical medical file (in paper or electronic format) contains records and documents belonging to the facility and should *never be removed* from the facility. Sending photocopied medical chart notes or data, CDs, videotapes, and even reading medical record information on the telephone to anyone outside the treatment facility requires permission and a **release of information form** signed by the patient or his or her authorized, or legal, representative. Releasing information to the patient in the form of photocopies of notes or reports also requires that a release of information be signed and filed. Any photocopies of pages from the medical record that contains any type of identifying information should be limited to in-house use, unless it is explicitly requested and released by the patient or his or her authorized, or legal, representative. Facilities have policies that guide any release of information and standard "release of information" forms. Additionally, most facilities ask that any queries or requests for medical records that come from an attorney be referred to their Legal Affairs Department or Risk Management office.

XIV. MEDICAL ETHICS AND ETHICAL REVIEWS

The principles of **biomedical ethics** apply to everyone who works in a medical setting. Issues such as abortion, euthanasia, and the right to refuse treatment have prompted us to look to ethical principles for guidance in many health care decisions (Strand, Yorkston, & Miller, 2007). Strand et al. provide a review of the basic principles of medical ethics (autonomy, beneficence and nonmaleficence, justice, veracity, confidentiality, and fidelity) as they specifically apply to medical SLP. Professions also have **codes of ethics** that direct the conduct of their members. The Code of Ethics of the American Speech-Language-Hearing Association (ASHA) is provided to every ASHA member, and references are available to elucidate the clinical application of the proscriptions and rules outlined in the current version of the ASHA Code of Ethics (ASHA, 2003; Miller, 2007). These codes are not merely suggested guidelines. They are the **ethical practice directives** that are aspirational and inspirational and set the behavioral expectations for members of the profession. Adherence to both the legal restrictions for practice within the state in which clinicians are licensed and the code of ethics of their profession will help them make appropriate decisions in patient care, client relationships, business practices, and so forth, but, occasionally, legal questions, ethical dilemmas, and conflicts arise. Consequently, most facilities have processes and programs in place for training and oversight of medical ethics. These programs may include the Risk Management office (which may be a part of the Compliance Office) and a medical ethics, or bioethics, committee that includes clergy members, facility attorneys, social workers, physicians, nurses, and community representatives. Further discussion of this topic is found in Chapter 14.

XV. CLINICAL COMPETENCIES

The learner outcomes, skills, and competencies gained from information contained in this chapter include the ability to:

- Read, interpret, and use terminology, abbreviations, and symbols routinely encountered in medical records.
- Describe how documentation is used in The Joint Commission's Tracer Methodology audits.
- List the common formats and organizational schema of medical records.
- Define the elements of a SOAP note.

- List the guidelines for SLP handwritten notes in the medical record.
- Define "ADC VAAN DISCL."
- Define HIPAA and PHI.
- Discuss the three types of names given to drugs.
- Identify where and how blood and renal lab panels are noted in physician's chart work.
- Differentiate between ICD and CPT codes.
- Discuss the importance of protecting confidentiality and security of medical records.

XVI. REFERENCES AND RESOURCES CONSULTED

American Speech-Language-Hearing Association. (2003). *ASHA code of ethics.* Rockville, MD: Author.

Avery, M., & Imdieke, B. (1984). *Medical records in ambulatory care.* Rockville, MD: Aspen.

Brown, J. E., & Pietranton, A. A. (2007). Current trends and issues in health care delivery: What speech-language pathologists need to know. In A. F. Johnson & B. H. Jacobson (Eds.), *Medical speech-language pathology: A practitioner's guide* (2nd ed.). New York: Thieme.

Burke, L. J., & Murphy, J. (1988). *Charting by exception.* New York: John Wiley & Sons.

Davies, J. J. (2008). *Essentials of medical terminology* (3rd ed.). Clifton Park, NY: Delmar Cengage Learning.

Flaherty, A. W. (2000). *The Massachusetts General Hospital handbook of neurology.* Philadelphia: Lippincott Williams & Wilkins.

Fromberg, R. (1990). *Medical records review.* Oak Brook Terrace, IL: The Joint Commission on Accreditation of Healthcare Organizations.

Jablonski, S. (2005). *Dictionary of medical acronyms and abbreviations* (5th ed.). Philadelphia: Elsevier Saunders.

Kelly, W. J. (Ed.). (1992). *Clinical skillbuilders: Better documentation.* Springhouse, PA: Springhouse.

Kummer, A. W., Johnson, P., & Zeit, K. (2007). Clinical documentation in medical speech-language pathology. In A. F. Johnson & B. H. Jacobson (Eds.), *Medical speech-language pathology: A practitioner's guide* (2nd ed.). New York: Thieme.

Leonard, P. C. (2007). *Quick and easy medical terminology* (5th ed.). St. Louis, MO: Saunders Elsevier.

Lewis, L. W., & Timby, B. K. (1988). *Fundamental skills and concepts in patient care* (4th ed.). Philadelphia: J. B. Lippincott.

Lubinski, R., Golper, L. A. C., & Frattali, C. M. (Eds.). (2007). *Professional issues in speech-language pathology and audiology* (3rd ed.). Clifton Park, NY: Delmar Cengage Learning.

Miller, T. D. (2007). Professional ethics. In R. Lubinski, L. Golper, & C. Frattali (Eds.), *Professional issues in speech-language pathology and audiology* (3rd ed.). Clifton Park, NY: Delmar Cengage Learning.

Rice, J. (1991). *Medical terminology with human anatomy.* Norwalk, CT: Appleton & Lange.

Strand, E. A., Yorkston, K. M., & Miller, R. M. (2007). Medical ethics and the speech-language pathologist. In A. H. Johnson & B. H. Jacobson (Eds.), *Medical speech-language pathology: A practitioner's guide* (2nd ed.). New York: Thieme.

The Joint Commission. (2008). *Accreditation and certification manuals.* Naperville, IL: Author.

University Hospital Pharmacy Service. (1992). *Hospital formulary.* Little Rock: University Hospital of Arkansas.

Vogel, D., & Carter, J. E. (1995). *The effects of drugs on communication disorders.* San Diego, CA: Singular.

Wolper, L. F., & Pena, J. J. (Eds.). (1987). *Health care administration.* Rockville, MD: Aspen.

CHAPTER 3

Vital Signs and the Physical Examination

Temperature, pulse, respiration, weight, and *blood pressure* are the vital signs and essential indicators of an individual's state of health. Significant deviations from normal vital parameters usually indicate illness. To function competently as a member of the health care team, medical speech-language pathologists (SLPs) should know how these vital signs are evaluated and monitored and how the physical examination contributes to a diagnosis.

I. CHAPTER FOCUS

This chapter outlines features of the physician's medical history interview, or "review of systems," the physical examination data, and vital signs measurements that are a part of medical care for adults and children. Terminology and abbreviations that are commonly found in a history and physical (H & P) examination report findings and many of the commonly ordered laboratory tests are described. Although much of what is discussed in this chapter applies across the age span, specific attention is given to the vital signs and physical examination of infants and children where needed. Additional terminology and further elaboration of diseases and procedures specifically related to respiration and circulation are found in Chapter 9. The mental status and neurologic examination of both children and adults are described in detail in Chapter 4 and discussed in Chapters 10 and 14.

II. VITAL SIGNS AND THE PHYSICAL EXAMINATION

A. Terminology

ABO blood group incompatibility. Hemolytic anemia in which maternal antigen-antibody reaction causes fetal blood cell destruction (also see Chapter 6, Medical Genetics).

Acrocyanosis. Peripheral cyanosis (blue discoloration) involving the hands, feet, and lips.

Adjusted age. Calculations made during the first 2 years of life after a premature birth. The adjusted age is calculated by subtracting the number of weeks of prematurity from a full-term, 40 weeks (e.g., 5 weeks premature equals 35 weeks) then subtracting that number from the child's chronological age in weeks (for age in months divide by 4). It is important to consider the adjusted age when evaluating growth (weight, length or height), and other age-referenced developmental data, for example, a CDC growth chart, see Figure 3–5.

APACHES scores. A computerized evaluation system for scoring severity of illness in the intensive care unit (ICU) to predict survival outcomes. APACHES scores take into account the acute condition and chronic illness variables. APACHES is an acronym for **a**cute, **p**hysiology, **a**nd **c**hronic **h**ealth **e**valuation **s**ystem.

Apical rate. The number of heartbeats occurring in 1 minute as monitored by auscultation (listening by stethoscope) over the apex (upper tip) of the heart.

Apical-radial pulse rate (A/R). The pulse rate obtained by two listeners when one obtains the apical pulse rate and the other obtains the radial (wrist) pulse rate.

Apnea. A period when there is no breathing.

Apnea monitor. Device for monitoring heartbeats and respiration.

Arrhythmia. An irregular pattern of heartbeats and pulse.

Arteriosclerosis. A loss of arterial wall elasticity.

Ascites. Effusion (collection) of serous fluid into the abdominal cavity.

Atherosclerosis. A narrowing of the inside of the arteries due to fat accumulations.

Auscultate. To examine by way of listening with a stethoscope.

Axilla. Armpit.

Axillary temperature. The measurement of body heat obtained from a thermometer placed in the axilla.

Babinski sign. Extension, instead of the normal flexion, of the large toe on stimulation of the plantar surface of the foot indicative of pyramidal disease that is noted as present or absent in the examination (see Chapter 4 for further discussion of neurologic findings in reflex testing).

Barrel chest. Expanded chest cavity sometimes seen in association with severe pulmonary disease.

Battle's sign. Ecchymosis (swelling due to a bruise) behind the ear associated with basilar skull fractures.

Bifurcation. Forking into two divisions; Y-shaped.

Blood gases. Blood gas analysis or, more accurately, *arterial blood gas* (ABG) analysis that provides the best means for establishing acid-base imbalances. Blood gases are abbreviated as PaO_2 (the level of dissolved arterial oxygen in the blood, with a normal range of 95 to 100 mmHg); $PaCO_2$ (the level of dissolved arterial carbon dioxide in the blood with a normal range of 35 to 45 mmHg); HCO_3 (the level of bicarbonate in the blood with a normal range of 23 to 25 mEq/L); SO_2 (the level of oxygen saturation, with a normal range of 90% to 100%); and pH (the acidity of the blood, with a normal range of 7.35 to 7.45).

Blood pressure (BP). The force of blood volume within a vessel or chamber.

Bounding, full pulse. A pulse that feels strong to the touch.

Bradycardia. Slow pulse; pulse that is below 60 beats per minute in adults.

Bradypnea. A slow respiratory rate.

Brazelton Neonatal Behavioral Assessment Scale (BNBAS). Tool used to assess a neonate's interactive and behavioral capabilities.

Bruit. An abnormal murmur heard on auscultation of a vessel.

Cachexia. State of malnutrition, emaciation, debilitation, and anemia (see Chapter 5 for further discussion of malnutrition).

Cardinal signs. Measurements of body temperature, pulse, respiration, and blood pressure; essentially synonymous with vital signs except for weight.

Carina. Ridge at the bifurcation to the main bronchi from the trachea.

Cellulitis. An inflammation that has spread within the tissues.

Chemosis. Connective tissue swelling near the cornea.

Chest tube. Drainage tube for removing fluid from the chest cavity after thoracentesis.

Cheyne-Stokes respirations (CSR). A gradually increasing then gradually decreasing depth of respirations followed by a period of apnea.

Chvostek's sign. Facial spasm brought on by tapping over the facial nerve indicative of hypocalcemic states.

Cicatrix. A scar left by the formation of new connective tissue over a healing wound.

Circumcision. Surgical removal of the prepuce (foreskin) of the glans penis.

Coloboma. Congenital incomplete development of the eye structures.

Congestive heart failure (CHF). A condition in which the heart is unable to pump adequately, thus allowing blood to accumulate in the lungs and liver.

Constant fever. Temperature that is consistently elevated above normal.

Crisis phase (in body temperature monitoring during fever). A dramatic return of an elevated body temperature to normal. Fevers may be recurring and several cycles of "crisis" and chills may occur at intervals until stability is reached.

Crock. Condescending reference to a patient felt to have an imagined, nonphysical, insignificant, or factitious/faked illness; a malingering patient.

Cullen's sign. Ecchymosis (swelling due to a bruise) in the flank associated with retroperitoneal hemorrhage.

Cyanosis. Generalized blue discoloration of the skin or mucous membranes due to reduced oxygen in red blood cell hemoglobin.

Diaphoresis. Profuse perspiration.

Diaphragmatic breathing. Respirations performed mainly by the diaphragm.

Diastole. The phase of a heartbeat when the ventricular heart muscle relaxes.

Diastolic pressure. The least amount of pressure detectably present in arteries when the heart muscle is in a relaxed state; the bottom number in a blood pressure recording.

Dubowitz assessment. System for examining physical and neurologic development of neonates to assess gestational age.

Ecchymosis. Extravasation of blood within and under the skin; swelling due to a bruise.

Epididymitis. Inflammation of the excretory duct of the testes.

Epulis. Nodular enlargement of the gums.

Erythema. A redness in areas of the skin or mucous tissues.

Erythema toxicum. A pink papular rash usually present in the first or second day of life in newborns.

Eschar. Slough of skin cells, or scab.

Etiology. Cause.

Exacerbation. Increased in severity.

Febrile. Having an elevated body temperature.

Feeble, or thready, pulse. Description of an abnormal, weak pulse volume to touch.

Fibrillation. Rapid, random, ineffectual, and irregular heart contractions.

Fissure. A crack split or groove in the skin or mucous membrane.

Fistula. A communication between two normally separated spaces.

Flutter. Rapid, regular, but ineffectual heart contractions.

Fontanelle. "Soft spots" on the skulls of infants.

Fox's law. A three-part maxim in which one predicts that: 10% of patients have 90% of the diseases; individuals with no redeeming qualities will survive; and nice people get terminal illnesses.

Gallop. A pathologic, extra heart sound that produces the auditory effect of a galloping horse. A gallop may be heard with severe myocardial disease. A ventricular gallop is indicative of congestive heart failure.

Gomer. A reference made to patients who refuse or are naive or unable to comply with medical management, making medical care difficult. The term may be an acronym for "Get out of my emergency room," or it may derive from the word "gummer," referring to the characteristic lesions in later-stage syphilis.

Hemangioma. Referring to a group of benign blood vessel tumors visible on the skin, including spider hemangiomas, port wine hemangiomas, and strawberry hemangiomas.

Hematemesis. Vomiting red blood or "coffee grounds" appearing blood.

Hematochezia. Bright red blood coming from the rectum.

Hemodynamic parameters. Peripheral arterial pressure, central venous pressure, pulmonary artery pressure, pulmonary capillary wedge pressure, left atrial pressure, cardiac output, cardiac index, and mixed venous oxygen saturation are hemodynamic parameters commonly used to assess and monitor critically ill patients.

Hemoptysis. Coughing up blood.

Hepatojugular reflex. Referring to pressure on the liver that results in an increase in cervicovenous pressure in patients who have right-side heart failure and causes a visible bulging of the jugular vein.

Hoffmann's sign. A neurologic sign elicited by flicking the palm surface on the end of a finger and causing the fingers to flex; indicative of pyramidal disease.

Hydroma. Fluid-filled sacs or cysts.

Hypertension. Abnormally high blood pressure.

Hyperthermia. Abnormally high body temperature.

Hyperventilation. Abnormally rapid, deep, and prolonged respirations.

Hypotension. Abnormally low blood pressure.

Hypothermia. Abnormally low body temperature.

Hypoventilation. Abnormally low amount of air entering the lungs.

Iatrogenic. A condition or problem resulting from medical treatment.

Idiopathic. Disease of unknown origin.

Induration. Hardened area.

Inspiration. Inhalation.

Intermittent fever. High body temperatures broken by periods of normal or subnormal temperatures.

Intermittent pulse. Periods of normal pulse rhythm broken by periods of irregular rhythms.

Interstitial edema. Collection of fluid within spaces in an organ or within tissues.

Invasion. The point at which fever begins.

Janeway lesion. Erythematous or hemorrhagic lesion on the palm or sole seen in association with subacute bacterial endocarditis.

Jaundice. A yellowish coloration to the skin resulting from excessive bilirubin.

Korotkoff's sounds. The blood flow sounds heard through a stethoscope when obtaining blood pressure readings.

Kussmaul's respiration. Deep, rapid respiration seen in some cases of coma or metabolic acidosis.

Lanugo. Thin, downy fine hair covering the infant's body.

Loculated. Enlarged small space or cavity; most often refers to fluid trapped in chambers or adjacent compartments that are difficult to drain.

Lymphadenopathy. Abnormal enlargement of the lymph glands due to infection or neoplasm.

Lysis (in body temperature monitoring). The gradual return of body temperature to normal; the term *lysis* may also refer to destruction or rupture of cells. Drugs or immune responses that cause tumors to break down are said to *lyse* tumors.

Melena. Black tarry stool usually indicative of an upper gastrointestinal hemorrhage.

Milia. Tiny white papules usually on the chin, nose, and forehead in newborns.

Mucopurulent. Containing pus and mucus.

Murphy's sign. Severe pain and inspiratory arrest occurring with palpation (touching) of the right upper quadrant associated with cholecystitis (gallbladder inflammation).

Neonate. Infant less than 28 days old.

Neurodermatitis. A skin lesion of neurologic origin.

Neutropenia. Abnormally low number of neutrophils (leukocytes that stain easily).

Nodal. Referring to lymph nodes.

Orchitis. Inflammation of the testes.

Orthopnea. A condition in which breathing is easier when the patient is in a sitting or standing position than when lying down.

Orthostatic hypotension. A fall in blood pressure when a person sits or stands too quickly; synonymous with *postural hypotension.*

Pallor. Pale skin.

Palpate. To examine by touch or feel.

Palpitation. Awareness of one's own heartbeat.

Patent. Open.

Patent ductus arteriosus. A congenital heart defect in which a small duct between the aorta and pulmonary artery, which normally closes by the time of birth, remains open.

Pathognomonic. Specifically associated with a given disease.

Pedal circulation. Circulation in the foot.

Percussion. A physical diagnostic procedure involving short, sharp blows to a body part.

Peripheral pulses. Pulse readings taken from sites distant from the heart.

Peritoneum. Membranous sac enclosing the abdominal and pelvic organs.

Petechiae. Small, pinpoint, nonraised, round purplish-red spots on the skin; small cutaneous hemorrhages.

Pleural effusion. Presence of fluid in the pleural space.

Polypharmacia, polypharmacy. The use of multiple, prescribed and over-the-counter, medications that has caused undesired drug interaction effects (see Chapter 14).

Premature contraction. A heart pulsation that occurs sooner than previous contractions.

Prostatism. Urinary difficulty caused by obstruction of the bladder by an enlarged prostate gland.

Pulse. A circulatory wave through the blood vessels set up by a contraction of the heart.

Pulse deficit. The difference between an apical (at the apex of the heart) and radial (at the wrist) pulse rate.

Pulse pressure. The difference between diastolic and systolic blood pressure.

Pulse rate. The number of pulsations felt per minute.

Pulse rhythm. The pattern of pulsations and pauses.

Pyrexia. Fever.

Quincke's sign. Alternating blushing and blanching of the fingernail following compression seen in aortic regurgitation.

Rales. Crackling sounds heard with a stethoscope indicative of fluid in the alveoli or respiratory passages.

Raynaud's phenomenon. Short episodes of pallor (whitening) followed by cyanosis (bluing) then erythema (reddening) and an associated numbness in the fingers and toes due to temporary constriction of the arterioles in the skin.

Remittent fever. A fever that fluctuates but does not come within the normal range.

Rhonchus. A low-pitched breath sound heard on auscultation indicating narrowed respiratory passages.

Rigors. Extreme chills.

Rub. The abnormal scratchy, grating sound made when two normally smooth internal surfaces rub against one another.

Sanguinous. Containing blood.

Sepsis. When infection is present; a patient is said to be **septic** when he or she has an infection or to have **septicemia** when there are bacteria in the blood.

Serum. The clear, noncellular component of blood after removal of the clotting proteins.

Serum enzyme tests. Tests for enzymes released in the blood following myocardial infarction; these tests include *creatine kinase* (CK), *lactic dehydrogenase* (LD), *troponins,* and *aspartate aminotransferase* (AST). The latter is also known as the *serum glutamic-oxaloacetic transaminase test* (SGOT).

Sign. An observation made by an examiner.

Sinus arrhythmia. An irregular pulse rhythm characterized by slowing on exhalation and increasing on inhalation.

Smith's minor anomalies. Physical abnormalities (such as abnormal dermal ridges) in newborns.

Sphygmomanometer. An instrument used to measure blood pressure.

Stertorous respirations. Noisy breathing; snoring.

Stethoscope. An instrument used to carry sounds from the body to the ear of an examiner.

Stool. Feces.

Stridor. Noisy breathing due to an obstruction in the upper (laryngeal) airway.

Symptom. An observation felt or described by the patient.

Systole. The phase in which the ventricular heart muscle is contracting.

Systolic pressure. The maximum pressure exerted on arterial walls when the ventricle is contracting (the top number in a blood pressure recording).

Tachycardia. A rapid heart rate.

Tachypnea. A rapid respiratory rate.

Tamponade (cardiac). Accumulation of excessive fluid in the pericardium (fibrous sac that surrounds the heart).

Telangiectasias. Hemangiomas that are flat, red, localized areas of capillary dilation.

Tetralogy of Fallot. A congenital malformation of the heart with the following distinct defects: *pulmonary artery stenosis, ventricular septal defect, shift of the aorta to the right,* and *hypertrophy of the right ventricle.*

Thoracic respiration. Using primarily the thoracic and intercostal muscles for respiration.

Thrill. A vibration perceptible on palpation (touch) due to surfaces rubbing together or to blood flow; for example, a thrill of the chest wall can be felt if there is friction between surfaces of the pericardium (fibrous sac surrounding the heart).

Tissue respiration, internal respiration. The exchange of oxygen and carbon dioxide between the body and blood cells.

Trousseau's sign. Carpal spasm produced when inflating the blood pressure cuff around the arm to a pressure above the systolic pressure. Trousseau's sign may indicate hypocalcemia.

Very low birth weight (VLBW). Neonate birth weight that is less than 1500 grams, or 3 pounds, 3 ounces; **extremely low birth weight** (ELBW) refers to a birth weight of less than 1000 grams, or 2 pounds, 2 ounces.

Vital signs (VS). Measurements of body temperature, weight, pulse rate, blood pressure, and respiratory rate.

B. Abbreviations

aa. Equal part of each

AA. Aortic aneurysm, age adjusted

AAA. Abdominal aortic aneurysm

AAO. Awake, alert, and oriented

AAS. Acute abdominal series

A&B. Apnea and bradycardia

AB, abd. Abdominal

ABGs. Arterial blood gases

ABN. Abnormal

abs. Absent

ABW. Actual body weight

ACC. Accident

ACG. Angiocardiography

ACLS. Advanced Cardiac Life Support

ACS. Acute coronary syndrome

AD. Right ear; *auris dexter* (write out "right ear"; AD can be mistakenly read as meaning "up to.")

AdmDx. Admitting diagnosis

ADM. Admission

AE (BE). Above the elbow (below the elbow)

A&E. Accident and emergency

AEIOU TIPS. Mnemonic for **a**lcohol, **e**ncephalopathy, **i**nsulin, **o**piates, **u**remia, **t**rauma, **i**nfection, **p**sychiatric, **s**yncope (in coma diagnosis)

AF. Afebrile, aortofemoral, or atrial fibrillation

AFB. Acid-fast bacilli, or in cardiovascular surgery, *aortofemoral bypass graft*

AFP. Alpha fetoprotein

AFVSS. Afebrile and vital signs are stable

AI. Aortic insufficiency

AIF. Aorto-ileo femoral (graft)

ALL. Acute lymphocytic/lymphoblastic leukemia

AK (BK). Above the knee (below the knee)

AKA, OKA. Also known as, otherwise known as

AKA (BKA). Above the knee amputation (below the knee amputation)

AKI. Acute kidney injury

ALARA. As low as reasonably achievable

AMA. Against medical advice

amb. Ambulatory

AMI. Acute myocardial infarction

AN. Admitting note

ante. Before

AO. Admitting office

A & O. Alert and oriented

AOB. Alcohol on breath

AODM. Adult-onset diabetes mellitus

AOR. At own risk

A-P. Anterior-posterior

A & P. Auscultation and percussion

ARD. Acute respiratory disease

ARDS. Adult respiratory distress syndrome

ARF. Acute renal failure

AS. Aortic stenosis; or left ear, *auris sinister* (write out "left ear"; AS can be mistakenly read to mean "as.")

ASA. Aspirin

A.S.A.1. Normal healthy patient

A.S.A.2. Patient with mild systemic disease

A.S.A.3. Patient with severe systemic disease

A.S.A.4. Patient with incapacitating systemic disease that is life threatening

ASAP. As soon as possible

ASD. Atrial septal defect; or in radiology, "airspace" disease

ASFAIK. As far as I know

ASH. Asymmetrical septal hypertrophy, synonymous with the older term *idiopathic hypertrophic subaortic stenosis* (IHSS)

ASHD. Arteriosclerotic heart disease

AST. Aspartate aminotransferase

ATC. Around the clock

AV. Atrioventricular

AVR. Aortic valve replacement

AVSS. Afebrile and vital signs are stable

A & W. Alive and well

AWOL. Absent without leave

AXR. Abdominal x-ray

BAL. Blood alcohol level

BBA. Born before arrival

BBB. Bundle branch block

BiPAP. Bilevel positive airway pressure

BM. Bowel movement, bone marrow

BM, BF. Black male, black female

BMI. Body mass index

BMT. Bone marrow transplant

BOT. Base of tongue

BP. Blood pressure

BPH. Benign prostate hypertrophy

BPM. Beats per minute

BRB. Bright red blood

BRBPR. Bright red blood per rectum

BRP. Bathroom privileges

BS. Breath sounds, bowel sounds, blood sugar

BTW. By the way

BUN. Blood, urea, nitrogen

BUO. Bleeding (or bruising) of underdetermined origin

BW. Birth weight, body weight

BWS. Battered wife or battered woman syndrome

Bx. Biopsy

C; Cau. Caucasian

CA. Cancer, carcinoma

CABG. Coronary artery bypass graft

CAD. Coronary artery disease

CAN. Cord around neck

CAPD. Continuous ambulatory peritoneal dialysis

Cath. Catheter

CBC. Complete blood count

CBG. Capillary blood gases

CC. Chief complaint

cc. Cubic centimeter (use "mL"; cc can be mistaken for "U," units)

CF. Cardiac failure, cystic fibrosis

C-Diff. *Clostridium difficile* (bacterium)

CFx. Compound fracture

C-GLMP. (Confirmed) gestational age by last menstrual period (+/−2 weeks)

Cl. Chloride

CHB. Complete heart block

ChemoTx. Chemotherapy

CHF. Congestive heart failure

CHI. Closed head injury

CK. Creatine kinase

CKD. Chronic kidney disease

CMPA. Cow's milk protein allergy

CN. Cranial nerve

CO. Cardiac output

c/o. Complains of

COAD. Chronic obstructive airway disease

COLD. Chronic obstructive lung disease

COPD. Chronic obstructive pulmonary disease

CP. Chest pain or cerebral palsy

CPAP. Continuous positive airway pressure

CPK, CK, CPMB. Creatine phosphokinase, creatinine kinase, creatine phosphokinase-myocardial band

CPR. Cardiopulmonary resuscitation

Cr. Cl. Creatinine clearance

C-R. Crown-to-rump (newborn measurement)

CR, DR. Computed radiography, digital radiography

CRF. Chronic respiratory failure, or chronic renal failure

Crit. Hematocrit

CSF. Cerebrospinal fluid

CT; CAT. Chest tube, computed tomogram; computed axial tomography

CTA. (Lungs) clear to auscultation

CT w C. Computed tomogram with contrast

CU. Cause unknown

CVA. Cerebrovascular accident

CVAC. Central venous access catheter

CVD. Cerebrovascular disease

CVL. Central venous line

CVC. Central venous catheter

CVP. Central venous pressure

c/w. Consistent with

CXR. Chest x-ray

DAT. Diet as tolerated

DC. Discontinue (write out "discontinue," because it can be mistaken for "discharge")

D/C. Discharge (write out "discharge," because it can be mistaken for "discontinue")

DD. Developmental delay

DDx. Differential diagnosis

Decub. Decubitus

DH. Drug history

DI. Diabetes insipidus

DIC. Disseminated intravascular coagulation

DJD. Degenerative joint disease

DM. Diastolic murmur; diabetes mellitus

DMFT. Decayed, missing, and filled teeth

DNKA. Did not keep appointment

DNR. Do not resuscitate (per family's or patient's request)

DNT. Did not test

DOB. Date of birth

DOE. Dyspnea on exertion

DP. Dorsalis pedis

DPT. Diphtheria, pertussis, tetanus

DTRs. Deep tendon reflexes

DTs. Delirium tremens

DU. Diagnosis unknown

D & V. Diarrhea and vomiting

DVTs. Deep vein thromboses

D/W. Discuss with

Dx. Diagnosis

EAHF. Eczema, asthma, hay fever

EBL. Estimated blood loss

EC-ASA. Enteric coated aspirin

ECC. Extracorporeal circulation

ECG, EKG. Electrocardiogram

ED. Emergency department, external device

Edent. Edentulous

EF. External fixation

EMT. Emergency medical technologist

EMV. Eyes, motor, verbal (Glasgow Coma Scale, see Chapter 4)

eod. Every other day

EOM. Extraocular movements/ muscles

ERV. Expiratory respiration volume

et. And

ET. Endotracheal, external

ETT. Exercise tolerance test

ETC. Emergency treatment completed

ETIO. Etiology

ETOH. Ethanol (alcohol)

FB. Foreign body

FBS. Fasting blood sugar

FD. Forceps delivery

Fem-pop. Femoral-popliteal

FEV. Forced expired volume

FH. Family history

FHR. Fetal heart rate

FHS. Fetal heart sounds

FLK. Funny looking kid

FME. Full mouth extraction

FNA. Fine needle aspiration

FOB. Fecal occult blood

FOM. Floor of mouth

FP. Floor procedure (done at bedside), full plate (denture)

FRC. Functional residual capacity

FT. Feeding tube

FTA-ABS. Fluorescent treponemal antibody–absorbed

FTR. Failed to report

FTT. Failure to thrive

F/U. Follow up

FUO. Fever of unknown/undetermined origin

Fx, fr. Fracture

G, grav. Gravida (pregnant)

GA. Gestational age, general anesthesia.

G1, G2, G3, G4, G5, G6. Grade one, two, etc. (extra heart sounds)

GB. Gallbladder, Guillain Barré (syndrome)

GC. Gonococcus (gonorrhea)

GCS. Glasgow Coma Scale

GI. Gastrointestinal

G.O.K. God only knows

G.O.R.K. God only really knows

Grade I, II, III, etc. Grade one, two, etc. (tumor histologic grades)

GREA. Generally regarded as effective

GRAS. Generally regarded as safe

G & S. Group and save

GSW. Gunshot wound

gt. Drops ("gutta")

G tube. Gastrostomy tube

GU. Genitourinary

GUS. Gestational age by ultrasound

HA. Headache

HAA. Hepatitis associated antigen

HAV. Hepatitis A virus

HBc. Hepatitis B core (antigen)

HBeAg. Hepatitis B e antigen

HBsAg. Hepatitis B surface antigen

HBV. Hepatitis B virus

HC. Hickman catheter

HCO_3. Bicarbonate

HCT. Hematocrit

HD. Hospital day

HDL. High-density lipoprotein

HEADS. *H*ome, *e*ducation/employment, *a*ctivities, *d*rugs, and *s*exuality (acronym guideline for taking an adolescent's history for triage purposes)

HEENT. Head, eyes, ears, nose, throat

HELLP. Hemolysis, elevated liver enzymes, low platelet count (syndrome)

HepB. Hepatitis B

Hgb. Hemoglobin

HH. Health history, hard of hearing

HIV. Human immunodeficiency virus

HJR. Hepatojugular reflex

HLTx. Heart and lung transplant

H & L. Heart and lungs

HO. History of

HOB. Head of bed

HOH. Hard of hearing

H&P. History and physical examination

HPF. High-power field

HPN, HPT, HBP, HTN. Hypertension(ive)

HR. Heart rate

HRT. Hormone replacement therapy

HSV. Herpes simplex virus

Ht. Height

HTLV-III. Human lymphotropic virus, type III (AIDS agent, HIV)

Hx. History

Hyperal. Hyperalimentation

ICT. Induced coma therapy

I & D. Incision and drainage

I & O. Intake and output, "ins and outs"

I.A.O. Immediately after onset

IDDM. Insulin-dependent diabetes mellitus

ILV. Independent lung ventilation (system)

IMP. Inpatient multidimensional psych (scale)

Imp. Impression

IPD. Intermittent peritoneal dialysis

IPPB. Intermittent positive-pressure breathing

IPOP. Immediate postoperative period

IR. Inspiratory reserve

IRDM. Insulin-resistant diabetes mellitus

IRDS. Infant respiratory distress syndrome

IRV. Inspiratory reserve volume

IV. Intravenous

IVC. Intravenous cholangiogram, inferior vena cava

IVH. Intraventricular hemorrhage

IVP. Intravenous pyelogram

JODM. Juvenile-onset diabetes mellitus

K. Potassium

KOR. Keep-open rate

KUB. Kidneys, ureters, bladder

L (R) A. Left (right) atrium

LBBB. Left bundle branch block

LBW. Low birth weight

LD. Lactic dehydrogenase

LDL. Low-density lipoprotein

LE. Lupus erythematosus

LFTs. Liver function tests

LGA. Large for gestational age

L (R) LE. Left (right) lower extremity

L (R) LL. Left (right) lower lobe

L (R) LQ. Left (right) lower quadrant

LMD. Local MD, family doctor

LOC. Loss of consciousness

LOS. Length of stay

L (R) UE. Left (right) upper extremity

L (R) UL. Left (right) upper lobe

L (R) UQ. Left (right) upper quadrant

L (R) V. Left (right) ventricle

LWCT. Lee-White clotting time (coagulation time)

Lymphs. Lymphocytes

lytes. Electrolytes

m.a.s. Patient is disagreeable and uncooperative

MAS. Meconium aspiration syndrome

MAST suit. Military antishock trousers

M1, M2. Mitral valve sounds

MBC. Minimum bacteriocidal concentration, maximum breathing capacity

MCH. Mean cell hemoglobin

MCHC. Mean cell hemoglobin concentration

MCV. Mean cell volume

Med-Surg. Medical and surgical

Mets. Metastases

MHB. Maximal hospital benefits

m.g.r. Murmurs, gallops, rubs (heart sounds)

MI. Myocardial infarction

MIC. Minimum inhibiting concentration

mL. Milliliter

MOC. Maintenance of Certification

MODY. Maturity onset diabetes of youth

MOSF. Multiple organ systems failure

mm. Muscles, muscular

MM. Mucous membrane

MmR. Mumps, measles, rubella

M & R. Measure and record

MRGT. Murmur, rub, gallop, thrill

MRSA. Methicillin-resistant *Staphylococcus aureus*

MS. Mitral stenosis, mental status, medical student, multiple sclerosis

MSL. Midsternal line

MSR. Muscle stretch reflexes

MSU. Midstream urine

MVA. Motor vehicle accident

MVC, MCH, MCHC. Mean cell volume, mean cellular hemoglobin, mean cellular hemoglobin concentration

MVit. Multivitamin

MVP. Mitral valve prolapse

MVR. Mitral valve replacement, mitral valve regurgitation

MX. Mastectomy

Nl. Normal

Na. Sodium

N/A. Not applicable

NA. Not available

NAD. No acute distress; no active disease

NANDA. North American Nursing Diagnosis Association

NB. Newborn

NBC. Non bed care

NBS. Normal breath sounds, normal bowel sounds

NE(R)D. No evidence (of recurrent) disease

NEC. Necrotizing enterocolitis (inflammatory bowel disease)

NI. No insurance

NIDDM. Non-insulin-dependent diabetes mellitus

NIP. No infection present, no inflammation present

NKA. No known allergies

NKDA. No known drug allergies

NOK. Next of kin

NOMS. Not on my shift

NOS. Not otherwise specified

NPD. No pathologic diagnosis

NPO. Nothing by mouth (*nil per os*)

NSA. No significant abnormality

NSAID. Nonsteroidal anti-inflammatory drug

NSR. Normal sinus rhythm

NT/ND. Nontender/nondistended (abdomen)

NTG. Nitroglycerin

N & V. Nausea and vomiting

N & W. Normal and well

OD. Officer of the day, overdose, right eye (*oculus dexter*)

Ox3. Oriented times 3 (person, place, date)

O_2. Oxygen

O & E. Observation and examination

OM. Otitis media

O & P. Ova and parasites (stool examination)

OOB. Out of bed

OS. Left eye (*oculus sinister*)

OSA. Obstructive sleep apnea

OTC. Over-the-counter (drugs)

OTW. Off the wall, bizarre

OU. Both eyes

p. Post, para, per

P & A. Percussion and auscultation

$PaCO_2$. Arterial carbon dioxide (blood gases)

PaO_2. Arterial oxygen (blood gases)

Palp. Palpable

PAT. Paroxysmal atrial tachycardia

PB. Piggyback

PCP. Primary care physician

PDA. Patent ductus arteriosus

PDx. Primary diagnosis

PDR. *Physicians' Desk Reference*

PDQ. Pretty darn quick

PEEP. Positive end-expiratory pressure

PEERLA. Pupils are equal (in size) and equally reactive to light and accommodation

PERLA. Pupils are equal and reactive to light and accommodation

PERRLDAC. Pupils are equal, round, and reactive to light directly and accommodation consensually

PHC. Post-hospital care

PI. Present illness, pulmonary insufficiency

PKU. Phenylketonuria

PM, PPM. Pacemaker, permanent pacemaker

PMH. Past medical history

PMD. Private MD

$\bar{p}$ MN. After (post) midnight

P-MVA. Pedestrian in a motor vehicle accident

PND. Postnasal drip, paroxysmal nocturnal dyspnea

PO. By mouth

POC, POT. Plan of care, plan of treatment

POD. Postoperation (surgical) day

POMR. Problem-oriented medical record

Post OP. Postoperation

PP. Partial plate (denture), pulsus paradoxus, or postprandial

P & PD. Percussion and postural drainage

PPD. Purified protein derivative

ppd. Packs (of cigarettes) per day

PPE. Personal protective equipment

PRN. As needed (*pro re nata*)

Pre Op. Preoperative

Pr.Tx. Prior treatment (or therapy)

PSH. Past surgical history

PSVT. Paroxysmal supraventricular tachycardia

P.Sz. Paranoid schizophrenia

Pt. Patient

PTA. Prior to admission; percutaneous, transluminal angioplasty

PTH. Parathyroid hormone

PUD. Peptic ulcer disease

PVC. Premature ventricular contraction

PVD. Peripheral vascular disease

PWB%. Partial weight bearing (at a stated percent)

Px, Phys. Physical examination, physical

Q. Each (*quaque*)

q/s. Each shift

QNS. Quantity not sufficient

RBBB. Right bundle branch block

RBC. Red blood cell, red blood count

REP. Renal electrolyte profile

RIND. Reversible (or resolving) ischemic neurologic deficit

RLW. Routine laboratory work

RO. Renew order

R/O. Rule out

ROP. Retinopathy of prematurity

ROS. Review of systems

RPG. Retrograde percutaneous gastrostomy

RPN. Resident progress note

RRR. Regular rate and rhythm (heart)

RTC. Return to clinic

RUA. Reduced under anesthesia

RV. Right ventricle, residual volume

Rx. Recipe, prescription, treatment

Rx'd. Prescribed

S1, S2, S3. Sound one, two, etc. (heart sounds)

SA. Sinoatrial

SB. Stillborn

SBE. Subacute bacterial endocarditis

SBFT. Small bowel follow-through (radiology study)

SCD. Sudden cardiac death

SDx. Secondary diagnosis

SG. Swan-Ganz (catheter)

SGA. Small for gestational age, subjective global assessment

SGOT. Serum glutamic-oxaloacetic transaminase

SIDS. Sudden infant death syndrome

sl. Sublingual

SMA. Sequential multiple analysis

SO. Significant other

SOAP. Subjective, objective, assessment, plan

SO_2. Oxygen saturation

SOB. Shortness of breath; short of breath

SOC. Start of care

SOL. Space-occupying lesion

S/P. Status post

SR. Slow release (medication), sinus rhythm, or "see report"

Ss. Half

SS. Soap suds, Social Security

Stat. Immediately (*statim*)

STD. Sexually transmitted disease

Sub ling. Sublingual

Sub q. Subcutaneous

SVT. Supraventricular tachycardia

Sx. Symptoms, signs

Sz. Seizure

T_1, T_2, T_3, T_4. Type 1, 2, 3, 4 rankings for cleft palates

T & A. Tonsillectomy and adenoidectomy

TAA. To all areas

TB, LC. Term birth, living child

TBI. Traumatic brain injury, total body irradiation

TBSB. Total body surface burn

T & C. Type and crossmatch

TENS. Transcutaneous electrical nerve stimulator

TIA. Transient ischemic attack

TIBC. Total iron-binding capacity

TKO. To keep open

TM. Tympanic membrane

TNJ. Tongue, neck, jaw

TNTC. Too numerous to count

t/o. Telephone order

TPO. Time postonset

TPR. Temperature, pulse, respiration

TSH. Thyroid-stimulating hormone

TTN. Transient tachypnea of the newborn

TURB. Transurethral resection of the bladder

TURP. Transurethral resection of the prostate

TV. Tidal volume

Tx. Treatment, therapy, traction

Type 1 DM, Type 2 DM. Type 1 diabetes mellitus, type 2 diabetes mellitus

U. Units (of)

UA. Urine analysis/urinalysis, uric acid

UCD, UCHD. Usual childhood diseases

UFN. Until further notice

USA. Unstable angina

USOH. Usual state of health

VC. Vital capacity

VDRL. Venereal Disease Research Laboratory

VF. Visual field

Viz. Namely

VLDL. Very low-density lipoprotein

Vol. Volume

v/o. Verbal order, or voice order

V & P. Vagotomy and pyloroplasty

VS. Vital signs

VSD. Ventricular septal defect

V-tach. Ventricular tachycardia

W/A. While awake

WBC. White blood count or white blood cell

WC. Wheelchair

WD. Well-developed

Wk. Week

WN. Well-nourished

WM/WF. White male/white female

WNL. Within normal limits

wrt. With respect to

Wt. Weight

W/U. Workup

WYSIWYG. What you see is what you get

x. Times (multiplied by)

XRT. X-ray therapy

XX. Female chromosomes

XY. Male chromosomes

YO. Years old

III. MEDICAL HISTORY, REVIEW OF SYSTEMS, AND PHYSICAL EXAMINATION

When patients are admitted to the hospital, they normally undergo a thorough **history and physical (H & P) examination**, which includes a medical and social history, **review of systems (ROS)**, and physical examination.

A. Medical History

The medical history interview usually addresses the following areas:

- Chief complaint (CC) (a statement, in the patient's own words, describing the current problem)
- History of the present illness (HPI)
- Past medical history (PMH)
- Family medical history (FMH)
- Psychosocial history

B. Review of Systems

After the medical history has been taken, the physician interviews the patient with questions related to organ systems. This review of systems normally follows a standard interview format similar to that outlined below.

1. General

Queries related to any recent weight gain or loss, complaints of fatigue, fever, chills, nocturnal sweats, or appetite changes.

2. Skin

Queries related to any rashes, pruritus, lesions, or bruising noted by the patient.

3. Head

Queries related to any trauma, headache, scalp/head tenderness, or dizziness.

4. Eyes, Ears, Nose, and Throat

Queries related to vision and hearing changes, tinnitus, pain, discharge, vertigo; sinus problems, polyps; teeth, tongue, gums, dentures, hoarseness, or sore throat.

5. Respiratory

Queries related to cough, dyspnea, or history of pulmonary problems.

6. *Cardiovascular*

Queries related to chest pain, dyspnea on exertion, claudication (pain when walking), and edema.

7. *Gastrointestinal (GI)*

Queries related to dysphagia, heartburn, nausea, vomiting, hematemesis, indigestion, diarrhea, abdominal pain, melena, red blood in the stool, hemorrhoids, change in stool appearance, and jaundice.

8. *Genitourinary (GU)*

Queries related to urinary frequency, urgency, hesitancy, hematuria, dysuria, nocturia, incontinence, discharge, or sexually transmitted diseases.

9. *Gynecological*

Queries related to birth and deliveries, including gravida, abortions, age of menarche, dysmenorrhea, and forms of contraception.

10. *Endocrine*

Queries related to polyuria, polydipsia, polyphagia, temperature intolerance, hormone therapy, or changes in the skin or hair.

11. *Musculoskeletal*

Queries related to arthritis, trauma, and bony deformities.

12. *Hematologic*

Queries related to anemia, bleeding tendency, easy bruising, or lymphadenopathy.

13. *Neuropsychiatric*

Queries related to seizures, memory problems, syncope, weakness, dyscoordination, problems with mood, sleep disorders, emotional problems, or substance abuses.

C. Physical Examination

Following the medical history and the review of systems, the physician's physical examination will follow a format, similar to that listed below, with infants, children, and adults. Abdominal quadrants and region referents are illustrated in Figure 3–1.

1. *General*

Race, gender, development, mood and mental status, remarkable characteristics, and state of distress.

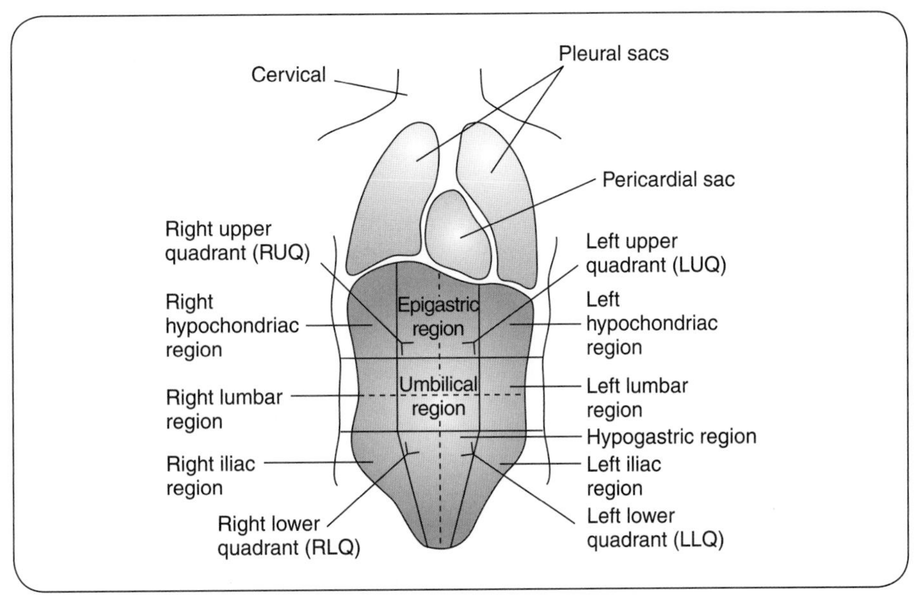

FIGURE 3–1 Body site referent in the physical examination. Source: Delmar Cengage Learning

2. *Vital Signs*

Temperature, pulse, respirations, blood pressure, weight, and height.

3. *Skin*

Rashes, scars, moles, hair distribution and pattern, and eruptions.

4. *Nodes*

Location of any enlarged nodes (cervical, supraclavicular, axillary, inguinal) and their size, mobility, and tenderness.

5. *Head, Eyes, Ears, Nose, and Throat*

Head – Fontanel suture line (pediatric patients), size, shape, tenderness, trauma, and bruits (pronounced "brew-eez," referring to sounds or murmurs in blood flow with auscultation of head and neck vessels). *Eyes* – Pupil size, relative shape of the pupils in each eye; reactivity to light and accommodation, extraocular muscular movements; acuity; extent of the visual fields; conjunctiva; sclera; eyelids; enophthalmos (recessed eyeball) or exophthalmos (bulging eyeball) positioning; and *fundus* (disc color, size, margins, cupping, venous patterns, and pulses). *Ears* – Hearing, discharge, tinnitus, external auditory canal, tympanic membrane appearance, position of the ears and appearance. *Nose* – Symmetry, tenderness, lesions, and obstructions. *Throat* – Lips, teeth, gums, tongue, tonsils, and pharynx; noting the appearance, swelling, lesions, symmetry, shape of the palatal vault, and clefts.

6. *Neck*

Range of motion, jugular venous distention (JVD), tenderness, nodes, masses, thyroid, larynx (vocal fold movement), bruits (see definition), and hepatojugular reflex.

7. *Chest*

Shape, movement during respiration, and breath sounds.

8. *Heart*

Regularity of rate and rhythm; thrill; auscultation at the apex, lower sternal border, and right and left second intercostal spaces (listening for murmurs, rubs, gallops, and clicks).

9. *Breast*

Surgeries, shape, nipple, discharge, masses, dimpling, or tenderness.

10. *Abdomen*

Shape (flat, distended, obese, scaphoid); scars; bowel sounds; tenderness; masses; guarding; rebound; size or span of the liver; tenderness; and adenopathy.

11. *Genitals* (Male) and *Pelvic* (Female)

Swelling, lesions, drainage, or masses.

12. *Rectum*

Fissures, skin tags, hemorrhoids, sphincter tone, masses, prostate, presence of stool, and presence of occult (not obvious) blood.

13. *Extremities*

Range of motion, deformities, joint tenderness or swelling, amputations, hair pattern, pulses, cyanosis, clubbing, nails, and edema.

14. *Neurologic and Mental Status Examination*

Orientation, memory, speech and language, cranial nerves, motor functions of extremities, cerebellar functions, sensory functions, reflexes, and neurologic tests and studies (see Chapter 4).

D. Characteristics of Masses

Abnormal bumps and body masses are of particular interest in the physical examination. These masses are described by their *mobility* (fixed or mobile); *shape* (irregular, round, tubular, ovoid); *consistency* (nodular, granular, spongy, hard, or edematous); *tenderness*; *size* (indicated in centimeters); and *location*.

E. Disease Staging

Some diseases, particularly certain forms of cancer, are ranked by the stages of the disease. These are a part of the taxonomy of medical conditions and are especially important in clinical treatment trials when assessing outcomes with different severities of diseases. In staging some types of cancer, for example (see Chapter 12, TNM system), disease staging is included in the description, but other disorders (diabetes, AIDS, appendicitis) also will be "staged" as follows: *Stage 1*, No complications; *Stage 2*, Local complications limited to a single organ or system; and *Stage 3*, Multiple site involvement or systemic involvement and complications.

F. Burns

Thermal injuries require close examination of the extent and depth of the wounds. The severity of the burn is evaluated by the amount of the **body surface area (BSA)** involved, applying a system known as the "rule of 9s," as shown in Figure 3–2. With this rule the percent of damage is estimated by assigning values (mostly multiples of 9) to particular body areas. Burns may be limited to the superficial epidermal layer of the skin, called **first-degree burns**, which typically heal within a week. **Second-degree burns** may be superficial or deep. **Third-degree burns** are full-thickness wounds involving all layers of the skin and usually require grafting.

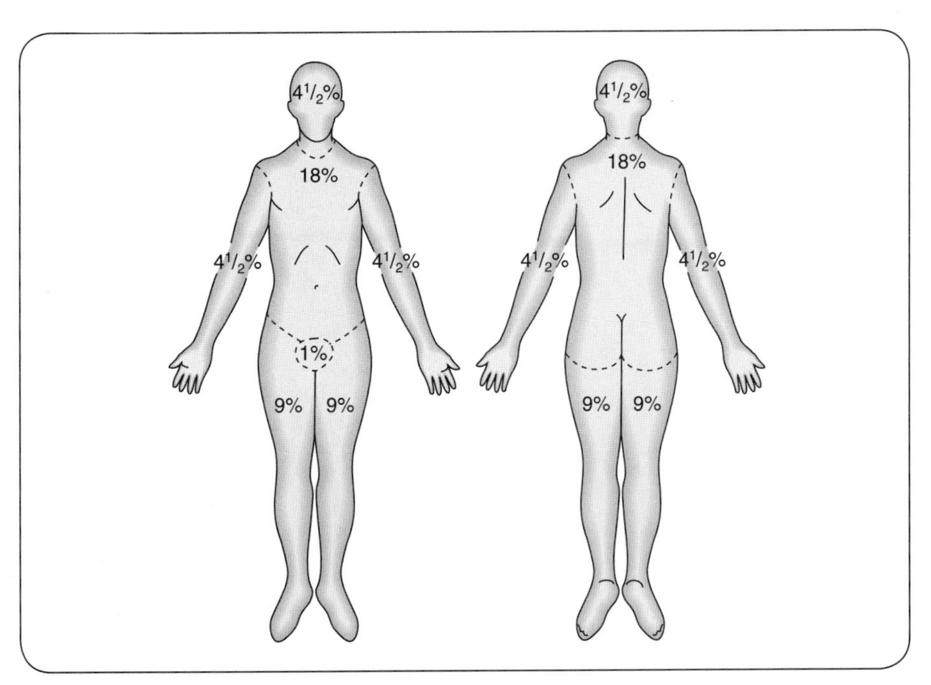

FIGURE 3–2 Rule of Nines *(continues)*

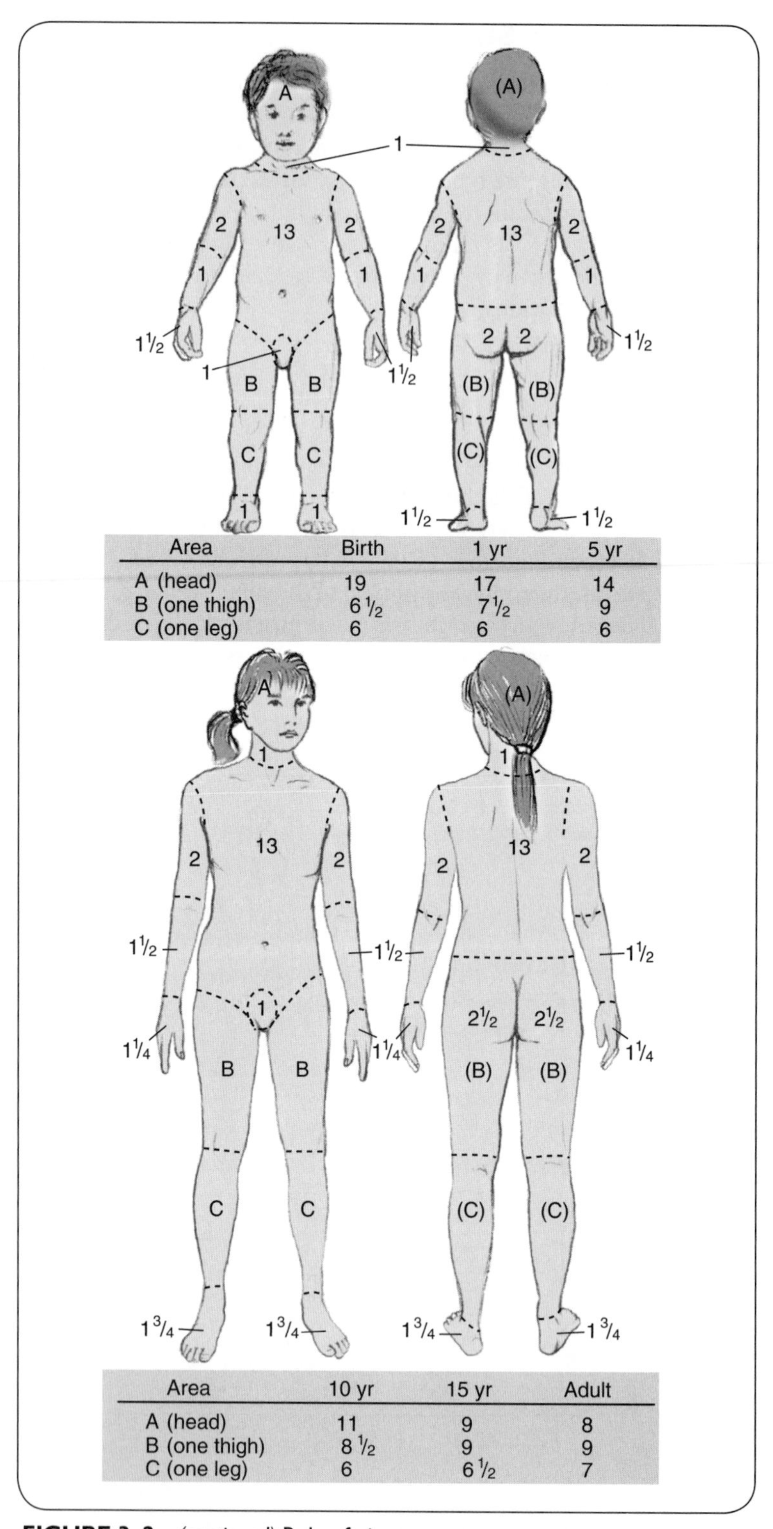

Area	Birth	1 yr	5 yr
A (head)	19	17	14
B (one thigh)	$6\frac{1}{2}$	$7\frac{1}{2}$	9
C (one leg)	6	6	6

Area	10 yr	15 yr	Adult
A (head)	11	9	8
B (one thigh)	$8\frac{1}{2}$	9	9
C (one leg)	6	$6\frac{1}{2}$	7

FIGURE 3–2 *(continued)* Rule of nines. Source: Delmar Cengage Learning

IV. COMMONLY ORDERED TESTS AND PROCEDURES

Findings on the physical examination will indicate which laboratory tests should be ordered. This section summarizes tests that are commonly ordered as part of the diagnostic workup and baseline assessments and to assess changes in medical status. Typically, normal laboratory values and the range for normal values are printed on the patient's laboratory report data form. Laboratory data should be compared to the range of values that are *normal for the reporting laboratory.* Acceptable levels for "normal" can be adjusted according to several factors, for example, age, body mass, sex, existing diseases, and medications taken. The importance, or clinical significance, of values outside the normal range is determined by the patient's physician. Some laboratory test results are influenced by factors that require consideration in interpretation. For example, factors such as recent immunizations, current drugs, food recently ingested; the age, sex, and body mass of the patient; medications taken; diseases; and pregnancy status can affect laboratory results. Figure 2–1 illustrates one of the shorthand methods used to record laboratory (blood and renal) values in the patient's progress notes (refer to the normal values listed in Appendix A).

Standard laboratory tests include a **complete blood count** (white blood count, hemoglobin, hematocrit, platelets, types of cells, and the volume and concentration of hemoglobin); **electrolytes** (sodium, chloride, potassium, and bicarbonate ratios); and a standard **blood chemistry panel**, which provides an analysis of renal function. The latter series may or may not include a **creatinine analysis**, and it may be labeled in various ways depending on the facility and the laboratory it uses. Typically, renal electrolyte findings are *profiled* as: *ASTRA-7, sequential medical analysis* (SMA-6), or *renal electrolyte profile.*

A. Laboratory Tests and Assays to Identify Specific Conditions or Factors

Acid-fast bacilli stain (AFB smear). Test for microorganisms, specifically mycobacterium, of which tuberculosis is the most common.

Acid phosphatase. Indicators for carcinoma of the prostate.

Adrenocorticotrophic hormone (ACTH). Adrenal gland function, pituitary insufficiency.

Acucheck. Blood glucose with a fingertip stick.

Albumin. Nutritional status, renal disease, Hodgkin's disease, leukemia, alcoholic cirrhosis, inflammatory bowel disease, hyperthyroidism, collagen disease.

Aldosterone. Adrenal and pituitary function.

Alkaline phosphatase. Hyperparathyroidism, hyperthyroidism, bone tumors, osteomalacia, liver disease, malnutrition, excessive ingestion of vitamin D.

Alpha-fetoprotein (AFP). Spina bifida (when found in the mother's serum), testicular tumor, hepatoma.

Ammonia. Reye's syndrome, liver disease.

Amylase. Pancreatitis or duct obstruction, alcohol ingestion, liver damage, renal disease, mumps, parotiditis, gallbladder disease, peptic ulcers, intestinal obstruction, mesenteric thrombosis.

Antinuclear antibody (ANA). Systemic lupus, lupus-like syndromes, scleroderma, rheumatoid arthritis.

Antistreptolysin O. Streptococcal infections, rheumatoid arthritis.

Aspartate aminotransferase (AST). Myocardial infarction; also see **serum glutamic-oxaloacetic transaminase** (**SGOT**).

B_{12}. Polycythemia rubra vera, malabsorption, pregnancy, pernicious anemia, leukemia.

Bilirubin. Liver damage, obstruction, or dysfunction; biliary obstruction; hemolytic anemia; jaundice of the newborn.

Bleeding time. Thrombocytopenia, defective platelet function in aspirin therapy.

Blood serum test. Analysis of certain proteins to determine if cancer synthesis is present.

Blood urea clearance. Renal function.

Blood urea nitrogen (BUN). Renal failure, decreased renal profusion due to congestive heart failure and other causes, starvation, drugs, overhydration or dehydration.

C. Peptide. Diabetes.

Calcitonin. Anemia, chronic renal sufficiency, carcinoma of the thyroid.

Carbon dioxide, bicarbonate. Acidosis and ketoacidosis (from various causes), dehydration, severe diarrhea, drugs, adrenal insufficiency, starvation.

Carboxyhemoglobin. Smoke or exhaust exposure.

Catecholamines. Neural crest tumors, pheochromocytoma.

Cholesterol. Hypercholesterolemia, biliary obstruction, nephrosis, hypothyroidism, diabetes, malnutrition, anemia, steroid therapy.

Cold agglutinins. Atypical pneumonia, cirrhosis, infections.

Complement C3. Rheumatoid arthritis, rheumatoid fever, systemic lupus, glomerulonephritis, sepsis, subacute bacterial endocarditis, hepatitis.

Complement C4. Rheumatoid arthritis, systemic lupus, hepatitis, cirrhosis, glomerulonephritis.

Complete blood count. Includes a *white cell count*, *red cell count*, *hemoglobin*, *hematocrit*, *mean corpuscular hemoglobin* (MCH), *mean corpuscular hemoglobin concentration*, *mean corpuscular volume* (MCV), and *red cell distribution width* (RDW). These studies are done as a part of routine, diagnostic assessment with multiple medical conditions and prior to surgeries.

Coombs' test. Incompatible blood transfusion, hemolysis.

Cortisol. Adrenal adenoma, adrenal carcinoma, Cushing's disease, ACTH-producing tumor, pituitary insufficiency.

Creatine phosphokinase (CPK, CK, CKMB). Muscle damage due to acute myocardial infarction, myocarditis, muscular dystrophy trauma; brain trauma, rhabdomyolysis, and hypothyroidism.

Enzyme-linked immunosorbent assay (ELISA). Screening assay for human immunodeficiency virus (HIV) and other viruses; this assay is confirmed by a Western blot test.

Ferritin. Iron deficiency.

Fibrin degradation products (FDP). Deep vein thrombosis, pulmonary embolism, myocardial infarction, disseminated intravascular coagulation.

Fibrinogen. Sepsis, amniotic fluid embolism, surgery, hematologic conditions, snake bite, acute severe bleeding, burns.

Fluorescent treponema antibody absorbed (FTA-ABS). Syphilis.

Fungal serologies. Antibodies to various fungi.

Gastrin. Pyloric stenosis, pernicious anemia, atrophic gastritis, renal insufficiency, ulcerative colitis.

Glucose, glucose tolerance test. Diabetes mellitus, Cushing's syndrome, pancreatitis, glucagonoma and other pancreatic tumors, liver disease, endocrine disorders, hypothyroidism, hypopituitarism, malnutrition, sepsis, infant born to a diabetic mother, prematurity, and other inborn metabolic disorders.

Glycosolated hemoglobin. Diabetes mellitus, renal failure.

Gonococcal (GC) cultures. Gonorrhea.

Gram stains. Tests for types of bacterial growth.

Guaiac test. Blood in the feces, gastrointestinal bleeding.

Haptoglobin. Liver disease.

Hemoccult. Gastrointestinal bleeding.

Hemogram. Referring to an order for a standard blood chemistry study.

Hepatitis HBsAG, anti-HBc, anti-HbcIgm, HbeAg, anti-HBe, anti-HBs, anti-HAV, anti-HAV IgM. Tests for antigens and antibodies in viral hepatitis.

High-density lipoprotein (HDL) cholesterol. High cholesterol, obesity, diabetes, liver disease, uremia, assessment for coronary artery disease risks.

HIV tests. Tests of body fluids, usually saliva or serum, examining for the presence of human immunodeficiency virus.

Kline test. Blood test for syphilis.

Lactate dehydrogenase (LDH). Acute myocardial infarction, anemia, malignant tumors, pulmonary embolus, renal infarction, muscle injury, liver disease.

Lactic acid. Hypoxia, hemorrhage, shock, cirrhosis, carcinoma, and sepsis.

Lee-White clotting time. Plasma clotting factor deficiency, heparin therapy.

Leukocyte alkaline phosphatase (LAP) score. Leukemia, nephrotic syndrome, acute inflammation, Hodgkin's disease.

Lipase. Acute pancreatitis or duct obstruction, fat embolus syndrome.

Low-density lipoprotein (LDL) cholesterol. Endocrine disease (hypothyroidism, diabetes); hypercholesteremia; excessive saturated fats in the diet; biliary cirrhosis; liver disease; malabsorption; hyperlipoproteinemia.

Lupus erythematosus (LE) preparation. Systemic lupus erythematosus, rheumatoid arthritis, scleroderma.

Magnesium. Renal failure, severe dehydration, lithium intoxication, hypo- or hyperthyroidism, malabsorption, alcoholism, hypophosphatemia, respiratory or metabolic acidosis, response to chronic dialysis or diuretic use, response to hyperalimentation or nasogastric suctioning, acute pancreatitis.

Mantoux. Skin test for detecting tuberculosis exposure.

Methylene blue test. Test for kidney function in which an injection of blue dye is expected to appear in the urine after 30 minutes if the kidneys are functioning normally.

Monospot. Lymphoma, viral hepatitis, rheumatoid arthritis, mononucleosis.

Myoglobin (urine analysis). Acute myocardial infarction, severe hyperthermia, electrical burns, crushing injury, severe muscle injury.

5' Nucleotidase. Liver disease.

Parathyroid hormone (PTH). Hyper- or hypoparathyroidism.

Partial thromboplastin time (PTT). Heparin therapy, defect in blood clotting mechanisms.

Phosphorus. Hyper- or hypoparathyroidism, renal failure, alcoholism, diabetes, response to hyperalimentation, gout, vitamin D deficiency, acidosis, alkalosis, response to diuretics, hypokalemia, hypomagnesemia.

Prostate-specific antigen (PSA). Prostate cancer.

Protein electrophoresis. Nutritional disorders, liver disease, collagen disease, hypoglobulinemia or macroglobulinemia, alpha-1 antitrypsin deficiency, cancer.

Prothrombin time (PT). Blood-clotting mechanisms.

Retinol-binding protein (RBP). Malnutrition, vitamin A deficiency, chronic liver disease.

Rheumatoid factor. Rheumatoid arthritis, systemic lupus erythematosus, chronic inflammation, subacute bacterial endocarditis, pulmonary disease, syphilis.

Sedimentation rate (ESR). Infections, inflammation, rheumatic fever, myocardial infarction, neoplasm.

Serum calcium. Hyper- or hypothyroidism and hyper- or hypoparathyroidism, metastatic bone tumors, response to thiazides, Paget's disease, chronic renal failure, acute pancreatitis, insufficient vitamin D, hypomagnesemia.

Serum chloride. Diabetes with ketoacidosis, renal disease with sodium loss, excessive vomiting, diarrhea, renal tubular acidosis, response to hyperalimentation.

Serum creatinine. Renal failure, acromegaly and gigantism, loss of muscle mass.

Serum foliate. Malabsorption, malnutrition, neoplasm, anemia.

Serum gamma-glutamyl transpeptidase (SGGT). Liver disease, pancreatitis.

Serum glutamic-oxaloacetic transaminase (SGOT). Acute myocardial infarction, brain damage, liver disease, muscle trauma, pancreatitis, burns, renal failure, Reye's syndrome, severe diabetes with ketoacidosis. This test is now referred to as aspartate aminotransferase (AST).

Serum glutamic-pyruvic transaminase (SGPT). Liver disease, pancreatitis.

Serum osmolality. Alcohol ingestion, hyperglycemia, response to mannitol, response to diuretics, poor fluid balance management, disorders of sodium and water balance.

Serum potassium. Renal failure, acidosis, massive tissue damage, vomiting, nasogastric suctioning, diarrhea, metabolic alkalosis.

Serum protein. Myeloma, macroglobulinemia, hypergammaglobulinemia after an acute inflammatory process, sarcoidosis, malnutrition, inflammatory bowel disease, leukemia, Hodgkin's disease.

Serum sodium. Nephrotic syndrome, congestive heart failure, cirrhosis, renal failure, response to antidiuretic hormone, response to mannitol, excessive sweating, Cushing's syndrome, vomiting, diarrhea, pancreatitis, hyperlipidemia, hyperglycemia, multiple myeloma.

Sputum cytology. Abnormal (cancerous) cells in the bronchi and lungs.

Stool cultures. Infections, Crohn's disease, gastrointestinal (GI) hemorrhages, ulcerative colitis, tuberculosis.

Sweat chloride. Cystic fibrosis.

T3 triiodothyronine (RIA). Thyroid functions.

T3 resin uptake (RU). Thyroid functions.

T4 total thyroxine. Thyroid functions.

Thrombin time. Response to heparin therapy, fibrinogen deficiency.

Thyroglobulin. Graves' disease, thyroid carcinomas, nontoxic goiter; presence of abnormal levels of testosterone or steroids.

Transferrin. Iron deficiency, poor nutritional status, acute inflammation, liver disease.

Thyroid-stimulating hormone (TSH). Thyroid functions.

TORCH battery. Toxoplasmosis, "other," rubella, cytomegalovirus, and herpes simplex; sometimes the acronym **STORCH** is used, referring to *syphilis*, "other," toxoplasmosis, rubella, cytomegalovirus, and herpes simplex.

Total iron, iron-binding capacity (TIBC). Anemia, hemochromatosis.

Troponins. Heart enzymes for ischemic cardiac events.

Uric acid. Gout, renal failure, response to diuretics, anemia, toxemia, hypothyroidism, lactic acidosis, Wilson's disease.

Urinalysis (UA) studies. Most commonly include an examination of the appearance, specific gravity, and pH of the urine and tests for bilirubin, blood, acetone, glucose, protein, nitrite, leukocyte esterase, urobilinogen, epithelial cells, hyaline cases, bacteria, and crystals. Like the CBC, the UA is done for routine and preoperative assessments and as a part of the diagnostic workup with multiple medical conditions. The UA is used to detect the presence of urinary tract infections, renal disease, drugs, and diabetes. Creatinine clearance and urine output are indicators of renal disease and fluid imbalances.

Venereal Disease Research Laboratory (VDRL) screen. Syphilis.

Viral cultures and serology. Viral infections (such as herpes simplex).

Wayson stain. Bacterial infections.

Western blot analysis for AIDS. Confirmation following positive antigens for acquired immune deficiency syndrome.

B. Diagnostic Procedures

This section lists some commonly ordered special examinations and procedures performed as part of the physical examination (see Chapter 4 for descriptions of neurologic studies, Chapter 5 for procedures related to nutrition and hydration, and Chapter 7 for more detailed descriptions of x-ray and other imaging studies).

Angiography. Radiologic examination of blood vessels.

Barium enema. A lower GI x-ray study using both air and barium (double contrast) introduced through an enema to examine for obstructions, growths, and abnormalities on the surface of the lower intestine lining.

Biopsy. Excision and removal of a tissue specimen for microscopic analysis. An **excisional biopsy** involves removing a piece of tissue from a suspicious mass. An **incisional biopsy** refers to a surgical incision to remove a wedge of tissue from a suspicious tumor. A *needle biopsy* removes a core of tissue through a special needle lumen. A *punch biopsy* removes a plug of tissue, usually from the skin. A *stereotaxic needle biopsy* involves a precise placement of a needle for aspiration of tissue, a methodology used in some brain tumor biopsies.

Bronchoscopy. Examination of the trachea and bronchi with either a rigid or a flexible (fiberoptic) endoscope.

Chemstick. Examination for levels of sugar in blood.

Chest x-ray (CXR). A still x-ray study of the chest to examine the lungs, heart, ribs, and upper spine.

Cholecystography. Examination of the gallbladder with x-ray.

Cystoscopy. Examination of the urethra and bladder with an endoscope.

Echoradiography. Ultrasound imaging procedures in which deep body structures are visualized from reflections of sound pulses.

Endoscopy. Examination with an endoscope, which can be a rigid instrument or a flexible (fiberoptic) tube, introduced into a hollow cavity, tube, or duct.

Gastric analysis. Examination of secretions aspirated (suctioned) from the stomach.

Intravenous pyelography (IVP). An x-ray examination of the urinary tract using a contrast medium to delineate the structures.

Kidneys, ureters, and bladder (KUB). A plain x-ray film of the kidneys, ureters, and bladder.

Laparoscopy. Endoscopic examination of the abdomen.

Lumbar puncture. A procedure in which a needle is inserted below the arachnoid layer of the meninges between the fourth and fifth or third and fourth lumbar vertebrae to remove cerebrospinal fluid for analysis.

Panendoscopy. Endoscopic examination with a complete exploration of the cavity.

Paracentesis. Removal of fluid from the abdominal cavity through a procedure that uses a piercing instrument (trocar) or needle with an outer cannula for draining fluids into rubber tubing. The fluids are removed to reduce pressure and for microscopic analysis.

Sigmoidoscopy and proctoscopy. Examination of the lower colon with a flexible (fiberoptic) scope.

Thoracentesis. Removal of fluid from the plural cavity for the purpose of examining for infection, tumor cells, and pulmonary diseases.

Thyroid scan. A radiology study using radioactive iodine administered to the patient orally or by injection. After allowing time for absorption by the thyroid gland, a scanning device is used to detect any alterations in the rate or symmetry of absorption.

Upper GI series. X-ray studies using barium to study the esophagus, stomach, and duodenum for evidence of dysmotility, tumors, strictures, ulcers, and potential causes of reflux.

V. MONITORING AND RECORDING VITAL SIGNS

Nurses monitor vital signs and record findings graphically at the patient's bed or with online electronic monitoring and recording. Vital signs are usually measured and recorded at least once per shift (day, evening, and night shifts). Unless specifically ordered, weight is measured at admission and discharge, and blood pressure is usually measured once a day. Measurements and recordings are made of the patient's temperature, pulse, and respiration three times a day. In addition, nurses note the patient's level of activity, appetite, and urine and stool elimination ("ins and outs"). Vital signs may be reported using both numeric values and descriptive data.

A. Pulse Rates and Heart Sounds

Pulse rate ranges decrease with age (Table 3–l). Pulses can be taken from different peripheral sites (Figure 3–3) and are recorded by noting the site(s) used (e.g., "femoral pulse," "carotid pulse," "brachial pulse," etc.).

The sounds heard during *stethoscope auscultation* of the heart are described using four basic heart sound types: *S1* (sound occurring at the onset of **systole** when the mitral and bicuspid valves close); *S2* (sound attributed to the closure of the aortic and pulmonary valves); *S3* (difficult to hear sound associated with ventricular filling); and *S4* (nearly impossible to hear sound associated with ventricular filling and atrial contraction). Usually only the S1 and S2 sounds are described (the "lub dub" sounds, respectively). The notation *M1* and *M2* denotes a "split" sound heard during S1.

Extra heart sounds are also described usually as *snaps*, *clicks*, *murmurs*, and *rubs* (see previously). The timing and intensity of the extra heart sounds are graded as *grade 1* (softest audible murmur); *grade 2* (murmur of medium intensity); *grade 3* (loud murmur without thrill); *grade 4* (murmur with thrill); *grade 5* (loudest murmur requiring a stethoscope to hear); and *grade 6* (murmur that is audible without a stethoscope on the chest).

B. Respiration

In intensive care units (ICUs), respiration may be monitored continuously with special devices (see Figure 11–1); however, when respirator monitors are not used, respiration may be described by observing breathing characteristics. Respiratory rates, like pulse rates, tend

TABLE 3–1 Normal pulse rates

AGE	AVERAGE RANGE (HEARTBEATS/MIN.)
Neonate	120–160
2-year-old	80–40
5 to 12 years old	75–100
Adolescent and adult	60–100

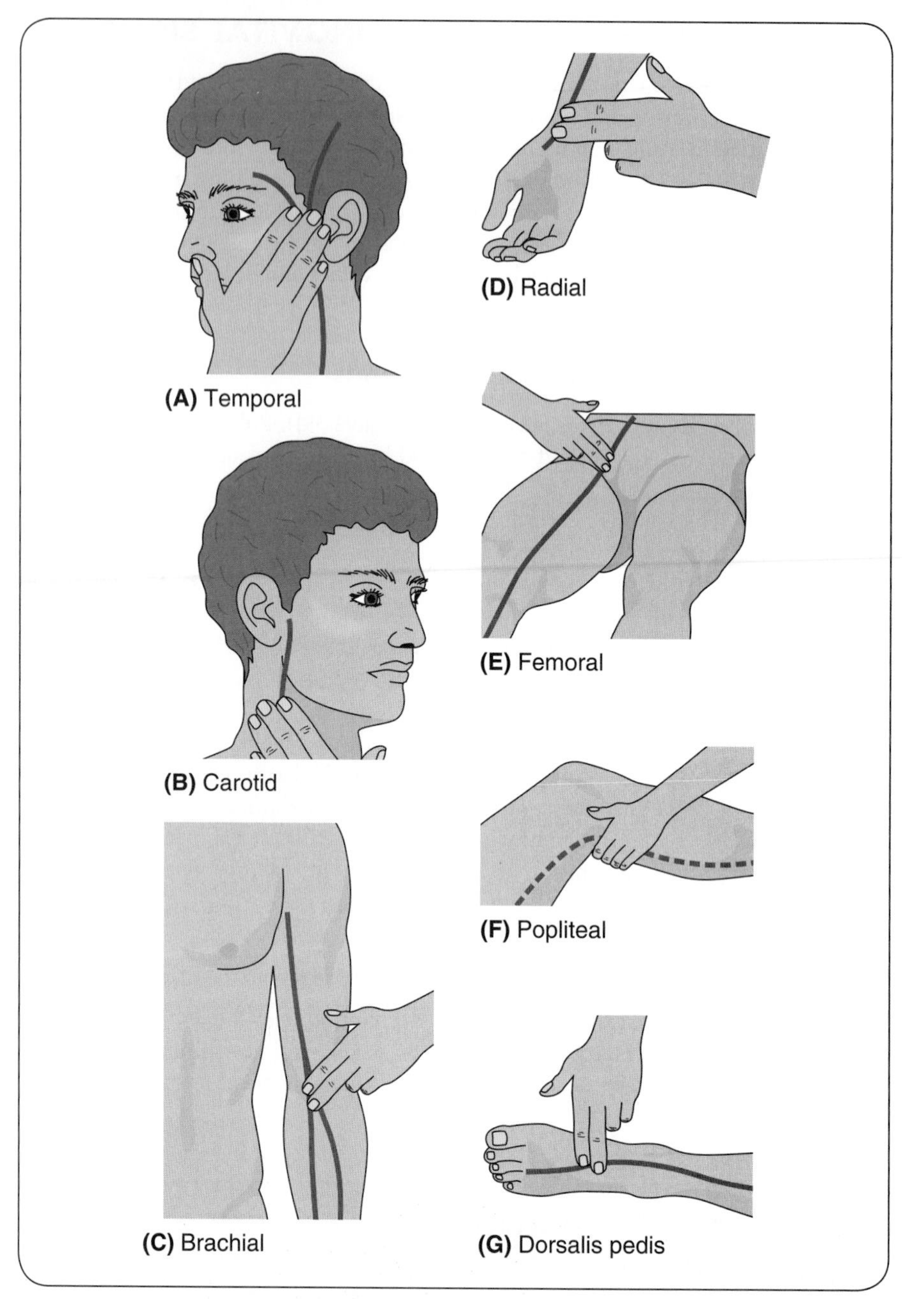

FIGURE 3–3 Pulse points. Source: Delmar Cengage Learning

to decrease with age. Newborns have a respiratory rate ranging from 30 to 80 respirations per minute, whereas adult respirations range from 14 to 20 per minute. Adult patients who are breathing quietly (with an average tidal volume of 500 mL) at the average rate of 16 respirations per minute breathe about 8 liters of air per minute. Chapter 9 contains descriptive terminology used for respiration observations. Table 3–5 provides a summary of normal respiration rates for children.

C. Temperature

Temperature is usually measured with a clinical thermometer (oral, rectal, or axillary). Heat-sensitive paper, tape, or patches are sometimes used to obtain temperature. Electronic thermometers with disposable probes are preferred in hospitals. Most thermometers display temperature in degrees Celsius (C) and degrees Fahrenheit (F). Celsius temperature refers to a *centigrade scale* referenced by the freezing point for water (0°C) and the boiling point for water (100°C). *Fahrenheit scale*, in which the freezing point for water is 32°F and the boiling point for water is 212°F, is not commonly used in medical settings. To compute Celsius from Fahrenheit temperatures, subtract 32 from the Fahrenheit temperature, multiply that number by 5, and divide by 9.

D. Weight

In medical settings, weight is commonly measured in kilograms (kg) than in pounds (lb) and height in centimeters (cm) rather than in inches (in). Table 3–2 provides a translation table for kilograms and pounds. Increasingly, weight is reported along with a calculation known as the **body mass index (BMI)**. The BMI formula is the same for children as it is for adults. To calculate BMI multiply weight in pounds by 703 and divide that number by height in inches squared. In the metric system, multiply weight in kilograms by height in meters squared. Because height is commonly measured in centimeters, divide height in centimeters by 100 to obtain height in *meters*.

TABLE 3–2 Comparison of kilograms to pounds

Kilograms (kg)	Pounds (lb)
1	2.2
5	11
10	22
15	33
20	44
25	55
30	66
40	88
50	99
60	132
70	154
80	176
90	198
100	220

E. Blood Pressure

The force produced by the volume of blood pressing on the walls of the arteries is called *blood pressure.* Blood pressure measurements reflect the elasticity of the arteries, the volume of the blood circulating in the body, and the efficiency of the heart's pumping action. Blood pressure is measured in millimeters of mercury (mmHg) with the **systolic pressure** (representing ventricular contraction) as the top number and the **diastolic pressure** (representing the ventricular relaxation) as the bottom number. The average normal ranges for blood pressure readings increase with age. Children at 1 year of age have an average normal blood pressure of around 95/65 mmHg, whereas adults over age 18 have an average blood pressure of around 120/80 mmHg. With aging, the normal range increases.

F. ICU Vital Sign Monitors, Lines, Tubes, and Catheters

In Chapter 11, Acute and Critical Illness, Figure 11–1 provides an example of the typical array of lines, catheters, tubes, and monitors encountered in an ICU with patients with traumatic brain injury. Patients in ICUs require continuous nursing observations and electronic monitoring of vital signs. Vital signs are monitored with hemodynamic and cardiovascular monitors, respiratory and pulmonary function monitors, spectrometry and capnography, blood gas and oxygen saturation monitoring (oximetry), and assessment of nutritional status by measuring the production of carbon dioxide (CO_2) and consumption of oxygen (O_2). Patients with neurologic dysfunction related to increased intracranial pressure require **intracranial pressure (ICP)** monitoring, which is described later. The following list describes some of the procedures for monitoring and managing patients in an ICU.

Antiembolism stockings. Long white stocking used to prevent blood from pooling in the legs; frequently called **TEDS.**

Arterial catheters. Catheters used for continuous monitoring of blood gases and blood pressure. Pulmonary artery catheters (balloon-tipped catheters inserted through the right side of the heart into the pulmonary artery for cardiac monitoring) are frequently referred to as Swan-Ganz catheters, which are described later.

Cardiac monitors. On-line cardiac rhythm and conductivity monitoring equipment for cardiac functions are at each bedside in the ICU. Cardiac monitoring includes a central console at the nurses' station, slave oscilloscopes for visualization of the patient's heart rhythms, rhythm strips at a central station and at bedside, and memory and alarm circuitry with visual and auditory signals.

Central venous pressure (CVP), Swan-Ganz catheters. Manometric measures of right atrial pressure.

Dobbhoff feeding tube (DHFT). Virtually any nasogastric tube can be used as a feeding tube, but usually the physician will use one of the mercury-weighted tubes, such as the Dobbhoff feeding tube, DHFT, or similar tube (Keogh tube, Duo-tube) for enteral feeding. This variety of feeding tube is inserted when feeding is the main requirement for a gastrointestinal (GI) tube insertion (there is no need for gastric aspiration or decompression). Because the DHFT is a small-bore tube, it is less irritating to the pharynx, and the weighted tip makes it easier to pass beyond the pylorus into the duodenum or through to the small intestine (jejunum). Placing the feeding tubes further into the GI tract is sometimes felt to be preferable for reduced aspiration risks (also see *nasogastric tubes* [NGTs] and *nasointestinal tubes* [NITs] later) or when there is concern for gastric pooling and reflux.

Drains. Surgical drains or catheters to remove unwanted body fluids may be in place. Drain types include Penrose drains, the cigarette drain, **Foley catheters** (for urine drainage), and double lumen sump catheters.

Intracranial pressure (ICP) monitoring. ICP monitors are placed with a subarachnoid screw and inserted by way of a burr hole through the cranium and dura into the subarachnoid space. In some cases, a fiberoptic device with a pressure transducer-tipped catheter is used instead of the subarachnoid screw. Other methods for intracranial monitoring include an Ommaya reservoir (a mushroom-shaped capped tube placed into one of the lateral ventricles that can be left in place to sample cerebrospinal fluid) and a *ventricular drain* (see later).

Nasogastric (NG) tubes. Nasogastric tubes are used mainly for aspiration and gastric decompression, as well as administration of medications, gastric lavage, or feedings. *Nasointestinal tubes* (NITs) are sometimes preferred because they are felt to have lower risks for aspiration (see Dobbhoff feeding tubes). **NG/nasojejunal tubes (NGJ)** are tube feeding systems with two outlets. The gastric outlet is used for bolus feeding while the other outlet goes directly into the small bowel for continuous tube feeding via a pump.

Nasotracheal, endotracheal (orotracheal), or tracheostomy tubes. These devices are used for patients requiring airway or air supply support.

Oximeters, pulse oximeters. These devices provide continuous measurements of oxygen saturation and may be either indwelling intravascular devices or less invasive devices worn on the finger, earlobe, or foot (in infants) in which monitoring of oxygen levels is done transcutaneously by way of a light shining through the body part.

Oxygen therapy. Patients with conditions requiring oxygen therapy are given some sort of oxygen delivery system. This can include a Venturi mask, which is driven by pure oxygen, or a nasal cannula, which has nasal prongs and permits oral breathing augmented by oxygen.

Pacemakers. External pacemakers provide temporary or permanent correction of cardiac arrhythmias.

Pleur Evac (chest) tube. Pleural chest tubes are used to evacuate blood, pus, air, and fluid from the thoracic cavity to reestablish negative pressure in the intrapleural space and thereby expand the lungs following a collapse (usually resulting from surgery or trauma).

Pulmonary artery catheters. These are manometric monitors of left heart filling pressures and cardiac output.

Sengstaken-Blakemore tubes. This tube has a balloon and lumen for aspiration of stomach contents and is used to treat esophageal or gastric bleeding.

Sequential compression stockings. Plastic leg wraps with inflating and deflating air channels that prevent blood pooling in the legs; frequently called *Kendalls*.

Ventilator monitoring. Patients on mechanical ventilators (respirators) have suction equipment at bedside, and the ventilator is equipped with alarms for oxygen, apnea, low pressure, high pressure, and tidal volume. The ventilator has settings for *tidal* *volume*; *ventilatory rate*; *positive end-expiratory pressure* (PEEP); and mode of function (*intermittent mandatory ventilation* [IMV] and *controlled mandatory ventilation* [CMV] or *synchronous intermittent mandatory ventilation* [SIMV]).

Ventriculostomy drain. ICP line to drain excessive fluid from the ventricles of the brain. Typically a No. 8 pediatric feeding tubing is placed in the lateral ventricles for drainage.

VI. APGAR SCORES AND ESTIMATION OF GESTATIONAL AGE

A. Apgar (APGAR) Scores

Apgar scores refer to the standard numerical rating of the vital signs of infants observed at 1 minute and 5 minutes following delivery. Although "Apgar" is an eponym referring to Virginia Apgar, who introduced the scoring system in the early 1950s, the five areas examined are often listed by use of the acronym APGAR (Table 3–3). This is a slight modification of Apgar's original terminology, but the categories are essentially the same. Apgar ratings are made at 1 minute postdelivery, because that is considered the time of maximal stress to the infant. Newborns with Apgar scores of 4 to 6 usually require resuscitation. Scores of 0 to 3 indicate acute distress.

B. Gestational Age Estimates

Estimating gestational age and neonatal development is important for determining risk for post delivery complications. Figure 3–4 illustrates a method for determining the neurologic maturity of newborns, and Table 3–4 explains the ratings. This method, developed by Dubowitz and colleagues nearly 4 decades ago (Dubowitz, Dubowitz, & Goldberg, 1970) has undergone revisions and refinements since the initial publication (also see Dubowitz, Dubowitz, & Goldberg, 1998). Higher scores indicate a greater gestational maturity. The neurologic maturity ratings also may be applied in postneonates when there is a question of delayed neurologic development. Facilities differ with regard to their preferred standard scales for estimating neurologic and physical maturity, and instruments have been expanded to include extremely premature infants (Ballard et al., 1991).

TABLE 3–3 Agar scores

	SCORES		
SIGN	**0**	**1**	**2**
Appearance	Blue or pale	Blue extremities	Pink
Pulse	Absent	Less than 100/min	More than 100/min
Grimace	No response	Grimace	Cough or sneeze
Activity	Limp	Some flexion	Active
Respirations	Absent	Slow, irregular	Good, crying

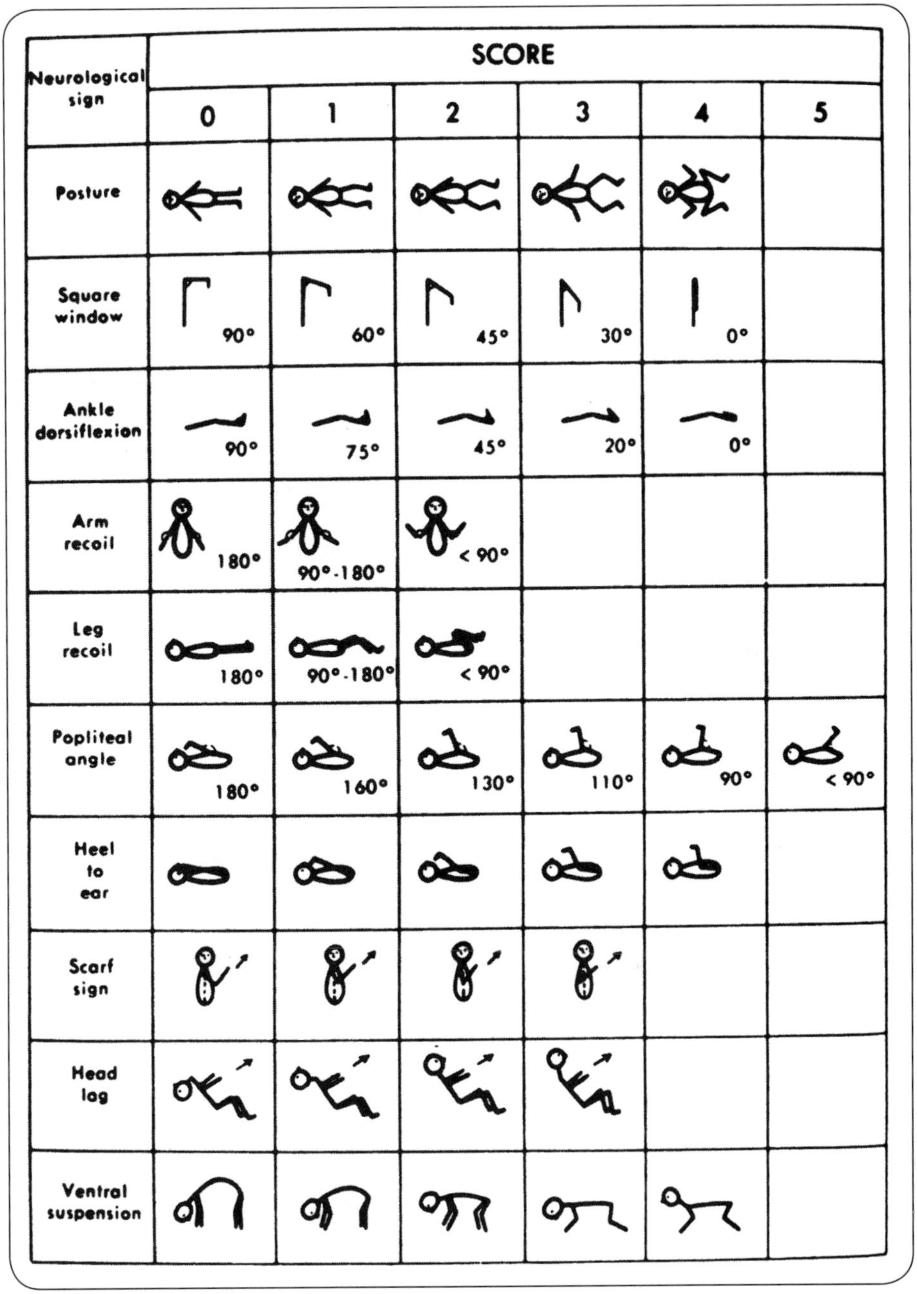

Neurological sign	SCORE 0	1	2	3	4	5
Posture						
Square window	90°	60°	45°	30°	0°	
Ankle dorsiflexion	90°	75°	45°	20°	0°	
Arm recoil	180°	90°-180°	< 90°			
Leg recoil	180°	90°-180°	< 90°			
Popliteal angle	180°	160°	130°	110°	90°	< 90°
Heel to ear						
Scarf sign						
Head lag						
Ventral suspension						

FIGURE 3–4 Illustration of neurologic scoring system. "Reprinted from Dubowitz, L.M.S., Dubowitz, V., & Goldberg, C., 1970. Clinical assessment of gestational age in the newborn infant. *Journal of Pediatrics*, 77, pp. 4–5, with permission from Elsevier."

TABLE 3–4 Newborn neurologic maturity assessment[a]

SIGN	SCORES	FINDINGS
Posture	0	Arms and legs extended
	1	Slight to moderate flexion of LEs
	2	Strong flexion of LEs
	3	Slight flexion of UEs, strong flexion of LEs
	4	Full flexion of arms and legs
Square window	0	Flexing the hand at the wrist produces a 90° angle
	1	60° angle
	2	45° angle
	3	30° angle
	4	0° angle
Ankle dorsiflexion	0	Flexing the ankle produces a 90° angle
	1	75° angle
	2	45° angle
	3	30° angle
	4	0° angle
Arm recoil	0	Flexing the arm for 5 seconds followed by pulling the arms and releasing produces a recoil posture at 180°
	1	90 to 180°
	2	less than 90°
Leg recoil	0	Flexing the legs and hips for 5 seconds then pulling the legs to a full extension produces no response recoil
	1	90 to 180° recoil
	2	less than 90° recoil
Popliteal angle	0	Fully flexing the thigh produces a 180° angle
	1	160° angle
	2	130° angle
	3	110° angle
	4	90° angle
	5	less than 90° angle
Heel to Ear Maneuver	0	Movement of the infant's foot toward the head is fully possible
	1–4	See Figure 3–4

SIGN	SCORES	FINDINGS
Scarf sign	0	Infant's hand can be drawn across its neck and shoulder fully to the opposite side
	1–3	See Figure 3–4
Head lag	0	When lifting infant by the arms the head shows no evidence of support
	1	Slight support
	2	Partial support
	3	Fully supported
Ventral suspension	0	When lifting the infant by the hand under the chest from a prone position, there is no truncal support
	1–4	See Figure 3–4

[a] Refer to Figure 3–4.

Based on: Dubowitz, L.M.S., Dubowitz, V., & Goldberg, C., 1970. Clinical assessment of gestational age in the newborn infant. *Journal of Pediatrics*, 77, pp. 4–5, with permission from Elsevier.

VII. NORMAL GROWTH, RESPIRATORY RATES, AND BLOOD PRESSURE IN CHILDREN

In neonates, respirations are typically abdominal and range from 30 to 60 per minute. Respiratory rates, shown in Table 3–5, gradually slow through the age of 16 when adult rates are reached (17 per minute at rest). Weight is an important vital and development sign in children and is usually

TABLE 3–5 Respiration rates from newborn through 20 years

AGE	RESPIRATION RATE
New born	60 bpm
1 year	30 bpm
2 years	25 bpm
3 years	24 bpm
5 years	20 bpm
10 years	18 bpm
15 years	18 bpm
20 years	17 bpm

Based on: Valadian, J., & Porter, D. (1977). *Physical growth and development.* Boston: Little, Brown, p. 311.

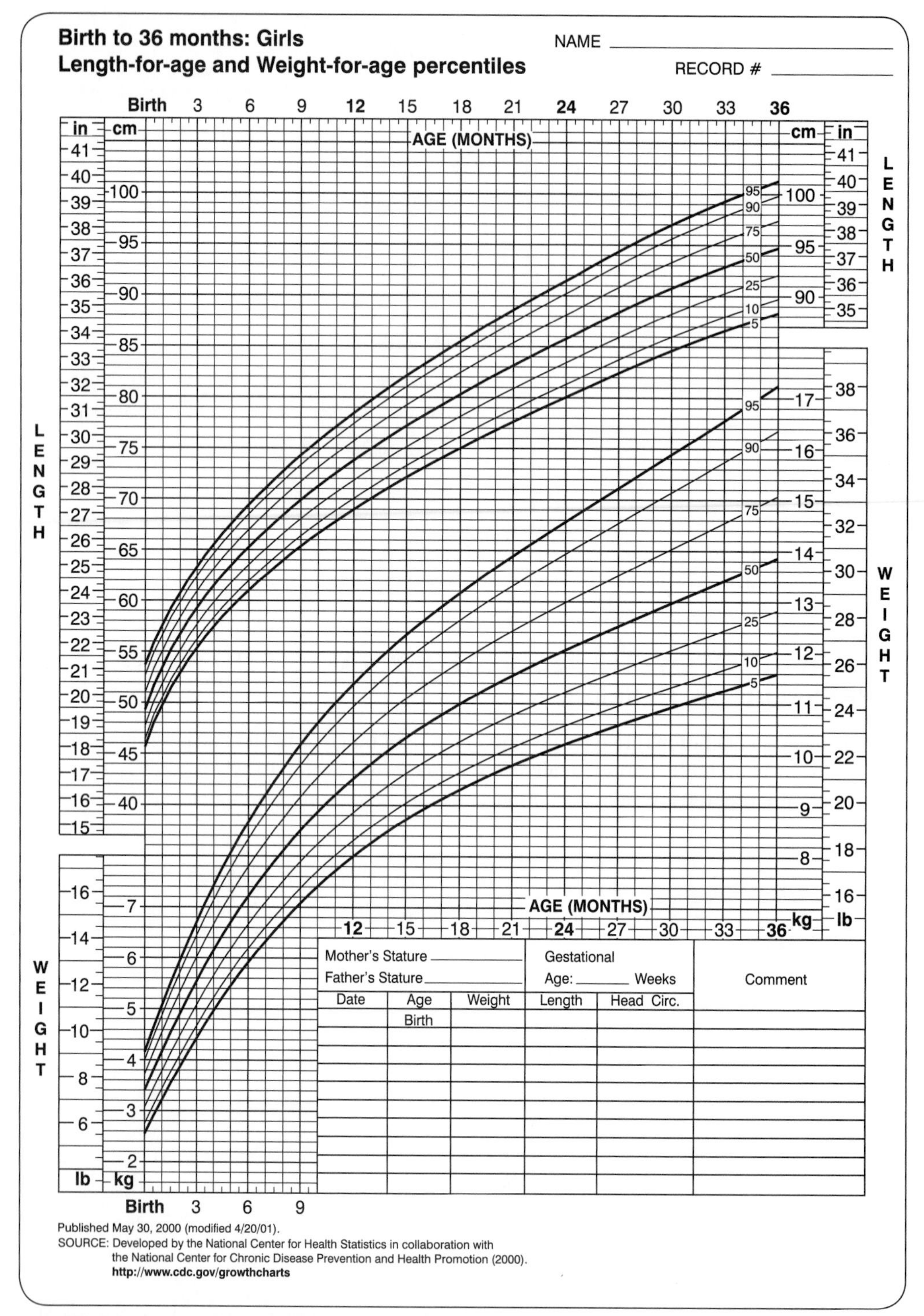

FIGURE 3–5 Physical growth chart for children (females). Source: Developed by the National Center for Health Statistics in collaboration with the National Center for Chronic Disease Prevention and Health Promotion. (2000). Retrieved August 2008, from http://www.cdc.gov/growthcharts

measured as a ratio of weight to length/height (Figure 3–5). Blood pressure measurements are taken immediately after birth and followed to detect cardiac abnormalities. Normal blood pressures for infants and children are variable, and physicians typically take measurements over time to look for trends toward high or low ranges. The normal ranges for young children aged 2 to 6 are considerably lower than those of adults. A systolic pressure between 80 and 110 mmHg and diastolic pressure of 50 to 80 mmHg would be considered normal in very young children. Normal ranges gradually increase through adolescence and teenaged years to adult values.

VIII. CLINICAL COMPETENCIES

The learner outcomes, skills, and competencies gained from information contained in this chapter include the ability to:

- Read, interpret, and use terminology and abbreviations related to the physician's history and physical and diagnostic procedures.
- List the essential elements of a medical history.
- List the areas of inquiry that comprise a "review of systems."
- Describe the typical format for the physical examination.
- Define the "rule of nines."
- Describe some of the commonly ordered laboratory tests and what they measure.
- Describe some of the commonly performed diagnostic procedures and their purpose.
- List the "vital signs" and how they are typically measured.
- List some of the lines, drains, and monitors that are used in ICUs.
- Describe how gestational age is determined.
- Describe the areas evaluated when determining an Apgar score.

IX. REFERENCES AND RESOURCES CONSULTED

Anderson, D. (Ed.). (2003). *Dorland's illustrated medical dictionary* (30th ed.). Philadelphia: W. B. Saunders.

Andreoli, T. A., Carpenter, C., & Grigg, R. C. (Eds.). (2007). *Cecil essentials of medicine* (7th ed.). Philadelphia: W. B. Saunders.

Andreoli, T. A., Carpenter, C. J., Plum, F., & Smith, L. H. (Eds.). (1990). *Cecil essentials of medicine* (2nd ed.). Philadelphia: W. B. Saunders.

Apgar, V. (1953). A proposal for a new method of evaluation of the newborn infant. *Anesthesia and Analgesia, 32*, 260–264.

Arvedson, J. C., & Brodsky, L. (2002). *Pediatric swallowing and feeding: Assessment and management* (2nd ed.). San Diego, CA: Singular, Thomson Learning.

Ballard, J. L., Khoury, J. C., Wedig, K., Wang, L., Ellers-Waisman, B. L., & Lipp, R. (1991). New Ballard Score, expanded to include extremely premature infants. *Journal of Pediatrics, 119*, 417–423.

Ballard, J. L., Novak, K. K., & Driver, M. (1979). A simplified score for assessment of fetal maturation of newly born infants. *Journal of Pediatrics, 95*, 769–774.

Berkow, R. (Ed.). (1990). *The Merck manual* (15th ed.). Trenton, NJ: Merck Sharpe and Dohme.

Boggs, R. L., & Wooldridge-King, M. (1993). *AACN procedure manual for critical care* (3rd ed.). Philadelphia: W. B. Saunders.

D'Angelo, H. H., & Welsh, N. P. (1988). *The signs and symptoms handbook.* Springhouse, PA: Springhouse.

Daniels, R., Nosek, L., & Nicoll, L. (2007). *Contemporary medical-surgical nursing.* Clifton Park, NY: Delmar Cengage Learning.

Davis, M. A., Gruskin, K. D., Chiang, V. W., & Manzi, S. (Eds.). (2005). *Signs and symptoms in pediatrics: Urgent and emergent care.* Philadelphia: Elsevier Mosby.

Davies, J. J. (2008). *Essentials of medical terminology* (3rd ed.). Clifton Park, NY: Delmar Cengage Learning.

DeGowin, E. L., & DeGowin, R. L. (1987). *Bedside diagnostic examination* (4th ed.). New York: Macmillan.

DeGowin, R. L., LeBlond, R. F., & Brown, D. O. (2004). *DeGowin's diagnostic examination* (8th ed.). New York: McGraw-Hill Medical Publishing Division.

Detmer, W. M., McPhee, S. J., Nicoll, D., & Chou, T. M. (1992). *Pocket guide to diagnostic tests.* Norwalk, CT: Appleton-Lange.

Dubowitz, L. M. S., Dubowitz, V., & Goldberg, C. (1970). Clinical assessment of gestational age in the newborn infant. *Journal of Pediatrics, 77,* 1–6.

Dubowitz, L. M. S., Dubowitz, V., & Goldberg, C. (1998). An optimal score for the neurologic examination of the term newborn. *Journal of Pediatrics, 133,* 406–416.

Fuchs, A. (2007). *Pediatrics pocketcard set.* Hermosa Beach, CA: Börm Bruckmeier.

Gomella, L. G. (Ed.). (1989). *Clinician's pocket handbook* (6th ed.). East Norwalk, CT: Appleton & Lange.

Gomella, L. G. (Ed.). (1993). *Clinician's pocket reference* (7th ed.). East Norwalk, CT: Appleton & Lange.

Keir, L., Wise, B., Krebs, C., & Kelley-Arney, C. (2008). *Medical assisting: Administrative and clinical competencies* (6th ed.). Clifton Park, NY: Delmar Cengage Learning.

Kelly, W. J. (Ed.). (1992). *Clinical skillbuilders: Better documentation.* Springhouse, PA: Springhouse.

Kenner, C. A. (1992). *Nurse's clinical guide: Neonatal care.* Springhouse, PA: Springhouse.

Leonard, P. C. (2007). *Quick and easy medical terminology* (5th ed.). St. Louis, MO: Saunders Elsevier.

Melonakos, K. (1990). *Saunders pocket reference for nurses.* Philadelphia: W. B. Saunders.

National Center for Health Statistics in collaboration with the National Center for Chronic Disease Prevention and Health Promotion. (2000). *Physical growth chart for children (females).* Retrieved August 2008, from http://www.cdc.gov/growthcharts

Seikel, J. A., King, D. W., & Drumright, D. G. (2005). *Anatomy and physiology for speech, language, and hearing* (3rd ed.). Clifton Park, NY: Delmar Cengage Learning.

Valadian, J., & Porter, D. (1977). *Physical growth and development.* Boston: Little, Brown.

Willett, M. J., Patterson, M., & Steinbock, B. (1986). *Manual of neonatal intensive care nursing.* Boston: Little, Brown.

CHAPTER 4

Mental Status and the Neurologic Examination

Physicians and other health care professionals make an assessment of mental status as a routine part of the neurologic aspects of the physical examination of adults, especially in cases with decreased alertness or when there is some reason to suspect the presence of a psychiatric disorder, delirium, or dementia. Geriatric patients are more likely to undergo a formal mental status examination than younger persons. Patients with notable impairments in mental (cognitive) functions are likely to be seen by a neurologist and, in some cases, a psychologist or psychiatrist will be consulted. Any communication-related deficit should prompt a referral to a speech-language pathologist (SLP) (Strub & Black, 1993). Mental status is an important indicator of a patient's *medical* status, and abrupt changes in mental status of any patient, regardless of age, mandate immediate medical attention. If mental status is determined to be impaired, the staff is likely to monitor and comment on the alertness, orientation, memory, responsiveness, and quality of the patient's verbalizations in the medical record at each visit; for example, "Pt. is awake, alert, oriented x 3, introduced this examiner to family members present and explained relationships; able to recall what he had for lunch today."

I. CHAPTER FOCUS

This chapter reviews the essential elements of a mental status examination and other aspects of the neurologic examination. A glossary of the terminology, abbreviations, and frequently ordered tests and procedures in the neurologic workup are provided. Examples of the questions and tasks used in mental status assessment, the areas covered, and a typical format for the neurologist's history and physical are reviewed. Reference figures and tables are provided. Discussions of the assessment of **coma**, **confusion**, **delirium**, **depression**, and **dementia** are included. These disorders are addressed again in Chapter 10, along with other neurologic and psychiatric disorders. Most of the information provided in this chapter generally applies across the age span. Where appropriate, age-specific tests or measures are described in this chapter and elsewhere (see Chapters 3 and 14). Issues related to behavioral neurology related to rehabilitation and geriatric care are addressed in Chapter 14, and neuroradiologic imaging studies are discussed in Chapter 7. An example of a neonatal neurologic maturity assessment is illustrated in Table 3–4.

II. TERMINOLOGY AND ABBREVIATIONS

A. Terminology

Abduction. Motion away from the center.

Abulia. Slowness, apathy, psychomotor retardation.

Acalculia. Impaired ability to perform arithmetic operations.

Accommodation. Adjustments in the lens, pupil, and position of the eye in response to objects held close to the eye; near vision reflex.

Achromatopsia. Lack of color vision.

Acrophobia. Fear of high places.

Adduction. Motion toward the center.

Adductor tenotomy and obturator neurectomy (ATON). Surgery performed on children with cerebral palsy to release the adductor muscles of the hips and reduce partial dislocation (subluxation).

Afferent. Impulse traveling toward the nerve body.

Agnosia. An impairment, unrelated to sensory loss, in the ability to recognize a sensory stimulus despite relatively preserved primary sensory input.

Akathisia. The inability to remain still; motor restlessness.

Akinesis. Lack of motor movement not attributable to paresis or paralysis.

Amaurosis fugax. Temporary episode of unilateral visual loss often characterized by a gradual visual field loss from the top-down as if a window shade were being pulled down over the eyes.

Amnesia. A loss of memory.

Amusia. A loss of musical ability or recognition of musical features, or both.

Analgesia. Lack of pain.

Anencephaly. Lack of brain and cranium development.

Anesthesia. Loss of sensation.

Aneuploidy. An abnormal number of chromosomes.

Anisocoria. Unequal pupil size.

Anomic aphasia. Aphasia type characterized by a predominant impairment in naming, word-finding, and semantic abilities.

Anosmia. A loss in the sense of smell.

Anosodiaphoria. Tendency to minimize or joke about the extent of paresis or paralysis of an affected limb; occasionally seen in patients with right hemisphere cerebral dysfunction.

Anosognosia. An inability to recognize the presence of one's illness or to exaggerate the residual function of the affected limb.

Aphasia. An acquired loss of language abilities.

Apraxia. An inability to initiate, imitate, coordinate, or perform a previously learned skilled movement despite an intact motor and sensory system.

Argyll Robertson pupil. An impairment in the pupillary reflexive reaction to light with a retained near vision (accommodation) reflex. Argyll Robertson pupils are found in chronic degenerative diseases of the nervous system, such as diabetes, late-stage Alzheimer's disease, viral encephalitis, Wernicke's encephalopathy, and cerebrovascular disease.

Astereognosis. A type of agnosia characterized by an inability to recognize objects placed in the hand. *Oral astereognosis* refers to the inability to recognize objects or shapes placed in the mouth.

Asterixis. A rapid palmar flapping when the wrists are dorsiflexed, which is seen in association with metabolic encephalopathies (as in liver or renal failure).

Astrocyte. A star-shaped neuroglial cell.

Asymmetrical tonic neck reflex (ATNR). In infants, as the head is turned the arm and leg extend in the same direction; "fencer's posture."

Ataxia. Broad, jerky, dyscoordinated movements. This is often due to proprioceptive disturbances, causing what is sometimes called **sensory ataxia**, or to cerebellar lesions (or lesions within the cerebellar circuitry), producing a so-called **cerebellar ataxia**.

Atelencephaly. Incomplete development of the cerebral hemispheres.

Atelomyelia. Incomplete spinal cord development.

Athetosis. A movement disorder characterized by slow, writhing movements of the distal extremities, face, or trunk muscles; a feature of chorea, dystonia, and ballismus.

Atrophy. Decrease in muscle mass due to denervation or disuse.

Automatism. Compulsively performed or repetitive behaviors.

Autonomic dysfunction. Neurologic disorders manifested in dysfunction of autonomic regulations (e.g., orthostatic hypotension, syncope, impotence, pupillary abnormalities, or urinary and gastric disorders).

Autonomic nervous system (ANS). Pertaining to the nerves that maintain the internal environment of the body, including heart rate, digestion, and bowel and bladder control. Breathing is an autonomic function controlled by the central nervous system. The ANS is divided into two divisions, sympathetic and parasympathetic, which have counteractive functions serving to maintain the body's homeostasis.

Autotopagnosia. A form of agnosia in which there is a failure to recognize a body part.

Axon. Long fiber extending from the neuron carrying messages away from the cell body.

Babinski's sign. An abnormal reflexive response to stroking the plantar surface of the foot in which there is extension of the great toe and fanning of the toes instead of the normal flexion response. This "protective sign" usually indicates an abnormality of the central nervous system involving the pyramidal tracts (upper motor neurons).

Ballismus. A movement disorder characterized by an abrupt flinging motion of a body part, usually associated with lesions of the subthalamic nucleus.

Basal ganglia, basal nuclei. Referring to the subcortical gray masses (caudate and lentiform nuclei of the corpus striatum, the amygdaloid body, and the claustrum) deep within each hemisphere.

Bell's palsy. Weakness of the upper and lower hemiface caused by irritation to the facial nerve or nerve sheath.

Biogenic animes. Neurotransmitters (e.g., epinephrine, norepinephrine, acetylcholine, dopamine, and serotonin).

Bite reflex. A jaw-closing reflex elicited with stimulation of the teeth or surfaces within the mouth.

Blood-brain barrier. A neurophysiologic mechanism that regulates the entry of certain serum substances to brain tissues. The blood-brain barrier is a physical barrier formed by the basement membrane of the capillaries of the brain and foot processes of the astrocytes.

Bradykinesia. Movement disorder characterized by slowness or lack of movement independent of rigidity and tremor, often associated with Parkinson's disease and other states, such as drug toxicities and multi-infarct dementia.

Bradyphrenia. Slowed cognitive processes.

Brain stem. Base of the brain consisting of the pons and medulla.

Brain stem auditory evoked responses (BAER, BSER). A computerized, evoked potential study used to detect an interruption in the synapses in the central auditory system to determine a site of lesion.

Broca's aphasia. A type of aphasia (acquired language disorder) usually corresponding to anterior, left, middle cerebral artery lesions characterized by dysfluent (nonfluent) verbal expression with relatively intact auditory comprehension.

Cacogeusia. Sensation of a disagreeable taste. **Ageusia** refers to a *loss* in taste sensation, and **dysgeusia** refers to a disordered taste sensation.

Capgrass syndrome. A visual agnosic disorder in which a familiar person is thought to be an impostor.

Carpal tunnel syndrome. Intermittent numbness and paresthesia of the median nerve distribution in the wrist due to disease or injury, causing compression of the nerve.

Cauda equina. "Horse tail," fanlike, nerve roots exiting from the thecal sac of the spinal cord. In most adults, the spinal cord ends at the second lumbar vertebra, which is the level where the cauda equina originate.

Causalgia. Burning pain that radiates distally to an injured nerve.

Central nervous system (CNS). Pertaining to the functions and structures of the spinal cord, brain stem, midbrain, and the cerebellar and cerebral hemispheres.

Central pontine myelinolysis. Condition occurring mainly in alcoholics, menstruating women, and patients who have had rapidly corrected hyponatremia; manifested by quadriparesis and gaze palsy, dysarthria, and obtundation leading to coma.

Cerebellar nystagmus. Although there are several forms of cerebellar nystagmus, if horizontal gaze nystagmus is more obvious when the patient looks laterally toward the side of lesion, the nystagmus is felt to be cerebellar in origin.

Cerebellum. Portion of the brain lying dorsal to the pons and medulla oblongata, consisting of two lateral hemispheres and the vermis, a narrow middle portion, which are attached to the brain stem by three pairs of fiber bundles. The cerebellum controls synergistic skeletal muscle activity and coordination of voluntary movement.

Cerebral cortex. The surface gray matter of the brain.

Cerebromalacia. Softening of the brain tissue.

Cerebrum. The largest part of the brain including two hemispheres separated by a deep longitudinal fissure with a surface characterized by *gyri* (folds) and *sulci* (fissures) and containing *white matter tracts* and *deep gray masses* (basal ganglia) within the hemispheres. The cerebrum receives sensory information, controls motor activity, and is the center of higher cognitive abilities.

Cervical spondylosis, cervical osteoarthritis. Degenerative diseases of the cervical spine.

Chorea. A hyperkinetic movement disorder characterized by abrupt writhing movements.

Chronic pain. Discomfort lasting more than 6 months.

Clonus. Sustained series of rhythmic jerks.

Cogwheel rigidity. Movement pattern in which the fluidity of movement is lacking with intermittent resistance present during passive stretching motions often associated with Parkinson's disease.

Coma. Condition in which there is little or no evidence of mental or motor response to vigorous, persistent, and noxious external stimulation. Although terms such as "stupor," "obtundation," and so forth are found in medical documents, coma is best rated by one of the objective scales, which are described later.

Conduction aphasia. Type of aphasia (acquired language disorder) characterized by a predominant impairment in verbal repetition with relatively intact auditory comprehension and oral expression said to be due to a disruption of the sensory-to-motor white matter connections of the language dominant hemisphere.

Confusional state. Clouded state of consciousness characterized by incoherent, inappropriate, or nonmeaningful verbal expression; misperceptions of surroundings and others; and nonpurposeful or inappropriate behaviors.

Conjugate and dysconjugate gaze movements. Eye movements occurring in unison are termed *conjugate gaze* movements. *Dysconjugate gaze* deviations refer to eyes that do not move in one direction. Conjugate gaze deviations can occur *toward the side of a unilateral destructive hemispheric* lesion (opposite the side of the hemiparesis), "looking at the lesion"; *away from the side of a unilateral irritative lesion* (away from the seizure focus); *away from the side of a destructive lesion in the brain stem* (at the oculomotor decussation lesions cause gaze to deviate toward the side of the paralysis); or there may be a **vertical deviation** upward with an irritative lesion of the frontal lobes (e.g., "oculogyric crisis" in postencephalitic parkinsonism). Impaired voluntary gaze away from the side of the lesion is seen following disease of one side of the frontal lobes. Impaired smooth eye movements in visual pursuit are seen following diffuse disease of the hemispheres, particularly disorders involving the parietal lobes. *Ocular impersistence* (inability to sustain gaze on one object) is seen following diffuse disease of the hemispheres. Upward gaze or loss of gaze in either direction occurs following bilateral involvement of the corticobulbar tracts at the level of the midbrain. Conjugate gaze reflexes may be impaired with pontine lesions and multiple sclerosis. Dysconjugate eye movements may also be present, producing *diplopia* (double vision). Although not a gaze disturbance, accommodation responses also may be dysconjugate.

Constructional apraxia. Inability to plan and execute the production of graphic designs or three-dimensional structures.

Coprolalia. Bizarre, inappropriate, derogatory, or scatological utterances often described in patients with Gilles de la Tourette syndrome (GTS).

Corneal reflex. A reflex test in which bilateral blinks are elicited by a light touch to the cornea to examine the ophthalmic division of the trigeminal (V) nerve and the facial nerve (VII).

Cortical, or central, blindness. Loss of the ability to see resulting from bilateral lesions in the visual sensory cortex. Unlike other forms of blindness, the pupillary reflexes are preserved.

Cortical deafness. Loss of the ability to hear resulting from bilateral lesions to the auditory sensory cortex.

Cranial nerves (CN). Referring to the nerve bodies that provide motor and sensory innervation to head and neck structures and autonomic innervation of visceral organs.

Craniocele. Herniation of brain tissues.

Craniotomy. Opening into the cranium.

Decerebrate posture, decerebrate rigidity. Referring to the posture of a comatose patient in which the legs are stiff and extended, the arms are extended and internally rotated, the jaw is clenched, and the head is retracted. Decerebrate posture is associated with upper brain stem destructive lesions between the red nucleus and the vestibular nuclei (see Figure 4–6).

Decorticate posture. Referring to the posture of a comatose patient with a deep, hemispheric lesion at or above the level of the upper brain stem. In decorticate posturing the arms are flexed and adducted, the fists are clenched, and the legs are extended (see Figure 4–6).

Déjà vu phenomenon. Neurologic phenomenon sometimes associated with complex partial (psychomotor) seizures in which an individual has the intense feeling that he or she is reliving a past experience.

Delirium. Clouded state of consciousness characterized by difficulty in sustained attention, sensory misperceptions, disordered thinking, disturbances in sleep-wake cycles, and psychomotor unrest.

Delusion. False belief.

Dementia. Usually referring to a loss of multiple cognitive abilities as a result of diffuse damage or dysfunction of the central nervous system.

Dendrite. Tendrils extending from the neuron carrying input to the cell body.

Dermatome. Region innervated by a single segmental nerve.

Dialysis encephalopathy. A form of dementia characterized by personality changes, dysarthria, myoclonus, and seizures; felt to be a multisystem disorder in dialysis patients with end-stage renal disease.

Diffuse. Multifocal or widespread.

Diplegia. Bilateral lower extremity weakness.

Diplopia. Double vision.

Distant vision. Visual acuity tested from a distance of 20 feet.

Doll's eye phenomenon, oculocephalic reflex. Reflexive conjugate eye movements normally cause the eyes to move opposite to the direction of head movement, maintaining their position in relation to the environment. When present this reflex indicates integrity of the third, fourth, and sixth cranial nerves and their interconnections. No movement of the eyes, or an asymmetry of movement, indicates pontine-midbrain level destructive lesions. Barbiturate poisoning can also abolish this reflex.

Dorsiflexion. Upward flexion, or lifting.

Dysarthria. Speech disorder characterized by neuromotor paralysis, paresis, or dyscoordination of movement of the muscle groups that support speech.

Dysdiadochokinesia. Inability to perform rapidly alternating hand and/or articulatory movements.

Dysesthesia. Abnormal, unpleasant sensation in response to a sensory stimulus.

Dyskinesia. A movement disorder characterized by involuntary muscular movements, such as dystonias and tremors.

Dysmetria. Disturbed ability to judge range of motion. Dysmetria is demonstrated if there is "past pointing" when patients attempt to place a finger on an object held in front of them or touch their nose.

Dysphagia. Impaired ability to swallow.

Dysphasia. Term sometimes preferred in place of "aphasia" to denote a partial loss of language ability.

Dysthymia. Emotional or intellectual disorder usually referring to depression. Dysthymia may also imply a condition caused by a dysfunctional thymus gland.

Echoic memory. Short-term auditory memory.

Edinger-Westphal nucleus. Nucleus innervating the ciliary and pupillary sphincters of the eye. This nucleus is part of the parasympathetic innervation to the eye by the third cranial nerve (CN III).

Efferent. Going away from the neuronal cell body.

Empyema. Encapsulated collection of pus in a space (e.g., subdural or epidural in the brain, or pleural space in the lung).

Encephalitis. Inflammation of the brain.

Endorphins. Natural body substances with properties similar to morphine.

Epicritic sense. Ability to perceive fine degrees of touch, pain, or temperature from the skin or mucosa.

Epidural. Above or outside the dura mater covering of the brain.

Episodic memory. Memory processes related to temporal events (e.g., autobiographic information).

Evoked potentials. Electrical activity changes in the nervous system elicited by a sensory stimulus and detected by computerized averaging of responses to repeated sensory stimuli. Evoked potentials can be used to examine the visual, auditory, and somatosensory systems and the peripheral nerves and to conduct "brain mapping" with electroencephalograms (EEGs).

Expressive aphasia. A term sometimes used to denote a type of aphasia (acquired language disorder) characterized by a notable difficulty with verbal expression. Expressive aphasia is generally synonymous with "Broca's aphasia" but may be applied indiscriminately in medical settings whenever verbal output is impaired.

Extension. Movement away from the body.

Extraocular movements. Eye movements elicited in the cranial nerve examination for CNs III, IV, and VI.

Extrapyramidal movement disorder, extrapyramidal cerebral palsy. Movement disorder resulting from disorders of the nervous system not involving the pyramidal corticospinal and corticobulbar pathways. Extrapyramidal disorders include the cerebellar and basal ganglia movement disorders.

Falx cerebri. Fold in the dura mater that separates the cerebral hemispheres in the midsagittal plane. The falx cerebelli is the dura fold separating the cerebellar hemispheres.

Fasciculation. Irregular contractions and relaxations of muscle unit appearing as a twitch or ripple.

Febrile convulsion. Seizure in children associated with a high fever.

Fibrillation. Contraction of single muscle fibers that is detectable by monitoring the electrical activity of the muscle.

Flaccid. Paralysis characterized by a loss of muscle tone.

Flexion. Pulling toward the body.

Focal. Limited to a designated area.

Fundus. Back of the eye.

Glabellar reflex. Reflex elicited by gently tapping the forehead, causing momentary rhythmic eye blinks. This reflex normally extinguishes with repeated (2–3 taps) stimulation. Failure to extinguish this reflex is seen in parkinsonism.

Glia. Supportive tissues of the brain; includes astrocytes, microglia cells, and oligodendrocytes.

Global aphasia. Severe to profound loss of language ability across all modalities (i.e., speaking, listening, reading, gesturing, and writing).

Grand mal seizure. A generalized seizure characterized by loss of consciousness and tonic-clonic movements.

Graphesthesia. The ability to recognize shapes drawn on the palm.

Grasp reflex. One of the "frontal release" signs in which a reflexive grasp is elicited when the palm is stroked.

Hallucination. A perception or a sensation not founded on reality.

Halo brace. A ring and brace superstructure used to immobilize a patient with a high spinal cord injury (see Chapters 13 and 14 for additional discussions of orthopedic and rehabilitation bracing and devices).

Hemianopsia. Blindness for one-half of the visual field (see Figure 4–3).

Hemiparesis. Weakness (partial paralysis) of one side of the body.

Hemiplegia. Paralysis of one side of the body.

Herniation. The abnormal protrusion of an organ or tissue through an opening or space. Brain herniations include uncal herniation through the tentorial notch, cingulate herniation, upward cerebellar herniation through the tentorial notch, and cerebellar tonsil herniation through the foramen magnum.

Hoffman, or Tromner, sign. Indicates hyperreflexia of the upper extremities, with thumb flexion elicited by a brisk tapping of the distal digits (middle or index finger) of the hand.

Horner's syndrome. Neurologic syndrome characterized by unilateral ptosis (drooping of the eyelid), narrowing of the pupil, and diminished vasodilation and sweating present on the same side of the head as the brain lesion.

Hydrocephalus. An abnormal accumulation of fluid in the cranial vault (see "Disturbances in Cerebrospinal Fluid Circulation" in Chapter 10).

Hyperesthesia. A heightened sensitivity to sensory stimulation.

Hypnagogic. State of rest coming just before sleep.

Hypotonia. An absence of muscle tone; floppy.

Iconic memory. Visual memory.

Illusion. False interpretation of sensory perception.

Insight. Ability to observe and evaluate oneself and to appreciate the relationship between events.

Intention tremor. Coarse, rhythmic movements elicited by intentional hand movements (e.g., when reaching for objects).

Intractable pain. Constant, unrelenting pain.

Jaw jerk. A stretch reflex elicited by tapping the medial portion of the mandible.

Lambert-Eaton myasthenia syndrome (LEMS). An autoimmune disorder sometimes found in association with small-cell lung cancer; manifested by proximal leg or arm weakness and autonomic changes (e.g., dry mouth, impotence).

Lennox-Gastaut seizures. Variant of petit mal seizure having other associated seizure patterns (see "Seizure Disorders" in Chapter 10 for more in-depth descriptions of this and other types of seizures).

Leptomeninges. The pia mater and arachnoid.

Lethargic. Awake but drowsy, inactive, and indifferent to external stimulation.

Lissencephaly. Unconvoluted cerebral hemispheres associated with severe forms of retardation.

Logomania, logorrhea. Excessive, repetitious verbal output.

Long-term memory. Secondary memory; memory processes allowing for a large capacity of long-term storage of information (acquired knowledge).

Lordosis. Anterior curve of the spinal column.

Lower motor neuron (LMN) lesion. Lesions involving the motor neurons of the bulbar (cranial) and spinal nerves and their peripheral roots. The LMNs refer to the final common output pathway of the central nervous system consisting of the anterior horn cells and their axons, which form the peripheral nerves that innervate the muscles. LMN lesions are characterized acutely and chronically by *paralysis, hypotonia,* and *areflexia* in the distribution of the involved peripheral nerve(s) or nerve root(s). Chronic states are characterized by *fasciculations* and *atrophy* of the muscles innervated by that nerve.

Medulla oblongata. Bulblike lower portion of the brain stem; an enlarged extension of the spinal cord where it enters the foramen magnum of the occipital bone.

Meninges. The three membranes covering the brain: the dura mater, pia mater, and arachnoid.

Meningitis. Inflammation of the membranes covering the brain.

Miosis. Constriction of the pupil resulting from decreased or increased parasympathomimetic tone.

Misoplegia. Condition sometimes observed in patients with right hemisphere cerebral damage in which the patient expresses anger or hatred toward an affected limb.

Moribund. Near death.

Myelitis. Inflammation of the spinal cord.

Myokymia. Persistent irregular twitching of muscles, producing a "bag of worms" appearance.

Myotonia. Involuntary, painless delay in muscle relaxation after contraction.

Nasolabial fold. Crease running from the sides of the nose to the corners of the mouth. A "flattening" of the nasolabial fold noted during the neurologic examination may be an indication of weakness of that side of the face.

Near vision. Visual acuity tested at approximately 14 inches from the eye.

Neglect. A lack of awareness of or response to the environment or self on the side opposite a parietal lobe lesion.

Neonatal seizures. Seizures in the newborn usually caused by a metabolic abnormality or infection.

Neural tube defects/disease. The neural tube refers to the embryologic structure formed at approximately 23 days of gestation that closes to form the vestigial spinal cord and brain. Neural tube disorders arise from defects in this stage of human development (e.g., spina bifida).

Neuralgia. Pain in a particular nerve or its distribution.

Neurectomy. Surgical excision of a nerve.

Neuritis. Inflammation of a nerve.

Neuroleptic. Drugs that produce favorable tranquilizing and antipsychotic effects.

Neuron. The fundamental unit of the nervous system consisting usually of *dendrites* that receive messages, the *soma* (cell body), and the *axon* for transmitting messages.

Neurosis. A somewhat controversial term referring to a group of psychiatric disorders (e.g., certain forms of compulsions, phobias, anxiety, obsessions) in which mental or emotional dysfunction is present but *reality testing is intact.* Patients with *neuroses* do not have the delusions or hallucinations characteristic of most forms of *psychoses* (see Chapter 10).

Neurotransmitter. Neurochemical substance, such as norepinephrine, dopamine, acetylcholine, that is released when the axon terminal of a presynaptic neuron is excited.

Nominal aphasia. Term sometimes used to denote a type of aphasia (acquired language disorder) characterized by a primary difficulty with naming. The term "anomic aphasia" or "semantic aphasia" may also be applied. Patients with early- to middle-stage dementia are sometimes said to have "nominal aphasia," reflecting disintegrating lexicosemantic abilities.

Nuchal rigidity. Stiff neck; note, the "ch" in nuchal is pronounced like "k" as /nukɔ/.

Nystagmus. Abnormal, involuntary movement of the eyes reflecting an imbalance in the complex neuronal network involving the visual pathways, the labyrinthine proprioceptive influences from neck muscles, the vestibular and cerebellar nuclei, the reticular formation of the pontine brain stem, and the oculomotor nuclei.

Obtunded, obtunderate. Dull, indifferent, with responsiveness limited to little more than fleeting wakefulness.

Occupational, or pendular, nystagmus. A type of pendular nystagmus (slow, coarse movements in both directions) resulting from prolonged work in poorly lit surroundings (e.g., mines) in which rods are required for vision. Because there are no rods in the macula, the nystagmus is a temporary condition caused by the eyes' attempts to compensate for poor light.

Ocular bobbing. Brisk, downward bilateral, conjugate eye movements followed by a slow return to a normal position, which is indicative of cerebellar hemorrhages or caudal pontine lesions.

Ocular flutter. Rapid, rhythmic eye movements of decreasing amplitude on fixation.

Oculoplethysmography. Auscultation of intracranial arteries by placing the diaphragm of the stethoscope on the eyelid.

Opsoclonus. Random, clonic, conjugate eye movements usually felt to represent cerebellar lesions.

Optic chiasm. The location where optic nerve fibers for the temporal visual field cross to the opposite side (illustrated in Figure 4–3).

Optic radiation. The white matter tract looping laterally and posteriorly from the lateral geniculate body to the sensory nuclei in the calcarine fissure of the occipital lobe. The temporal section of the optic radiation is called the loop of Meyer.

Optic tract. The white matter tract from the optic chiasm to the lateral geniculate body of the thalamus.

Optokinetic nystagmus. A normal visual response to the landscape or objects moving rapidly in a horizontal plane in front of the eyes. This response may be lacking in patients having parietal lobe lesions.

Palilalia. Compulsive verbal repetitions.

Papilledema. Swelling of the optic disk, causing congestive changes in the optic nerve seen on fundoscopic examination.

Paralysis agitans. Parkinson's disease.

Paresthesia. Heightened response to sensory stimulation (e.g., touch, temperature, pain, etc.); or a "pins and needles" sensation.

Partial seizures. A seizure involving an abnormal electrical discharge in a focal brain area. This type of seizure may spread to become a *generalized seizure* (secondary generalization). Partial seizures may be *simple*, in which there is no impairment of consciousness, or *complex* (complex partial seizure), in which there is impaired consciousness. *Complex partial seizures* (or partial complex seizures) often arise in the temporal lobes.

Pattern-shift visual evoked response (PSVER). An evoked potential study widely adopted to examine for lesions in the visual system. It usually examines for any discrepancies between the left and right eyes, as might be found in patients with multiple sclerosis or retrobulbar neuritis.

Perception. Psychological awareness of a stimulus. Perception can occur without recognition and may be subliminal.

Percussion hammer. Small, rubber-tipped hammer used to elicit stretch reflexes during the neurologic examination.

Peripheral. In neurology, pertaining to the peripheral nervous system, as compared to the central nervous system (brain and spinal cord).

Persistent vegetative state. A state in which a person, although awake, shows no interaction with the environment. Such patients usually have suffered severe brain damage and are unable to speak or track objects visually and need to have all bodily functions cared for by others.

Petit mal seizure. A generalized seizure characterized by a momentary loss of consciousness; "absence spells."

Phantom limb pain. Pain felt after a body part has been amputated in which there is a sensation that pain is coming from the missing part.

Phobia. A persistent, irrational fear.

Photic stimulation, photic driving. The use of powerful stroboscopic light for evoked potential stimulation during EEGs.

Pons. Prominence on the ventral surface of the brain stem between the cerebral peduncles and the medulla. The pons, or "bridge," contains connections to and from the cerebrum and is the origin of the CN V (trigeminal), CN VI (abducens), CN VII (facial), and CN VIII (vestibulocochlear) nuclei.

Pontine. Pertaining to the pons.

Postconcussion syndrome. Referring to a wide variety of symptoms following mild head injury, such as headache, complaints of impaired memory, difficulty sustaining concentration, dizziness, depression, apathy, and anxiety.

Post-traumatic amnesia (PTA). Referring to the time period following brain trauma during which the patient lacks continuous memory of the events of daily life.

Post-traumatic stress disorder (PTSD). An emotional disorder resulting from a single or repeated frightening and life-threatening traumatic experience(s). PTSD sufferers may reexperience the traumatic event or events in some way; tend to avoid places, people, or other things that remind them of the event(s) (display avoidance); and are highly sensitive to normal life experiences (display hyperarousal). Patients may be diagnosed with **complex post-traumatic stress disorder (C-PTSD)** following repeated exposure to life-threatening events.

Primitive reflexes. One of the chief signs of *static encephalopathy* (cerebral palsy) is the persistence of primitive reflexes beyond 6 to 12 months of age, beyond the time when these reflexes normally disappear. Primitive reflexes may reappear in children or adults who have had head injuries or in association with *acute encephalopathies* or degenerative diseases of the central nervous system. Primitive reflexes include the **asymmetrical tonic neck reflex (ATNR)**; the **tonic labyrinthine reflex (TLR)**; the **positive support reflex**; and the **grasp**, **bite**, **snout/rooting**, and **sucking reflexes**. In the developing child, primitive reflexes normally diminish with a corresponding emergence of automatic movement reactions, such as the anterior protective response and lateral protective response.

Pronation. Medial rotation of the forearm (palm backward) or foot (sole backward).

Prosopagnosia. Impaired ability to recognize familiar faces.

Psyche. Mind.

Psychogenic. Not related to a physical cause.

Psychomotor agitation. Motor unrest.

Psychomotor retardation. Lack of movement and/or motor initiation without paresis.

Psychosis. Pertaining to major psychiatric disorders that may require psychiatric hospitalization treatment and pharmacologic therapies. Patients with psychoses will have impaired reality testing. Delusions and hallucinations are features of the majority of psychoses (see Chapter 10).

Ptosis. Weakness of the eyelid(s).

Pure word deafness, verbal agnosia. A type of agnosia in which there is a recognition impairment strictly limited to spoken words without an impairment in the ability to hear sounds or to recognize other sounds.

Quadriplegia, quadriparesis. Paralysis or paresis, respectively, of all four extremities.

Rachischisis. Disorders produced by a lack of fusion of the dorsal midline structures of the neural tube (e.g., spina bifida).

Receptive aphasia. Term sometimes used to describe an acquired language disorder in which there is a notable impairment of auditory comprehension; generally synonymous with "sensory aphasia" or "Wernicke's aphasia."

Resting tremor. Tremor present in a resting position. The "pill-rolling" tremor of the fingers characteristic of parkinsonism is a common example.

Retina. The location of receptors of visual stimuli in the back of the eye.

Retraction-conversion nystagmus. A nystagmus characterized by the eye adducting and jerking up into the orbit, associated with pretectal and tectal lesions of the midbrain.

Retrobulbar neuritis. Inflammation of the optic nerve.

Rigidity. Increased muscle tone that is present throughout the range of movement of a muscle.

Rinne test. Tuning fork test used by a neurologist or other examiner to compare air conduction (AC) versus bone conduction (BC) of sound. The vibrating tuning fork is first placed over the mastoid until the sound is no longer heard by the patient and then held near the external auditory meatus until the patient reports that he or she can no longer hear the sound. Because sound conducted by air is normally heard longer than sound conducted by bone, AC is usually longer than BC (AC>BC), unless there is conductive disease (BC>AC).

Romberg's sign. Clinical sign indicating a balance impairment due to a proprioceptive loss. A positive Romberg's sign is found when the patient, standing with feet together, has a loss of balance after closing his or her eyes.

Rotary nystagmus. Nystagmus characterized by circular eye movements.

Rotation. Turning or circular motion.

Rumination. The tendency to dwell on negative thoughts, events, and symptoms, such as fatigue and lack in initiative.

Scoliosis. Abnormal curvature of the spine.

Scotomata. Blind spots in the visual field. Sparks or shimmering spots in the visual field are called *scintillating scotomata.*

Seizure. Abnormal discharge of electrical activity in the central nervous system.

Semantic memory. Memory process not tied to temporal or spatial factors or sequences in which a schema of information containing related concepts, propositions, and sensations are stored and retrieved.

Sensory ataxia. A condition characteristic of patients with proprioceptive deficits.

Short-latency somatosensory evoked potentials (SSEP). A computerized evoked potential examination used in neurophysiology laboratories to confirm lesions in the somatosensory system, including the peripheral nerves, posterior column of the spinal cord, brain stem, and cortex. This test is useful in the evaluation of conditions such as cervical spondylosis, Guillain-Barré syndrome, or multiple sclerosis.

Short-term memory. Primary memory; a stage of memory processing in which a relatively small amount of information can be briefly retained (e.g., remembering a phone number you have just heard long enough to place a call).

Simultagnosia. Inability to perceive more than one stimulus at a time in a given modality.

Snout/rooting reflex. A normal response in infants, but in adults this reflex indicates bifrontal or diffuse cortical atrophy. The reflexive protrusion of the lips is elicited by tapping or touching the lips or corners of the mouth.

Soma. Body.

Somatic. Pertaining to the body.

Somatophrenia. Condition sometimes observed in patients with right hemisphere cerebral damage in which the patient denies ownership of a paretic limb, or attributes ownership of the limb to another person.

Somnolent. Sleepy, difficult to arouse from sleep, or demonstrating difficulty in sustaining alertness.

Spasmus nutans. A benign condition of childhood that usually appears in infancy and lasts for months to a few years, characterized by bilateral or monocular horizontal or vertical nystagmus, with rhythmic head nodding.

Spastic. A velocity-dependent increase in muscle tone, with exaggerated tendon reflex jerks, following upper motor neuron and pyramidal tract lesions.

Static encephalopathy. Another term for cerebral palsy (see Chapter 10).

Strabismus. Improper alignment of the visual axes.

Stupor. State of responsiveness in which the patient can only be aroused by vigorous and persistent external stimulation.

Subdural. Beneath the dura mater.

Supination. Lateral rotation of the forearm (palm forward) or foot.

Support reflex. Reflex elicited when an infant extends the legs to support weight when the feet are bounced against a surface.

Supratentorial. Above the sheath of the dura mater (tentorium cerebelli) that extends between the cerebellum and cerebrum. The term *supratentorial* is also sometimes used facetiously, as with the comment that the patient's complaint is "supratentorial," or "all in the head," not real.

Synapse. The junction between two neurons. Neurons communicate by passing chemicals (neurotransmitters) between each other. These chemicals may be *excitatory*, causing the receiving neuron to have an electrical discharge (impulse); *inhibitory*, preventing the receiving neuron from having an electrical discharge; or *neuromodulatory*, altering the response of the receiving neuron.

Syncope. Fainting; abrupt loss of conscientiousness usually from hemodynamic or neurologic causes.

Synkinesia. Involuntary muscle contractions associated with movement.

Tentorium. The fold of the dura mater that forms a partition *between the cerebrum and the cerebellum*. The **falx cerebri** is the dura fold in the *midsagittal separation* of the two cerebral hemispheres.

Tic. A movement disorder characterized by a repetitive, involuntary, or compulsive movement. Complex compulsive movements are called *habit tics*.

Tonic labyrinthine reflex (TLR). In infants, the arms and legs are pulled in toward the body when the head is flexed, and they extend when the head is held back and up.

Transcortical motor aphasia. A type of aphasia (acquired language disorder) characterized by mild or moderate dysfluency of speech that is improved during repetition tasks, well-preserved repetition, and relatively good auditory comprehension.

Transcortical sensory aphasia. A type of aphasia (acquired language disorder) characterized by fluently articulated, paraphasic speech, with much better auditory comprehension and relatively better repetition than typically found with Wernicke's aphasia.

Tremor. Rhythmic, alternating, oscillatory movements produced by repetitive patterns of muscle contraction and relaxation.

Trephination. Cutting a circular hole ("burr hole") in the skull; craniotomy.

Upper motor neuron (UMN) lesion. Lesions involving the motor cortex and/or corticobulbar or corticospinal tracts; lesions above the level of a lower motor nucleus. *Acute* motor consequences of upper motor neuron lesions can include *paralysis or paresis*, *hypotonia*, *hyporeflexia*, and the *Babinski's sign*. Postacutely motor responses are *hyperreflexia* and *hypertonicity* (evidence of spasticity) contralateral to the side of the lesion if the lesion is *above the decussation* of the corticospinal (pyramidal) tract.

Vertigo. A sensation of movement that is often, but not always, a sensation of rotating or spinning.

Vestibular nystagmus. Nystagmus, usually rotary nystagmus, resulting from diseases in the semicircular canals and their central connections.

Vestibulocephalic reflex. See *Doll's eye phenomenon, oculocephalic reflex.*

Visceral. Pertaining to the large internal organs of the three truncal cavities of the body.

Visual allesthesia. Phenomenon in which patients with hemi-inattention replace an image from the nonattended visual field to the attended visual field.

Wasting. Loss of muscle mass.

Weber test. Tuning fork test used by a neurologist or other examiner to test for a differential impairment in air conduction versus bone conduction of sound. With this test, the tuning fork stem, when placed on the midline of the forehead, will be heard louder on the side with conductive disease. When disease of the cochlea is present, the sound vibration will be reported to lateralize to the better, or nondiseased, ear.

Wernicke's aphasia. A form of aphasia (acquired language disorder) characterized by relatively poor auditory comprehension and fluently articulated verbal expression marked by paraphasic distortions ranging from occasional phonologic errors to jargon.

B. Abbreviations

ABI. Acquired brain injury

ACA. Anterior cerebral artery

ACDF. Adult children of dysfunctional families; anterior cervical (spine) diskectomy and fusion

ACh. Acetylcholine

AC<BC;AC>BC. Air conduction less than bone conduction; air conduction greater than bone conduction

AD. Alzheimer's disease

ADD-H. Attention-deficit disorder with hyperactivity

AKM. Akinetic mutism

ALS. Amyotrophic lateral sclerosis

AOS. Anterior operculum syndrome; apraxia of speech

ANS. Autonomic nervous system

BAD. Bipolar affective disorder

BAER (p). Brain stem auditory evoked response (potential)

C1, C2, etc. Cervical spine (vertebrae) number

CBS. Chronic brain syndrome

CJD. Creutzfeldt-Jakob disease

CN. Cranial nerve

CNS. Central nervous system

CPA. Cerebellar pontine angle

CPS. Complex partial seizure

CSF. Cerebrospinal fluid

CT, CAT, C CT. Computerized tomography, computerized axial tomography, contrast CT

CVA. Cerebrovascular accident

DAT. Dementia of the Alzheimer's type

DCS. Dorsal cord stimulation

DLB. Dementia with Lewy bodies

DSM-IV. *Diagnostic and Statistical Manual of Mental Disorders—Fourth Edition* (American Psychiatric Association, 1994); DSM-V is under development.

DTRs. Deep tendon reflexes

EEG. Electroencephalography

EMG. Electromyography

ENG. Electronystagmography

EOM. Extraocular movements

EST, ECT. Electroshock therapy, electroconvulsion therapy

F → N. Finger to nose

FOI. Flight of ideas

GII. General intellectual impairment

H → S. Heel to shin

HDS. Herniated disk syndrome

HNP. Herniated nucleus pulposus

ICP. Intracranial pressure

IMI. Isolated memory impairment

L1, L2, etc. Lumbar spine (vertebrae) number

LOA. "Looseness" of associations

LOC. Loss of consciousness

LP. Lumbar puncture

MAE. Moves all extremities; **MAEW,** moves all extremities well

MANSCAN. Mental activity network scanner (method of computerized EEG analysis)

MCA. Middle cerebral artery

MCI. Mild cognitive impairment

MG. Myasthenia gravis

MRA. Magnetic resonance angiogram

MRI. Magnetic resonance imaging; **fMRI** refers to "functional" MRI, in which the individual is engaged in some sort of mental task during the imaging study to determine which areas of the brain are activated by the task.

MRV. Magnetic resonance venogram

MS. Multiple sclerosis

MSA. Multiple system atrophy

MSLT. Multiple sleep latency test

ncCT. Noncontrast CT

NCV. Nerve conduction velocity

NDT. Neurodevelopmental therapy

NPH. Normal pressure hydrocephalus

O. Oriented, orientation

OPCD. Olivopontocerebellar degeneration

PCA. Posterior cerebral artery

PCS. Postconcussion syndrome

PD. Parkinson's disease

PDD. Primary degenerative dementia

PERLA. Pupils are equal and (equally) reactive to light and accommodation

PET. Positron emission tomography

PICA. Posterior inferior cerebellar artery

PNS. Peripheral nervous system

PSP. Progressive supranuclear palsy

P Sz. Paranoid schizophrenia

PTA. Post-traumatic amnesia

PTSD. Post-traumatic stress disorder; **C-PTSD** refers to "complex" PTSD

S1, S2, etc. Sacral spine (vertebrae) number

SCA. Spinocerebellar ataxia

SDAT. Senile dementia—Alzheimer's type

SIADH. Syndrome of inadequate antidiuretic hormone

SPECT. Single photon emission tomography

SzDis. Seizure disorder

T1,T2, etc. Thoracic spine (vertebrae) number

TBI. Traumatic brain injury; **mTBI** refers to "mild" TBI

TC. Tonic-clonic

TENS. Transcutaneous electrical nerve stimulator

V_1–V_3. Trigeminal (fifth) nerve and branches

VA shunt. Ventriculoatrial shunt; **VP shunt,** ventriculoperitoneal shunt

V-B A. Vertebrobasilar artery

V-B D. Vertebrobasilar disease

VBI. Vertebrobasilar insufficiency; vertebrobasilar ischemia

VER (p). Visual evoked response (potential)

III. MENTAL STATUS EXAMINATION

The neurologic examination usually begins with at least a brief mental status assessment, followed by examination of the cranial nerves, the motor system, coordination, reflexes, the sensory system, and gait and stability. While conducting the neurologic interview, subjective indicators of cognitive, emotional, mood, or psychiatric disturbances are noted. Psychiatric disturbances are identified from relatively subjective behavioral observations, whereas cognitive functions are more objectively examined with a series of tasks that compose a mental status screening. Patients with notable problems with cognition or with psychiatric disorders are referred for further evaluation (e.g., consultation with psychiatry or neuropsychology).

A. Subjective Psychiatric Observations

Part of the mental status examination includes observations of the patient's appearance and behaviors during the interview. When making subjective remarks about the patient's mood, affect, thinking processes, or content of thoughts in notes or reports, it is best to be as descriptive as possible and to **include verbatim examples of the patient's statements**. For example, it is better to report, "Pt. said, 'I don't know what the point of all of this is, I'm no good to anyone,'" than to say, "Patient seemed depressed." The following areas are typically noted.

- **Appearance.** Description of the patient's general habitus (e.g., grooming, hygiene, clothes, jewelry, etc.); use of gestures; any odd mannerisms, posture, or body language.
- **Motor activity.** The patient's rate and extent of initiation of movement, any excessive activity or notable inactivity, pacing, agitation, repetitive movements, or tremors.
- **Speech.** The rate of speech, any evidence of a flight of ideas, lack of coherence, any inappropriate content, and the characteristics of articulation and language.
- **Thought content.** Indicators of delusions, paranoia, hallucinations, low self-esteem, denial, worry, hypochondriasis, suspiciousness, panic, or irritability. Thought *content* refers to the ideas and preoccupations evident in the patient's language content.
- **Thought processes.** Any indicators of distractibility, evasiveness, displays of lapses or blocks, delayed or slow mental processing, impulsivity, or uncooperativeness. Thought *processes* refer to the progression of the patient's thinking patterns.
- **Insight.** Any indicators of the patient's lack of appreciation of his or her condition or situation. Insight refers to the patient's ability to interpret his or her condition or situation in a manner consistent with the perceptions of others.
- **Judgment.** Any indicators of an inability to form appropriate responses to everyday social situations. Judgment refers to the ability to *understand consequences* and to *form appropriate responses* to everyday situations.
- **Mood.** Any indicators of anger, sadness, euphoria, apathy, fear, or depression. Mood refers to the prevailing, general emotional state of the patient.
- **Affect.** Any notable affective displays, such as tearfulness, smiling, frowning, emotional lability, giddiness, or angry outbursts. Affect refers to the *fluctuating physical displays of emotions in facial expression, body movements,* and *voice.* Affect usually reflects a person's

mood, but mood and affect can also be out of synchrony, as in parkinsonism, where a flat, "masked" affect may fail to reveal the patient's underlying emotion.

B. Bedside Assessment of Mental Status and Higher Cortical Functions in Adults

The standard bedside mental status interview includes screening tasks for the following:

- **Language functions**. Assessing naming, repeating, reading, writing, and comprehension of verbal directions.
- **Orientation.** Determining if the patient knows his or her name, the place and location where he or she is currently, and the season and date.
- **Memory.** Asking the patient to recall digit strings or repeat sentences for *immediate memory;* recalling three unrelated words after 5 minutes for *short-term memory*; and asking if the patient can recall the names of the current and previous presidents or what he or she had for dinner the night before to assess *long-term* or *remote memory.*
- **Attention and calculation.** Asking the patient to subtract by 7s from 100.
- **Construction.** Copying designs, drawing a clock or daisy, copying a sentence.
- **Abstract reasoning.** Proverb interpretation.

The nature and extent of this screening mental status assessment should not be construed to be a "neuropsychological battery." Neuropsychologists use an array of standardized tests to elucidate perceptual, recognition, executive functions, memory, and language impairments associated with brain dysfunction.

Some of the published, brief tests of mental status are described in the next section. These instruments vary in the extent to which their reliability and validity have been determined. Because they are screening tests, they may not be sensitive enough to identify subtle problems (*false negatives*) or they may identify disorders that are not present (*false positives*). Also, because mental status screening tests require language facility to perform nearly all of the tasks, patients with mild or subtle aphasia could be inappropriately diagnosed to have a cognitive impairment (a false-positive finding).

C. Standardized Cognitive Screening Examinations

There are a number of published instruments for conducting standardized cognitive screening (Strub & Black, 1993). The following describes some of the more commonly used screening instruments in health care settings and the performance domains they assess.

1. *Mini-Mental State Examination (MMSE)* (Folstein, Folstein, & McHugh, 1975)

The MMSE is a brief examination that has been in use in psychiatry, neurology, and medicine for decades. The test includes items related to orientation; registration (short-term memory); attention; calculation; language (naming, repeating, reading, writing); and drawing. This test requires approximately 15 to 20 minutes to administer. It is

TABLE 4–1 Mini Mental State Examination sample items

Orientation to time

"What is the date?"

Registration

"Listen carefully. I'm going to say three words. You say them back after I stop. Ready? Here they are:

APPLE (pause), PENNY (pause), TABLE (pause). Now repeat those words back to me." [Repeat up to 5 times, but score only the first trial.]

Naming

"What is this?" [Point to a pencil or pen.]

Reading

"Please read this and do what it says." [Show examinee the words on the stimulus form.]

CLOSE YOUR EYES

probably the most frequently administered "standardized" mental status examination by physicians and nurses. The MMSE is used to screen for patients requiring further testing or as a means for longitudinal probes when progressive, dementing illness is suspected (Table 4–1).

2. *Short Portable Mental Status Questionnaire (SPMSQ)* (Pfeiffer, 1975)

This assessment is popular in bedside assessment because it is brief and simple to administer. The patient is asked:

What is the date today?

What day of the week is it?

What is the name of this place?

What is your telephone number?

How old are you?

When were you born?

Who is the president of the United States?

Who was the president just before him?

What was your mother's maiden name?

Subtract 3 from 20 and keep subtracting 3 from each new number, all the way down. Scoring: The total number of errors is interpreted to indicate the degree of cognitive impairment; extra points are allowed for decreased education and other potentially biasing factors.

3. *The Neurobehavioral Cognitive Status Examination (NCSE)* (Schwamm, Van Dyke, & Kiernan, 1987)

The screening items from this mental status examination can be administered in a brief time, but if the "metric" items (additional items of graded difficulty in each subtest) are administered, testing time is about 30 minutes. This test is seldom used in routine mental status screening because it requires pictures and other materials, (e.g., block design blocks) in its administration. However, this test enjoys some popularity in medical research as a quick cognitive assessment with populations having, or at risk for, central nervous system damage.

4. *Cognitive Capacity Screening Examination (CCSE)* (Jacobs, Bernard, & Delgado, 1977)

This cognitive screening instrument contains 30 items and requires about 10 to 20 minutes to complete. It can be administered by any health care professional. The CCSE tests orientation, concentration, attention, mental control, language (including concept formation), and short-term memory.

5. *Galveston Orientation and Amnesia Test (GOAT)* (Levin, O'Donnell, & Grossman, 1979)

This evaluation protocol is used mainly with patients who have had traumatic brain injuries. It evaluates orientation (time, place, and person) and memory functions.

D. Neurologic Interview

The neurologic examination attempts to answer the following questions: Where is the lesion? What diagnoses should be considered? What tests need to be ordered? What are the priorities and best avenues for management? The examination requires assessing both voluntary and involuntary neurologic signs from "head to toe." It begins with a neurologic history and *review of neurologic systems.* The patient will be asked to describe his or her concerns and experiences; if there is any decreased ability to perform everyday tasks; or if there are any associated headache, vision, hearing, tinnitus, vertigo, movement, numbness, bowel and bladder control, memory, and speech and language problems. This interview usually precedes the mental status examination and the rest of the neurologic physical examination.

E. Neurologic Physical Examination

1. *Domains*

The neurologic physical examination is organized by systems, generally in the following manner:

- Mental status
- Cranial nerves examination
- Motor and muscle strength assessment
- Coordination examination
- Station and gait examination
- Sensation assessment
- Reflex testing

2. *Cranial Nerves*

Table 4–2 lists the cranial nerves, their functions, and disorders associated with damage to particular cranial nerves. Figure 4–1 illustrates the anatomical location of cranial nerves. Figure 4–2 illustrates the tools that the neurologist uses during the cranial nerve examination and for sensory and motor testing of the extremities. Following is the list of cranial nerves:

- **CN I (Olfactory).** To test the olfactory nerve, the neurologist may present substances with odors (not noxious), such as coffee, lemon oil, and cloves, for the patient to smell.
- **CN II (Optic).** Visual acuity is examined with a Snellen chart or equivalent (Rosenbaum card). In addition, an ophthalmoscopic examination of the eyes is done to examine the fundus. Vision testing can locate sites of lesion along the visual pathway from the retina to the visual cortex (Figure 4–3). Visual field testing may be done grossly by asking the patient if he or she can see fingers wiggling in the upper, middle, and lower thirds of his or her left and right visual fields; or a precise mapping of the patient's area of vision can be made by an ophthalmologist using visual stimuli adjustments on a projection screen (Goldman fields). Neurologists may use a "Maddox rod," which is an instrument used to detect subtle evidence of double vision, in vision testing.
- **CN III (Oculomotor), IV (Trochlear), VI (Abducens).** Pupillary responses are mediated by CN II (afferent arc) and CN III (efferent arc). The neurologist stimulates pupillary responses (to test size, shape, and equality) with light and accommodation to objects near the eye. If pupils respond equally to contralateral light and accommodation stimulation, this finding is recorded as PERLA (pupils are equal and responsive to light and accommodation) or, equivalently, PERRLA and PEERLA. When pupils are dilated (widely open), as one sometimes sees in association with drug effects, the condition is referred to as **mydriasis**.

TABLE 4–2 Cranial nerves and their functions, and problems associated with their dysfunction

CRANIAL	NERVE	FUNCTION	DISORDERS ASSOCIATED WITH LESIONS
I	Olfactory	Smell	Anosmia
II	Optic	Vision	Vision loss
III	Oculomotor	Eye movements, pupillary constriction, and accommodation,	Ptosis, diplopia, loss of mydriasis accommodation
IV	Trochlear	Eye movement	Diplopia
V	Trigeminal	Facial sensation, mastication, and proprioception	Facial numbness and weakness
VI	Abducens	Eye movement	Diplopia
VII	Facial	Facial expression; taste; sensation of tonsils, soft palate, external and middle ear; salivation	Upper and lower facial weakness, loss of taste for anterior two-thirds of tongue, dry mouth, dysarthria
VIII	Vestibulocochlear	Equilibrium and hearing	Vertigo, nystagmus, disequilibrium, deafness
IX	Glossopharyngeal	Pharyngeal elevation; taste; sensation base of the tongue, epiglottis, uvula, pharynx, of auditory tube; parotid secretion	Dysphagia; dysarthria; loss of taste, posterior one of the third of tongue; anesthesia pharynx; dry mouth
X	Vagus	Taste; sensation of epiglottis,larynx, trachea, stomach, small intestine, transverse colon; muscles of deglutition and phonation; cardiac suppression; visceral movement and secretions	Dysphagia, hoarseness, palatal weakness, cardiac dysfunction, dysfunctions of the viscera
XI	Spinal Accessory	Phonation, head and shoulder movement	Hoarseness, weakness of head and shoulder muscles
XII	Hypoglossal	Tongue movements	Dysarthria, weakness or wasting of tongue muscles

Source: Adapted from Gilroy, J. (1990). *Basic neurology.* New York: Pergamon.

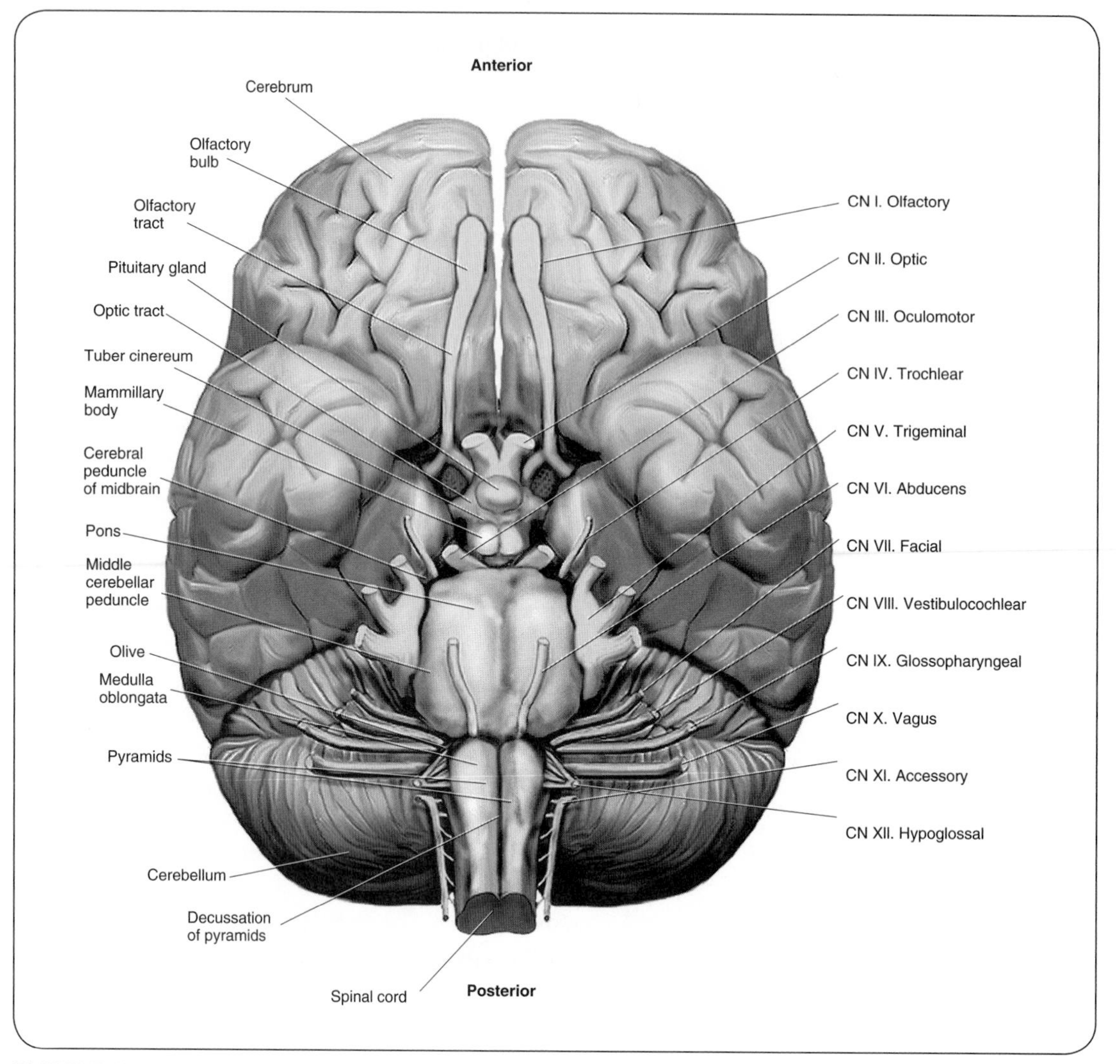

FIGURE 4–1 Location of cranial nerves. Source: Delmar/Cengage Learning

Figure 4–4 illustrates pupillary reactions in association with different lesions and disorders. This area of cranial nerve testing also examines volitional and pursuit eye movements or extraocular movements (EOMs). Cranial nerve III elevates the upper eyelid, and CN VII (facial nerve) closes the eyelid. CN IV provides some downward and outward movement, and CN VI provides lateral movement.

- **CN V (Trigeminal).** CN V is tested by assessing facial sensation, eliciting a corneal reflex (eye blink with light touch or air puff), checking for opening and closing the jaw against resistance; and examining for the jaw jerk reflex. (Afferent aspects are a part of CN V, and efferent aspects are a part of CN VII.)

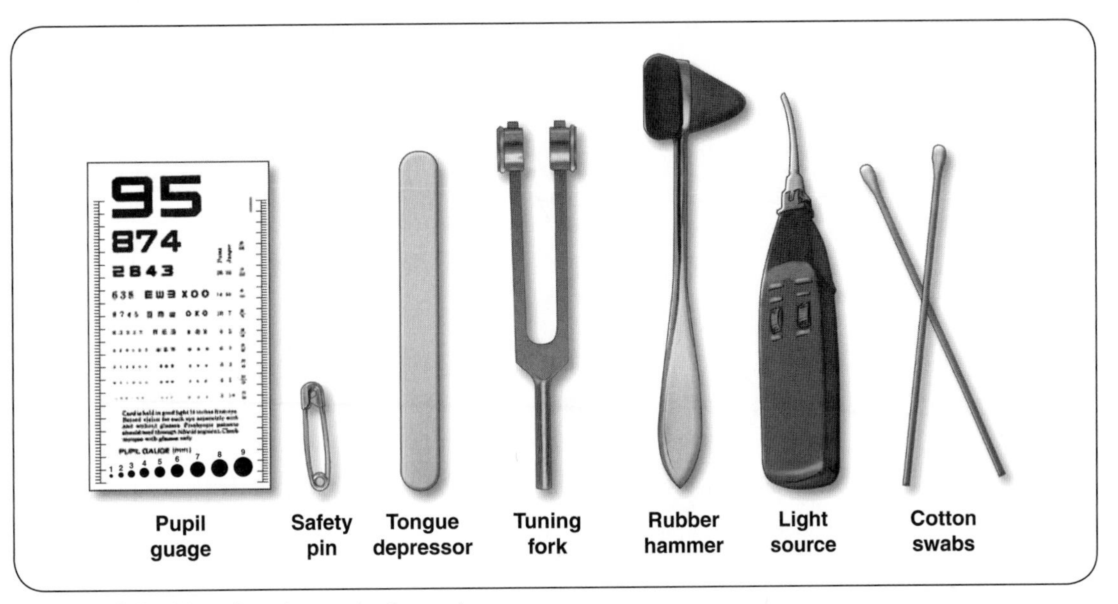

FIGURE 4–2 Neurologist's examination tools. Source: Delmar/Cengage Learning

- **CN VII (Facial).** To test CN VII, the neurologist will see if the patient can do such things as close the eyes, wrinkle the brow, show the teeth, smile, or whistle. A lower quadrant, facial weakness occurs with a contralateral upper motor neuron disease, and an upper and lower facial weakness will be found ipsilateral to disease involving the lower motor neuron. Figure 4–5 illustrates the innervation for the head and neck muscles.
- **CN VIII (Vestibulocochlear).** To test CN VIII, the neurologist will have the patient listen to a watch tick, conduct tuning fork tests, or request an audiologic evaluation. Vestibular testing might include a Barany test, caloric test, or posturography.
- **CN IX (Glossopharyngeal), X (Vagus).** These functionally integrated cranial nerves are tested mainly by listening to the patient speak. The neurologist will ask the patient to phonate and will examine the symmetry of palatal elevation with "ah," elicit a gag reflex, and ask the patient to swallow.
- **CN XI (Spinal Accessory).** To test CN XI, the patient will be asked to shrug the shoulders and push his or her head toward the left and right against resistance.
- **CN XII (Hypoglossal).** To test CN XII, the patient is asked to stick the tongue in and out of the mouth and to push against a tongue depressor to the left and right.

3. *Motor, Sensory, and Reflex Examination*

Motor testing. Motor testing may begin with an inspection of the patient's posture and movement in bed. If the patient is nonresponsive, the arm and leg posturing can help to determine the severity of neurologic damage. Decorticate or decerebrate posturing will be

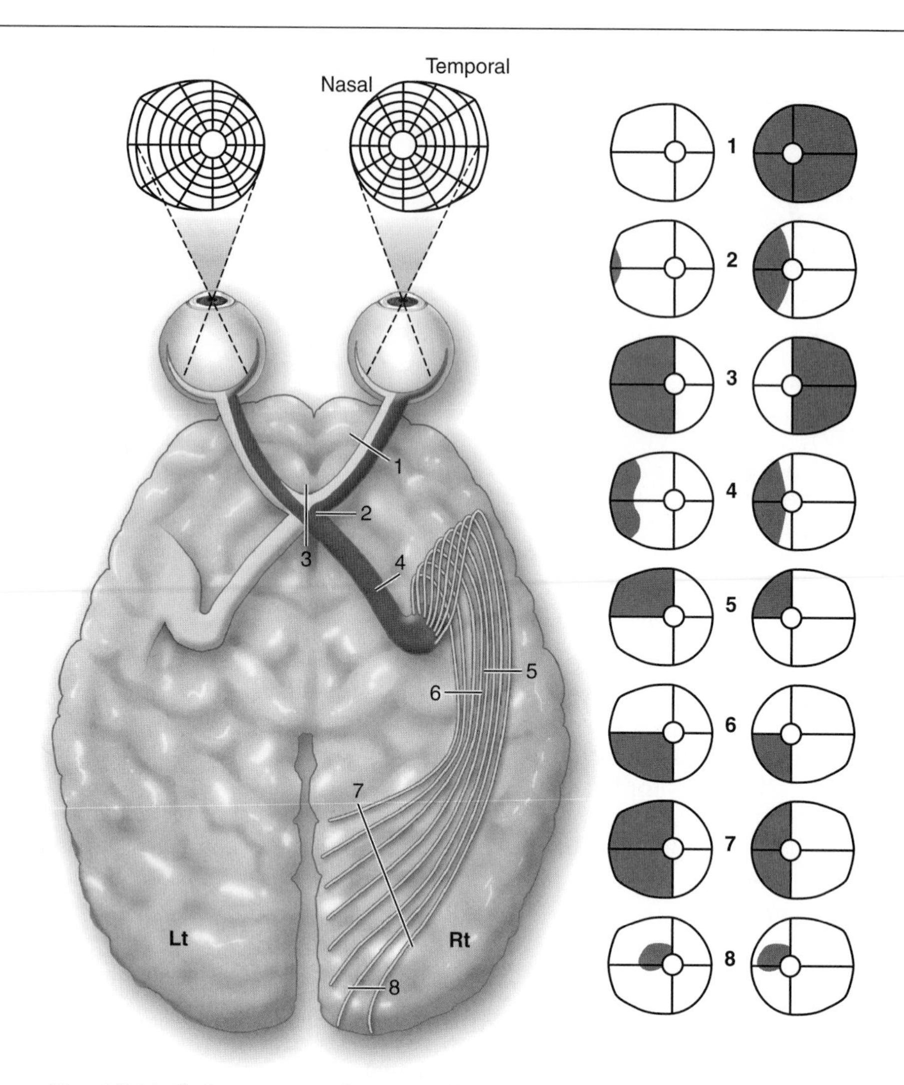

Visual fields that accompany damage to the visual pathways

1. **Optic nerve:** Unilateral amaurosis.
2. **Lateral optic chiasm:** Grossly incongruous, incomplete (contralateral) homonymous hemianopia.
3. **Central optic chiasm:** Bitemporal hemianopia.
4. **Optic tract:** Incongruous, incomplete homonymous hemianopia.
5. **Temporal (Meyer's) loop of optic radiation:** Congruous partial or complete (contralateral) homonymous superior quadrantanopia.
6. **Parietal (superior) projection of the optic radiation:** Congruous partial or complete homonymous inferior quadrantanopia.
7. **Complete parieto-occipital interruption of optic radiation:** Complete congruous homonymous hemianopia with psychophysical shift of foveal point often sparing central vision, giving "macular sparing."
8. **Incomplete damage to visual cortex:** Congruous homonymous scotomas, usually encroaching at least acutely on central vision.

FIGURE 4–3 Visual system lesions. Based on: Plum, F. [1985]. Neuro-opthamology. In J.B. Wyngaarden & L.H. Smith [Eds.], *Cecil textbook of medicine* [17th ed.]. Philadelphia: W.B. Saunders.

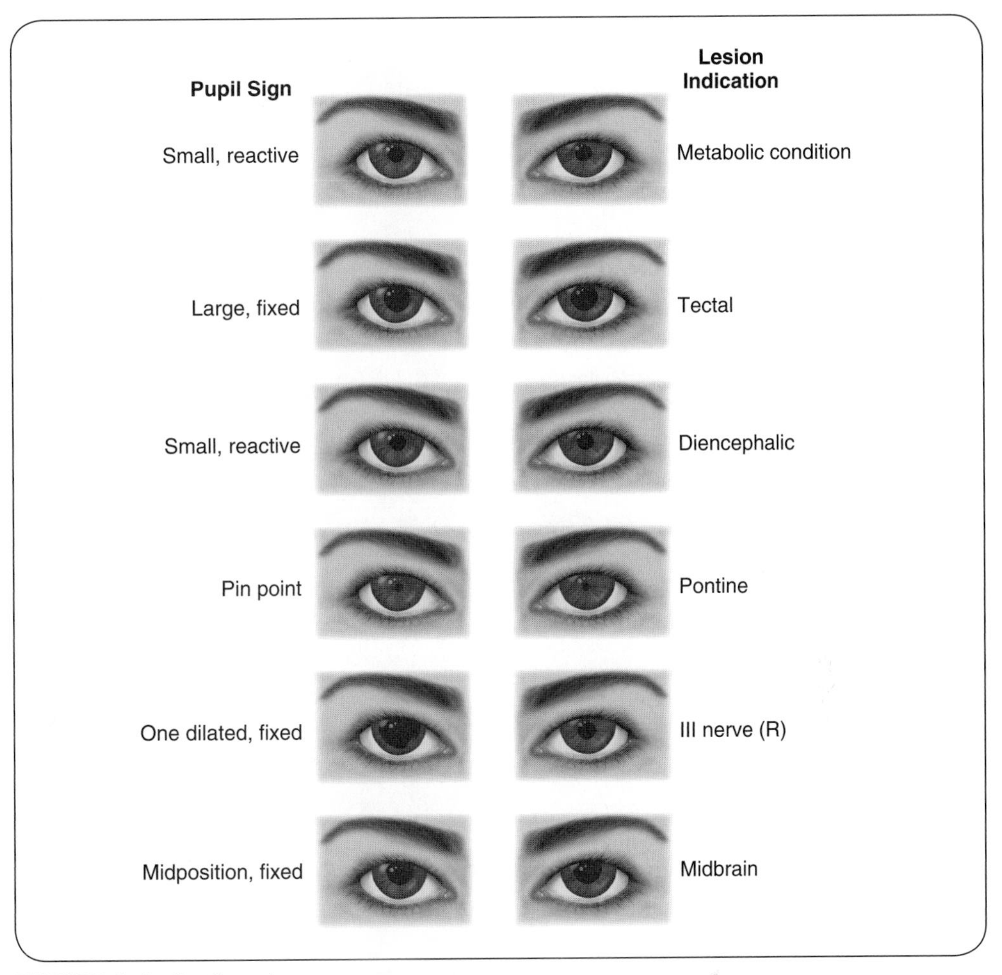

FIGURE 4–4 Pupillary signs. Based on: Plum, F., & Posner, J.B. [1980]. *The diagnosis of stupor and coma* (3rd ed.). Philadelphia: F.A. Davis.

noted (Figure 4–6). If the patient is able to sit or stand, muscle tone, range of movement, resistance, and strength in all extremities are tested.

Coordination and balance. Coordination is tested with rapid alternating movements, finger-to-nose test, heel-to-shin test, and standing with eyes closed.

Gait. Gait is examined by watching the patient walk and by asking the patient to walk on the toes and heels.

Sensation. Sensation testing examines responses to *touch, pain, temperature, vibration, proprioception* (position sense), *stereognosis* (ability to recognize objects by touch), *graphesthesia* (ability to recognize numbers drawn on the palm), and *two-point discrimination.* Sensation testing will reveal patterns of sensory loss within the distributions of segmental nerve roots and dermatomes (Figure 4–7).

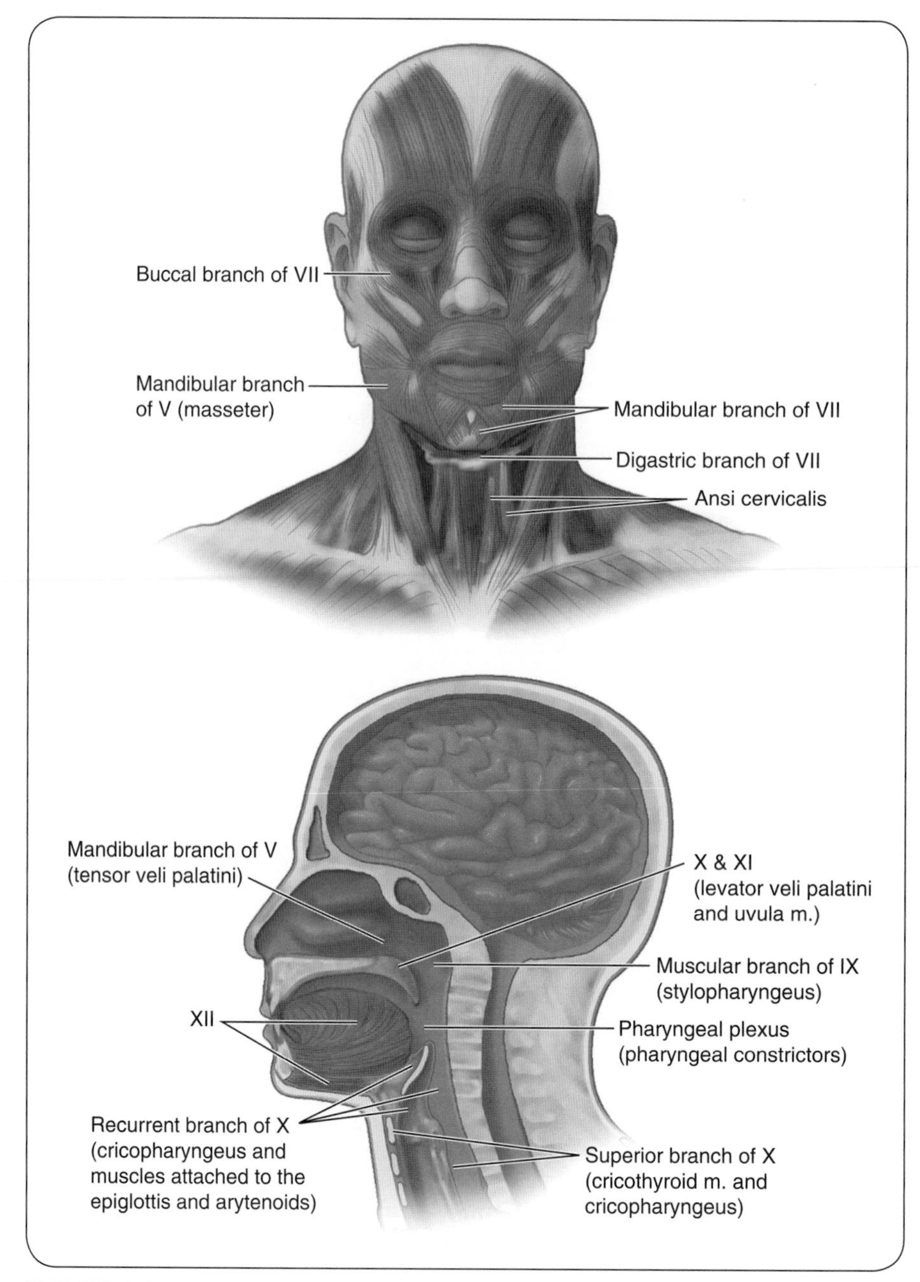

FIGURE 4–5 Innervation of the head and neck muscles. Source: Delmar/Cengage Learning

Reflexes. Reflex testing examines for normal, primary (pathologic), superficial, and deep tendon reflexes, and each is rated as normal, reduced, heightened.

- **Muscle stretch reflexes (MSRs).** Jaw jerk, CN V and CN VII; biceps, C5 and C6; triceps, C7 and C8; brachioradialis, C5 and C6; quadriceps, L3 and L4; ankle (Achilles tendon), S1 and S2; and patellar, L2, L3, and L4.

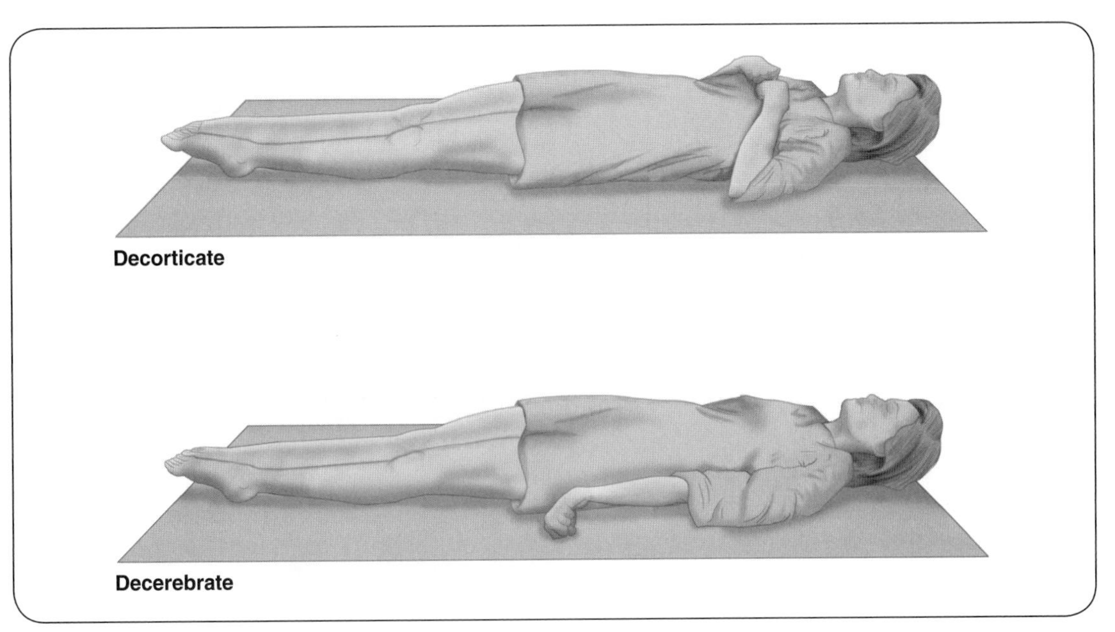

FIGURE 4–6 Decorticate and decerebrate postures. Source: Delmar/Cengage Learning

- **Urogenital reflexes.** Including the bulbocavernosal reflex, in which the anal sphincter contracts when the tip of the penis is grasped; the anal wink in which the anal sphincter contracts with stroking of the buttocks; and the cremasteric reflex (retraction of the testicles when stroking the inner thigh).
- **Cutaneous abdominal reflexes.** Abdominal wall contraction after stimulation of the skin over the abdominal quadrants.
- **Plantar reflex.** Flexion of the great toe when the plantar surface of the foot is stroked is normal; extension is abnormal and known as the Babinski's sign.
- **Thumb adduction reflex.** Hoffman, or Tromner, sign is elicited by briskly tapping the digits (middle or index finger) of the hands to elicit flexion of the thumb. Wartenberg hand signs include a reflex elicited by the examiner hooking his or her fingertips within those of the patient and then asking the patient to pull against the examiner's fingers. If the patient's thumb adducts across the palm into a simian grasp, then the abnormal thumb adduction reflex is demonstrated. Another sign includes the abduction of the little finger (extending away from the hand) when the fingers are fully flexed.
- **Other pathologic reflexes, or "release phenomena."** In adults, pathologic reflexes include the snout, or rooting, reflex; glabellar reflex; and bite reflex. In neonates, demonstrations of the Moro (startle) and suck reflexes are normal. During the first year of life the infant's primitive reflexes diminish, corresponding to an emergence of automatic movement reactions.

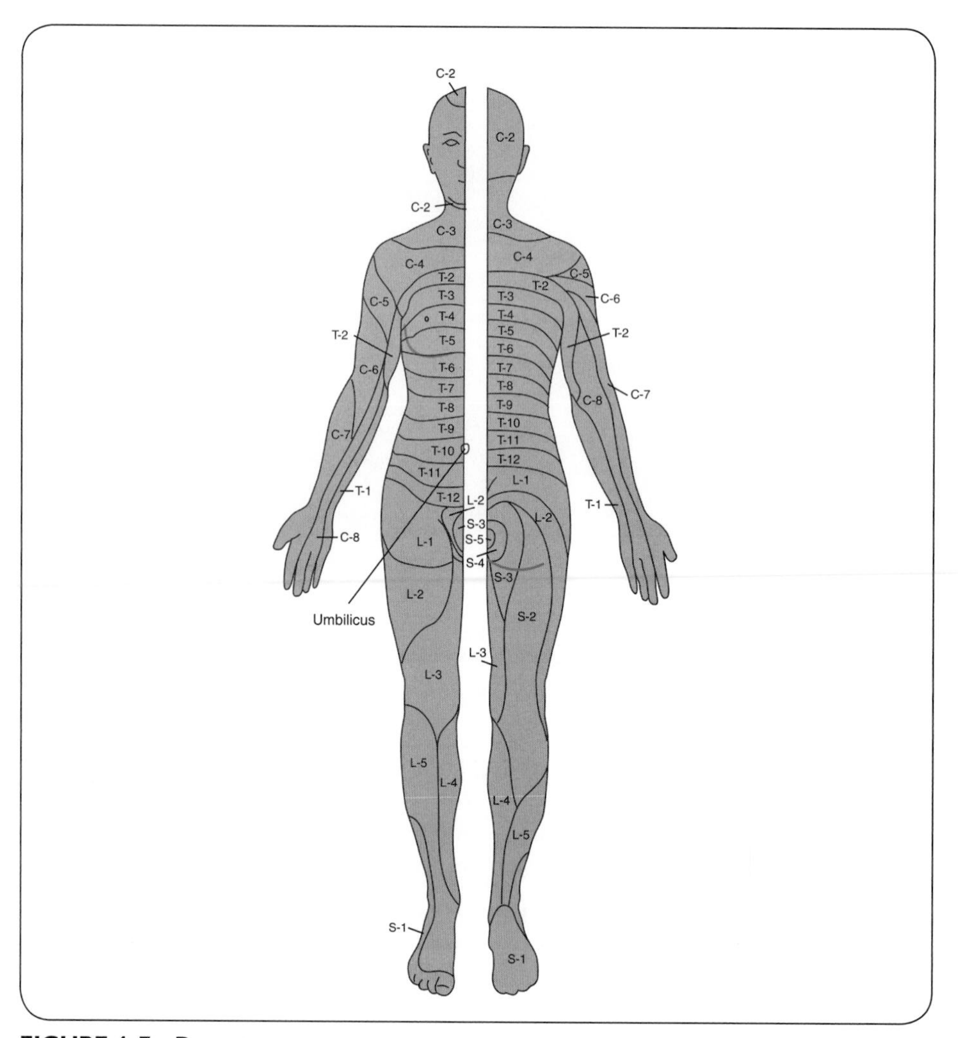

FIGURE 4–7 Dermatomes. Source: Delmar/Cengage Learning

4. *Reflex Grading*

Muscle stretch, or deep tendon, reflexes are numerically graded on a 0–4 (+) rating scale, as follows:

0 = absent

1+ = diminished

2+ = normal

3+ = increased

4+ = clonic

Mental Status

Alert, O×4, speech fluent, appropriate, repeats, follows directions, digits 6# ⇄, presidents, 3/3 5 minutes, serial 7s √

CNs

II – IX intact, PEERLA, EOMI, face/gag/palate symmetrical, $V_1 - V_3$ √, fundi ⊖

Motor

Strength 5/5, normal tone/bulk, Ø drift, F→N, gait heel/toe/tandem √, H→S

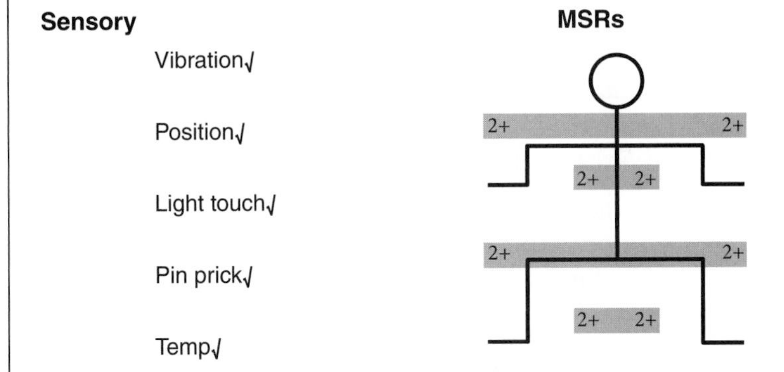

Interpretation: Patient is alert and oriented across four spheres; there is no apparent language impairment or dysarthria, memory functions for digit span for six digits backward and forward, presidents, proverbs, and serial 7 subtraction are intact; cranial nerve testing, motor and sensory functions are unremarkable; muscle stretch reflexes/deep tendon reflexes are normal, no pathologic reflexes.

FIGURE 4–8 Typical neurologist's note. Based on: Scott, T.F. (1999). The neurologic examination. In Shah, S.M., & Kelly, K.M. (Eds), *Emergency neurology; Principles and Practice.* Cambridge: The Cambridge Press.

Chart notes from the neurologic examination and MSR, or deep tendon reflex (DTR), testing will look similar to that shown in Figure 4–8, which is an illustration adapted from Scott (1999, p. 12) The findings from the reflex testing shown are illustrated by a stick figure to represent locations. This is an example of a normal examination.

5. *Muscle Strength Testing*

Muscle strength is usually graded subjectively on a 0 to 5 rating scale:

0 = Total paralysis, no muscle contraction is detectable

1 = Inability to contract against gravity

2 = Able to contract against gravity

3 = Active movement against gravity, no resistance

4– = Active movement against slight resistance

4 = Active movement against moderate resistance

4+ = Active movement against strong resistance

5 = Normal strength

6. Other Graded Scales

As illustrated in Figure 4–9, a facial grading system may be used to describe the characteristics and degree of facial weakness due to the fact that CN VII nerve damage may be of particular interest to SLPs, neurologists, neurosurgeons, and otolaryngologists.

The **House-Brackmann System** is commonly used by otolaryngologists in their examination of CN VII, or they may use a more refined instrument with good interrater reliability, such as that described by Ross et al. (1996) (see Figure 4-9 and Table 4-3).

F. Altered Mental Status in Children

Children who come to the pediatrician or emergency department with altered mental states, from mild confusion to coma, may require immediate cardiopulmonary stabilization and a differential diagnosis. The main categories for mental status changes in children include *primary brain insults* (trauma, cardiovascular accidents [CVAs], seizures, infections, ingestion of toxins, carbon monoxide exposure); *systemic illness* causing cerebral ischemia (such as hypoglycemia); illnesses known to cause general malaise and lethargy, for example, *dehydration* and *intussusception* (telescoping of one segment of the bowel into the immediately distal segment of the bowel); or *psychiatric disorders.*

Facial Grading System

Resting Symmetry

Compared to normal side

		Score
Eye (Choose one only)	normal	0
	narrow	1
	wide	1
	eyelid surgery	1
Check (naso-labial fold)	normal	0
	absent	2
	less pronounced	1
	more pronounced	1
Mouth	normal	0
	corner drooped	1
	corner pulled up/out	1
	Total	☐
Resting symmetry score	Total × 5	☐

Symmetery of Voluntary Movement — Degree of muscle EXCURSION Compared to normal side

Synkinesis — Rate the degree of INVOLUNTARY MUSCLE CONTRACTION associated with each expression

Standard Expressions	Unable to initiate movement/no movement	Initiates slight movement	Initiates movement with mild excursion	Movement almost complete	Movement complete		NONE: No synkinesis or mass movement	MILD: Slight synkinesis	MODERATE: Obvious but not disfiguring synkinesis	SEVERE: Disfiguring synkinesis/ Gross mass movement of several muscles	
Forehead Wrikle (FRO)	1	2	3	4	5	☐	0	1	2	3	☐
Gentle eye closure (OCS)	1	2	3	4	5	☐	0	1	2	3	☐
Open mouth Smile (ZYG/RIS)	1	2	3	4	5	☐	0	1	2	3	☐
Snarl (LLA/LLS)	1	2	3	4	5	☐	0	1	2	3	☐
Lip Pucker (OOS/OOI)	1	2	3	4	5	☐	0	1	2	3	☐
	Gross Asymmetry	Severe Asymmetry	Moderate Asymmetry	Mild Asymmetry	Normal Asymmetry	Total ☐					

Voluntary movement score: Total × 4 ☐

Synkinesis score: Total ☐

Patient's name ____

Dx ____

Date ____

Vol mov't score ☐ − Resting symmetry score ☐ − Synk score ☐ = Composite score ☐

Figure 4–9 Facial grading scale. Reprinted from Ross, B.G., Fradet, G., & Nedzelski, J.M. Development of a sensitive facial grading system. *Otolaryngology-Head and Neck Surgery, 114(3)*, 1996.with permission from Elsevier.

TABLE 4–3 House-Brackmann Facial Nerve Grading System

GRADE	DESCRIPTION	CHARACTERISTICS
I	Normal	Normal facial function in all areas
II	Mild dysfunction	Gross: slight weakness noticeable on close inspection; may have very slight synkinesis
		At rest: normal symmetry and tone
		Motion:
		Forehead: moderate to good function
		Eye: complete closure with minimum effort
		Mouth: slight asymmetry
III	Moderate dysfunction	Gross: obvious but not disfiguring difference between the two sides; noticeable but not severe synkinesis, contracture, and/or hemifacial spasm
		At rest: normal symmetry and tone
		Motion:
		Forehead: slight to moderate movement
		Eye: complete closure with effort
		Mouth: asymmetric with maximum effort
IV	Moderately severe dysfunction	Gross: obvious weakness and/or disfiguring asymmetry
		At rest: normal symmetry and tone
		Motion:
		Forehead: none
		Eye: incomplete closure
		Mouth: asymmetric with maximum effort
V	Severe dysfunction	Gross: only barely perceptible motion
		At rest: asymmetry
		Motion:
		Forehead: none
		Eye: incomplete closure
		Mouth: slight movement
VI	Total paralysis	No movement

Based on: House, J. W., & Brackmann, D. E. (1985). Facial nerve grading system. *Otolaryngology—Head and Neck Surgery,* 93.

TABLE 4–4 Primitive reflexes in neonates and infants

REFLEX	APPEARS BY	USUALLY GONE BY
Landau (head, trunk, leg extension when prone)	3 months	24 months
Asymmetric tonic neck reflex	2–3 weeks	4–6 months
Placing (when baby is upright and foot strokes the table)	1 day	2 months
Babinski	Birth	10 months
Crossed adductor	35 weeks	7 months
Automatic stepping when upright	35 weeks' gestation	2 months
Moro	34 weeks' gestation	3 months
Tonic neck (asymmetric)	34 weeks' gestation	4 months
Plantar grasp	34 weeks' gestation	10 months
Palmar grasp	34 weeks' gestation	6 months
Suck	34 weeks' gestation	4 months
Gag	32 weeks' gestation	persists

Based on: Flaherty, A. W. (2000). *The Massachusetts General Hospital handbook of neurology.* Philadelphia: Lippincott Williams & Wilkins.

G. Examining Infants and Children

A standard method for evaluating neonatal neurologic maturity and gestational age assessment is provided in Figure 3–4. The *pediatric neurology examination* includes some of the following procedures:

1. History

Queries regarding pregnancy history, weeks of gestation, Apgar scores, birth weight, postnatal problems, developmental milestones, school performance, appetite, behavior, and general health. (See Chapter 3 for additional discussion of gestational assessment.)

2. *Physical Examination*

- Measurement of the head circumference (with reference to standard growth chart).
- Assessment of closure of the fontanels (the posterior fontanel closes at 2 months, and the anterior fontanel closes at 2 years).
- General examination of face and limb morphology, skin, and vital signs.
- Check vision and eye movement; test eyes for a "blink" reflex.
- Check CN IX by pinching the nostrils closed, which should cause the tongue to protrude.
- Check for withdrawal to pin pricks.
- Examine movement of the extremities.
- Examine for age-appropriate developmental milestones (e.g., regards face, rolls over, coos).
- Reflex testing (Table 4–4).

IV. CONFUSION, COMA, DELIRIUM, AND DEMENTIA

A. Coma and Postcoma Cognitive Status

1. *Examination*

The physical examination of the comatose patient involves a neurologic appraisal to determine whether the disease is *supratentorial, subtentorial,* or *metabolic.* **Breathing patterns** are indicators of the level of lesion or type of disease. Hyper- and hypoventilation occur most often with metabolic disorders. *Cheyne-Stokes respirations* (see Chapter 9) are usually associated with hemispheric or pontomedullary disease. A **fundoscopic examination** of the eye will be made, looking principally for *papilledema* or *subhyaloid hemorraging,* which is the classic sign for a subarchnoid hemorrhage. Oculocephalic responses will be examined using the *doll's eyes maneuver* (see "Terminology," this chapter), unless there is reason to suspect a neck injury. *Pupillary reflexes* and *gaze positioning* will be examined. The extent and symmetry of muscle stretch reflexes and motor responses will be examined, and the limb, neck, and jaw posturing of the patient will be noted. Decorticate posturing, decerebrate posturing (see Figure 4–6), mixed posturing, or flaccid quadriplegia indicate different sites of lesions. The examination of a comatose patient and the patient emerging from coma will also include a rating of the level of consciousness and responsiveness.

2. *Ratings*

Coma is a state of unresponsiveness brought on by intracranial causes (supratentorial and infra/subtentorial), diffuse lesions, and metabolic disturbances. States of stupor and coma may be described with descriptive terms, such as *lethargic, obtunded, stuporous,* and *comatose*, but are better described by using a standardized rating scale. One of the most commonly used methods for rating coma levels is the **Glasgow Coma Scale (GCS)**, or Glasgow Rating Scale, shown in Table 4–5 for adults and in a modified version in Table 4–6 for infants and children (Flaherty, 2000). The **Rancho Levels of Cognitive Function (RLCF)**

TABLE 4–5 Glasgow Coma Scale for adolescents and adults

RESPONSE	SCORE
Eye Opening	
None	1
To pain	2
To speech	3
Spontaneous	4
Best Verbal Response	
None	1
Incomprehensible sounds	2
Inappropriate words	3
Confused conversation	4
Oriented conversation	5
Best Motor Response	
None	1
Abnormal extension (decerebrate rigidity)	2
Abnormal flexion (decorticate rigidity)	3
Withdrawal	4
Localizes pain	5
Obeys commands	6
Total GCS:	____

Based on: Teasdale, M. J., & Jennett, B. (1974). Assessment of command impaired consciousness: A practical scale. *Lancet, 11*, 81–84.

was originally developed as the "Rancho Los Amigos Cognitive Scale for Head Injury" in 1972, revised in 1974, and presented at the American Speech-Language-Hearing Association (ASHA) Convention in 1979 (Hagen & Malkmus, 1979). The original eight levels and their descriptions have recently undergone further revision by Hagen (personal communication, 2008). The latest version of this scale includes the addition of two new levels for higher functioning (purposeful, appropriate with assistance on request and appropriate without assistance). The Rancho Levels of Cognitive Function scale is not intended to be a diagnostic tool; rather, this scale is commonly used to rate or describe levels of cognitive responses during recovery from traumatic brain injury (Table 4–7) from admission through postacute recovery.

TABLE 4–6 Modified Glasgow Coma Scale for children and infants

RESPONSE	CHILDREN	INFANTS	SCORE
Eye Opening			
	None	None	1
	To pain	To pain	2
	To speech	To speech	3
	Spontaneous	Spontaneous	4
Verbal Response			
	None	None	1
	Incomprehensible nonspecific sounds	Moans in response to pain	2
	Inappropriate words	Cries in response to pain	3
	Confused	Irritable, cries	4
	Oriented	Coos and babbles	5
Best Motor Response			
	None	None	1
	Extensor response to pain	Abnormal extensor (decerebrate posture)	2
	Abnormal flexion response to pain	Abnormal flexion (decorticate rigidity)	3
	Withdrawal in response to pain	Withdrawal in response to pain	4
	Localizes painful stimulus	Withdrawal in response to touch	5
	Obeys commands	Moves spontaneously and purposefully	6
Total Modified GCS:			____

Based on: Nichols, D. G., Lappe, D. G., Haller, J. A., & Yaster, M. (Eds). (1996). *Golden hour: The handbook of advanced pediatric life support.* St. Louis, MO: Mosby Year Book; and Teasdale, M. J., & Jennett, B. (1974). Assessment of coma and impaired consciousness: A practical scale. *Lancet, 11*, 81–84.

TABLE 4–7 Rancho Los Amigos Cognitive Scale Revised

LEVEL	INDICATORS
I	No response: total assistance.
II	Generalized response: total assistance
III	Localized response: total assistance
IV	Confused/agitated: maximal assistance
V	Confused, inappropriate nonagitated: maximal assistance
VI	Confused, appropriate: moderate assistance.
VII	Automatic, appropriate: minimal assistance for daily living
VIII	Purposeful, appropriate: standby assistance
IX	Purposeful, appropriate: standby assistance on request
X	Purposeful, appropriate: modified independent

Source: Originally appeared in: Hagen, C., & Malkmus, D. (1979, November). Intervention strategies for language disorders secondary to head injuries. Paper presented at the American Speech-Language-Hearing Association Annual Convention, Atlanta, GA. Reprinted with permission of the authors.

B. Eye Movements in Pursuit and Gaze

Eye positions and movements can indicate sites of lesion in the poorly responsive patient. Coma can be caused by diffuse lesions in both cerebral hemispheres or by focal lesions of the midbrain and upper pons. Most comatose patients have roving **dysconjugate gaze** (unable to fix their vision on objects). This type of eye movement indicates that the brain stem is, to some extent, intact. Patients displaying a **forced downward gaze** may have had *thalamic hemorrhages*, lesions in the region of the pineal gland, or metabolic encephalopathies. A **forced upward gaze** occurs when the frontal eye fields (area 8 in the frontal cortex) exert a tonic effect on horizontal eye movements. With destructive lesions, the tonic control from the intact hemisphere forces the gaze toward the damaged hemisphere. **Forced horizontal gaze** can occur with brain stem lesions. Patients with **progressive supranuclear palsy (PSP)** often have difficulty with vertical and, later, horizontal gaze movements.

C. Delirium, Depression, and Dementias

1. *Differential Diagnosis*

When a patient presents with depressed mental functioning the neurologist will consider if the onset of the problem has been abrupt or acute or if mental changes were slowly progressive, if there is an indication of any underlying medical or emotional factor contributing to the disorder, and if there are any avenues for treatment.

2. *Delirium*

Delirium is an acute and transient condition characterized by fluctuating confusion, disorganized thinking, and difficulty maintaining and shifting attention. Delirium is usually reversible and it is directly associated with *systemic factors* (cardiovascular disease, infections, medications, neoplasm, metabolic disturbances, postoperative status, trauma, or substance abuse) and *central nervous system factors* (infection, neoplasm, trauma, vascular disorders, stroke, subdural hematoma, postictal status, subarachnoid hemorrhage, vasculitis, or arteriosclerosis).

3. *Delirium in the ICU*

Most patients in intensive care units (ICUs) have **decreased levels of consciousness** as a consequence of their acute medical condition, substance intoxication, or withdrawal, or due to the sedatives or other drugs they are receiving as a part of the medical care. Delirium can also develop as a consequence of prolonged stays in ICUs, and elderly patients (who make up the largest percentage of patients in ICUs) are particularly vulnerable to **ICU delirium**, especially if they have required prolonged intubation and ventilation. The ICU patient's clouded consciousness may fluctuate and is frequently worse at night. The facility may have developed standard assessments for their ICUs (MICU, SICU, CCU) or the medical staff may use their preferred published tools. A couple of the more frequently used published assessments have undergone validation studies: the **Richmond Agitation-Sedation Scale (RASS)** (Sessler et al., 2002) and the **Confusion Assessment Method for the ICU (CAM-ICU)** (Ely, 2002). The RASS rates alertness and agitation across a 10-point scale, with "0" representing *Alert and Calm.* Plus scores indicate agitation: "+1" *restless,* "+2" *agitated,* "+3" *very agitated,* and "+4" *combative.* Minus scores on this scale indicate decreased alertness: "−1" *drowsy,* "−2" *light sedation* (eye contact to voice), "−3" *moderate sedation* (movement or eye opening to voice), "−4" *deep sedation* (no response to voice but eye opening to physical stimulation), and "−5" *unarousable.* The CAM-ICU provides a worksheet that references the GCS or the RASS in the delirium and level of consciousness assessment, and it also examines for features related to **attention** (e.g., "I am going to read you a series of 10 letters. Whenever you hear the letter 'A' squeeze my hand") and **disorganized thinking** using verbal commands (e.g., "Hold up this many fingers") and yes-no questions ("Will a stone float in water?").

4. *Depression*

Although a formal assessment of depression is not routine, any indication of a depressed mental state, particularly in the elderly and teenagers, is a serious concern and essential feature of the differential examination of mental status. Depression can be associated with dementia, or depression alone can cause the patient to display cognitive deficits. In such cases pharmacologic, cognitive, and behavioral treatment for depression may reverse the cognitive deficits.

5. *Dementias*

Dementia is diagnosed when there is an acquired, persistent decline in cognitive ability across several domains without underlying psychiatric disease. Usually, the earliest and most prominent deficits are related to memory functions. The workup for dementia can be extensive and includes a complete blood count (CBC), SMA-20, vitamin B_{12} and folate assessment, thyroid function tests, brain imaging, and neuropsychology testing.

- **Reversible dementias.** Dementia is potentially reversible when the cognitive decline is related to treatable conditions such as depression, drug toxicity, normal pressure hydrocephalus, infection, nutritional deficiencies, cardiopulmonary disorders, or resectable brain lesions.

- **Irreversible dementias.** Causes of dementia that are not reversible include diagnoses such as acquired immunodeficiency syndrome (AIDS), Creutzfeldt-Jakob disease, Alzheimer's disease (AD), Pick's disease, alcoholic dementia syndromes, cerebro-cerebellar degenerations, Huntington's chorea, multi-infarction (see Chapter 9 for more elaboration), and certain types of parkinsonism. AD, multi-infarct dementia (MID), mixed AD and MID, and alcoholic dementia make up the majority of chronic dementing illnesses.

- **Multi-infarct dementia (MID).** MID can be found in conditions such as multiple lacunar infarctions in the central nervous system as seen with Binswanger's disease (hypertensive atherosclerotic disease leading to multiple subcortical lesions), large vessel atheromas, vasculitis, systemic hypoprofusion (due to occlusion of a major body vessel, such as the aorta, or heart attacks), and anoxic episodes.

- **Alzheimer's disease (AD).** AD is, at present, an irreversible, progressive disease resulting in profound dementia in its latter stages. The neuropathology includes degeneration and loss of nerve cells, particularly in those regions essential for memory and cognitive associations. It is characterized by neuritic plaques and neurofibrillary tangles. In addition, aggregates of amyloid protein can be found adjacent to and within blood vessels of patients with AD.

- **Frontotemporal dementia (FTD).** FTD refers to a group of dementing diseases, including Pick's disease, frontotemporal lobar degeneration, progressive aphasia/primary progressive aphasia, and semantic dementia, that are commonly misdiagnosed as AD. Patients with FTD have a markedly different clinical course and set of behavioral manifestations from AD. Some of the early signs of FTD may be confused with psychiatric disorders. Early in the onset of FTD patients display a lack of inhibition and an array of inappropriate social behaviors. There may be repetitive or compulsive behaviors and changes in eating and personal hygiene. Of particular significance to the SLP, these patients display difficulties with confrontational naming and progressively worsening word retrieval as well as reading and writing disorders. Research has shown different areas of the brain to be associated with the different forms of FTD, principally the frontal lobes, anterior temporal lobes, and left perisylvian cortex.

- **Alcohol-related dementia.** Alcohol-related dementia refers to a multifactorial disorder associated with long-term metabolic disruption, blows to the head following falls, poor nutrition, and other factors. **Wernicke-Korsakoff syndrome** is a form of dementia known to be associated with alcoholism, severe vitamin-impoverished diets, and anoxic or hemorrhagic cerebral ischemia, producing a selective, bilateral loss of neurons in the medial diencephalon and hypothalamus. Wernicke-Korsakoff syndrome usually reflects chronic thiamine depletion. **Wernicke's encephalopathy** is usually the acute manifestation, characterized by global confusion, ocular disturbances, apathy, and ataxia. **Korsakoff 's amnestic syndrome** (Korsakoff's disease, Korsakoff's psychosis, Korsakoff's dementia) is viewed as a chronic state, or later stage, of this syndrome. Korsakoff amnesics have a profound memory loss for recent events with spared language functions and relatively spared retrograde memory (memory for past events); a severe anterograde amnesia (impaired ability to acquire new information); and often, but not always, *confabulation,* which is the tendency to claim falsely to have seen, experienced, or done something.

V. COMMONLY ORDERED NEUROLOGIC STUDIES

For additional discussion of specific radiologic imaging studies, refer to Chapter 7.

A. Muscle and Nerve Conduction Studies

1. *Edrophonium (Tensilon) Testing*

Test done to diagnose an acetylcholine deficiency in myoneural junction disease (myasthenia gravis). This test requires introducing timed intravenous injections of edrophonium chloride (tensilon) and conducting tests of muscle strength improvements as an effect of this drug.

2. *Electromyography (EMG)*

EMG is an examination of the electrical impulses produced by a muscle. A needle electrode is inserted into a muscle, and the electrical wave pattern (frequency and amplitude of the electrical impulse) is read from an oscilloscope. The graphic copy is called the *electromyograph.* An EMG study can detect abnormalities in the muscle itself or the consequences of damage to the nerve innervating the muscle.

3. *Nerve Conduction Studies (NCS) or Nerve Conduction Velocity (NCV) Testing*

This test measures the velocity of electrical impulses along nerves. One electrode is placed along the course of the nerve to provide electrical stimuli, and a measurement is taken of the time required for the electrical stimuli to reach either a second electrode (for sensory nerves) or the time necessary to reach the muscle innervated by that nerve (for motor nerves). In NCV, *F-responses* refer to measures of conduction in the proximal portions of a motor nerve and ventral root. The *H-reflex* provides the equivalent of a stretch reflex in which sensory fibers of the posterior tibial nerve in the popliteal fossa are stimulated electrically, and the efferent evoked action potential from the soleus muscle is recorded.

B. Tests of Nystagmus, Balance, and Eye Movements

1. *Barany Test*

A labyrinthine nystagmus test in which nystagmus is induced by rotating the patient in a specially designed chair.

2. *Caloric Test*

A test used to examine the connections between the vestibular nuclei of the eighth cranial nerve and the oculomotor nerves. This test is performed by irrigating the external ear canal with water at a controlled temperature with the head at a 30° angle. In testing comatose patients, ice water is used. In the awake subject, temperatures of 30° F to 40° F are typical. Ice water in both ears simultaneously can be used to test vertical eye movement.

3. *Electronystagmography (ENG)*

Evoked potential test used as an alternative to, or to substantiate, caloric testing for nystagmus. This test is performed with the patient in a supine position with electrodes affixed with paste to the skin under the eyes. With the eyes closed, positional or caloric stimuli are introduced to elicit nystagmus. Eye movement recordings are made on an electronystagmograph. ENGs help to differentiate vestibular from nonvestibular balance disorders.

C. Neuroimaging Studies

Additional studies are described in Chapters 7 and 10.

1. *Cerebral Angiography/Arteriography*

An x-ray study of the brain done following the injection of a contrast dye into the major arteries.

2. *Computerized Tomography (CT) Scan*

This computerized x-ray study of the brain requires that the patient lie inside a large, donut-shaped scanner while x-ray beams make a complete circle through segments of the brain. As the beams pass through tissues, the scanner detects density differences, and the aggregate data are analyzed by a computer to construct a "picture" of the scanned segments. An intravenous infusion of an iodinated contrast agent (radiopaque dye containing iodine) is often injected into a vein prior to the study. This allows identification of vascular structures and disruption of the brood-brain barrier, providing enhancement; thus, when a contrast agent is used the study is called an "enhanced CT." Disruption of the blood-brain barrier is abnormal. Therefore, enhanced studies can delineate blood vessels, vascular malformations, vascular tumors, and regions in which the blood-brain barrier is lacking. Additional discussion of the CT scan is found in Chapter 8, and Figure 8–1 represents the anatomical areas demonstrated by CT scans. Figure 4–10 demonstrates the structures examined in a CT scan taken through the middle of the third ventricle.

3. *Myelography*

An x-ray study made of the subarachnoid space of the spinal cord with an injection of a contrast dye for the purpose of examining for impingement of nerve exits, intervertebral disc protrusions and herniations, or abnormal bony pressures on the cord or nerves.

4. *Magnetic Resonance Imaging (MRI)*

Like the CT scan, the MRI produces a computerized picture of the brain, or other body structures, but uses radio waves and magnetism instead of x-rays and does not require ionizing radiation. The MRI is based on the principle that all atoms have magnetic properties. This energy, when subjected to a radio wave, can be detected; and (like the CT scan) the detectors

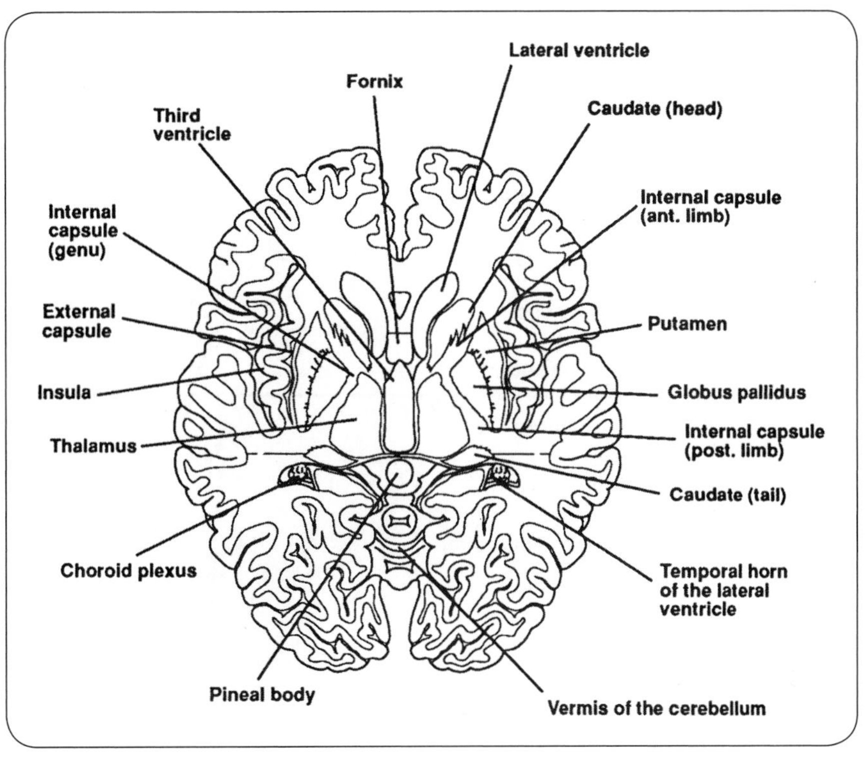

FIGURE 4–10 Anatomical structures revealed by a CT scan through the middle of the third ventricle. Source: Delmar/Cengage Learning

feed data to a computer to construct remarkably clear images, which are then interpreted by a neurologist or radiologist. Figure 4–11 provides an anatomical illustration corresponding to a midsagittal plane of the MRI. Additional discussion of the MRI is found in Chapter 7.

5. Functional Magnetic Resonance Imaging (fMRI)

Functional magnetic resonance imaging (fMRI) technology uses the principles and techniques of static nuclear magnetic resonance (NMR) imaging and earlier developed methods of imaging brain metabolic activity, PET scanning, SPECT scanning, and regional cerebral blood flow (rCBF) studies. fMRI is a safer, cheaper procedure than these nuclide scanning methods and the spatial and temporal resolution with fMRI and visualization of the brain when engaged in a mental activity are equivalent or better. fMRIs have been used experimentally to examine for areas of brain activity and evidence of networks of brain regions and structures involved in motor functions, sensory perceptions, language, and memory. The principles of fMRI involve the link between increases in regional metabolic functions during certain brain activities as shown by tracking oxygen consumption. The **blood oxygen level dependent (BOLD)** mechanism, in which the blood in an active region of the brain becomes more oxygenated, influences the brain's nuclear properties, and these changes are detected by NMR spectrography and analyzed by a computer to generate images of brain activity. MRI is also used in vessel studies throughout the body, for example, **magnetic resonance angiogram** and **magnetic resonance venogram**.

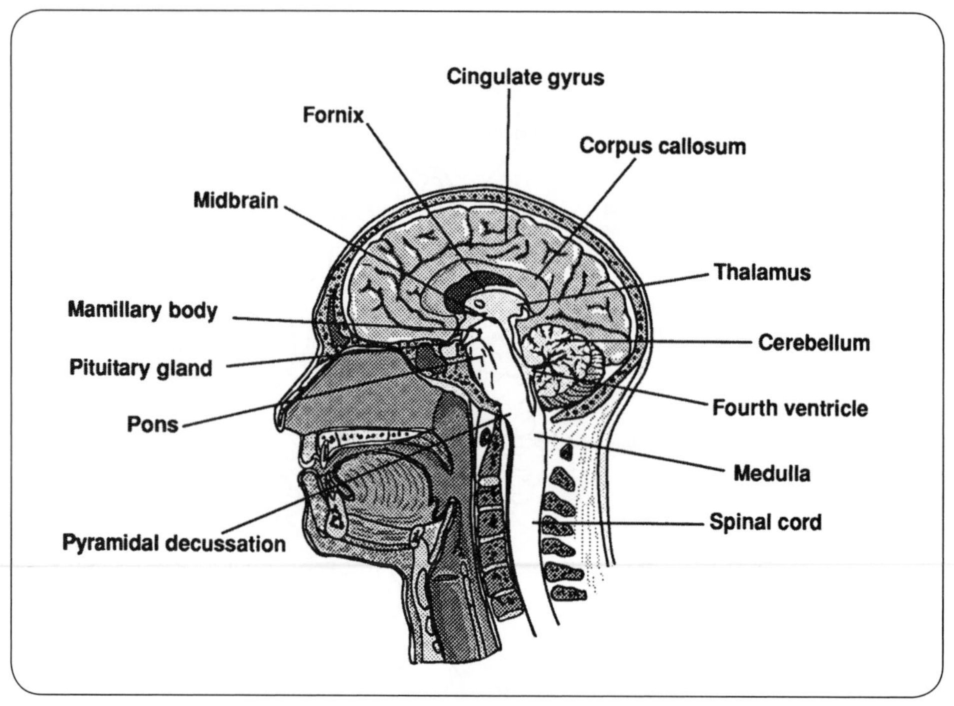

FIGURE 4–11 Anatomical structures revealed by MRI in a midsagittal section of the brain.
Source: Delmar/Cengage Learning

6. *Pneumoencephalography (PEG)*

This x-ray study involves the injection of air or gas into the subarachnoid space for the purpose of delineating the cisterns and the ventricular system. The PEG is especially useful for the evaluation of posterior fossa, suprasellar, and ventricular tumors.

7. *Single Photon Emission Control Tomography (SPECT) Scans*

SPECT is principally used in studies of the heart and brain. A radioactive substance, or tracer, is infused and then detected by a gamma camera to create three-dimensional images of these organs. SPECT may be used to determine seizure locus, referred to as a *seizure scan.*

8. *Skull Series*

Plain film radiograms taken in four views used to examine for bony and soft tissue abnormalities of the cranium.

D. Cortical Electrical Activity

1. *Electroencephalography (EEG)*

The EEG is a recording of electrical impulses in the brain made while the patient is awake, asleep, or receiving stimulation by staring at a pattern board or a flashing light (photic stimulation). The majority of EEG machines have 8, 12, 16, or 20 channels. Depending on the technique used, approximately 16 to 30 small chlorided silver electrodes are attached to the patient's scalp with a special paste, allowing a graphic recording of electrical impulses. The EEG tracings are *voltage versus time* graphs and record slow waveform (0.5–30 Hz) activity across specific areas of the brain. Studies require from 45 to 90 minutes. Findings can be analyzed *on line*, during actual examination, or *off line*, from recordings of the examination. The EEG is useful in studying seizure activity, to determine brain death, and to evaluate focal versus diffuse conditions (Table 4–8; Figure 4–12).

TABLE 4–8 EEG patterns

PATTERN	DESCRIPTION
Alpha	Frequencies of 8–13 Hz, but may be slower in children. An alpha frequency is often found as the posteriorly dominant rhythm present in the awake, alert individual with his or her eyes closed that disappears when the eyes are opened.
Beta	Symmetrical frequencies of 14–35 Hz of lower amplitude than alpha rhythms. Beta rhythms are normally found in the frontal areas and will be depressed over focal lesions.
Theta	Mild slowing with frequencies of 3–7 Hz. Slow waves are normal during sleep and are commonly seen in association with metabolic disorders and destructive lesions.
Delta	Severe slowing with frequencies less than 3 Hz. Normally seen in babies and in adults during sleep; associated with pathologic states in adults, including deep midline lesions, diffuse lesions, subcortical lesions, and metabolic encephalopathy.
Sharp	Waves showing a brief high-voltage electrical discharge from a focal area of the brain, often indicative of epilepsy. Also called "spike and dome" waves.
Negative	EEG pattern believed to represent a sudden burst of electrical activity from the brain surface, suggestive of epilepsy.
Asymmetric	EEG patterns corresponding to large areas of the left and right hemispheres are graphically displayed. The waves correspond to patterns of connections between the electrodes and the recording channels, known as **montages**. Location schematics of the montage reference sites and linkages are illustrated on the electroencephalogram tracing, as if you were looking at the top of the head. Asymmetric patterns reflect destructive lesions to one of the hemispheres.
Mu	Frequencies of 7–11 Hz located centrally or centroparietal that attenuate with movement.
Lambda	Transient waves from the occipital area occurring during visual scanning.

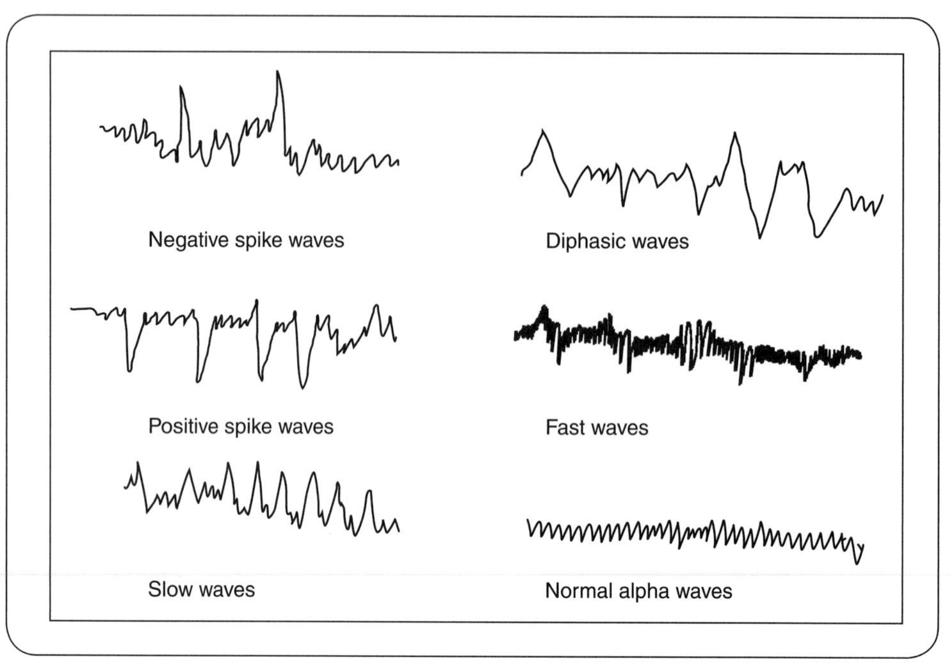

FIGURE 4–12 Illustration of EEG patterns. Source: Delmar/Cengage Learning

2. *Mental Activity Network (MAN) Scanning*

This is an example of a computerized analysis of EEG signals taken from 124 sites (instead of the usual 8 to 20). This technology is being used experimentally to examine patterns of electrochemical activity in the brain during various mental activities.

3. *Evoked Potential Studies*

Various methods are used to examine for synaptic responses to stimuli in the sensory and somatosensory pathways. **Visual evoked response (VER)** tests are used to diagnose sites of lesions within the visual system, principally problems with the optic nerve. Similarly, **brain stem evoked response (BAER) audiometry** is used by audiologists to determine hearing ability in a poorly responsive individual, or the site of lesion causing hearing impairment or dysfunction. **Somatosensory evoked response (SSER)** tests can determine the presence of spinal cord causes for numbness and weakness of the extremities.

E. Other Studies

1. *Intracranial Pressure (ICP) Monitoring*

Intracranial monitors may be placed when there is suspicion of cerebral edema, hemorrhage or hematoma, obstruction hydrocephalus, brain herniation, or clinical signs of a space-occupying or expanding lesion. The devices used for ICP include *intraventricular catheters, subarachnoid screws,* and *epidural fiberoptic sensors.* These devices measure pressure within the cranium, which is displayed on a monitor as pressure (mmHg) over time (minutes). ICP waves within normal parameters are referred to as "C-Waves."

2. *Neuropsychiatric and Neuropsychologic Testing*

Whenever appropriate, patients with emotional or cognitive deficits will be referred for neuropsychiatric or neuropsychologic evaluation. This testing may be an important part of the overall neurodiagnostic evaluation to examine for secondary emotional and cognitive deficits.

3. *Cerebrospinal Fluid (CSF) Analysis*

Laboratory analysis of CSF is done to determine if there are *changes in the normal constituents* (water, glucose, sodium chloride, and protein), which indicate brain disease; or if blood, which indicates hemorrhage; bacteria; or increased leukocytes, which indicate infection, are present. Appendix A contains a list of normal values in CSF analysis.

VI. DSM–IV CLASSIFICATION CODES

The American Psychiatric Association publishes a standardized classification system for psychiatric disorders called the *Diagnostic and Statistical Manual of Mental Disorders–IV,* indicating the fourth edition. A fifth edition is under development. DSM–IV classifications provide descriptive guidelines for psychiatric diagnoses. All DSM–IV codes are included in the International Classification of Disease codes (ICD-9, CM; ICD-10, CM). The DSM–IV classification system relies on what the patient says and does as indicators for how the patient thinks and feels. This system is *multiaxial.* The first three axes relate to the diagnostic assessment. *Axis I* codes clinical syndromes. *Axis II* codes personality disorders and developmental disorders. Axis III identifies relevant medical disorders and conditions. *Axis IV* codes the severity of the psychosocial stressors, and *Axis V* designates the **global assessment of function (GAF)**, based on a 100-point scale (*Quick Reference to the Diagnostic Criteria from DSM-IV*, American Psychiatric Association, Washington, DC, 1994). Classifications also include conditions not attributable to the disorders that are the focus of treatment (see further discussion in Chapter 10).

VII. PAIN AND SLEEP

A. Pain

Complaints related to pain are important factors in the neurologic examination. Pain is described relative to its *quality* (pulsing, sharp, tingling, dull, etc.); *intensity* (slight, mild, moderate, severe); *location*; and *duration* (acute, chronic, intermittent, and intractable). Pain and pain management are factors that health care providers are mandated to address in both inpatient and outpatient care settings. Any concerns about pain and discomfort are expected to be addressed in some manner by providers, including SLPs, at each visit.

B. Sleep

Sleep disturbances can be indicators of neurologic diseases. It is sometimes necessary to examine the patient's sleep patterns or to conduct EEG studies during sleep. Sleep centers use what are called **polysonograms** (on line recordings of EEG, ECG, EMB, respiratory airflow, earlobe oximetry, and abdominal and thoracic wall motion) to measure physiologic changes during sleep. A **Multiple Sleep Latency Test (MSLT)** is a measure of daytime sleepiness. Sleep patterns are described relative to "stages." Sleep has five stages: *sub-stage I* (relaxed, hypnagogic pre-sleep stage); *sub-stage II* (asleep but easily aroused); *sub-stage III* (aroused from sleep with difficulty); *deep (delta) sleep* (when brain waves are slow and metabolism slows), and *rapid-eye movement* (REM) stage sleep (when dreaming is present and respiration is irregular, there may be apnea during this stage and arousal is difficult).

VIII. CLINICAL COMPETENCIES

The learner outcomes, skills, and competencies gained from information contained in this chapter include the ability to:

- Read, interpret, and use terminology and abbreviations related to mental status testing and the neurologic examination.
- Understand notations used by neurologists to indicate findings on muscle strength and reflex testing.
- Describe the essential areas, or domains, that are evaluated and procedures for evaluation of those areas with a bedside, mental status screening assessment.
- Describe the neurologic review of systems.
- Discuss why any abrupt mental status changes in children require immediate attention.
- Describe pupillary and eye movement signs and what they indicate.
- List the cranial nerves and how the functions of those nerves are tested in the neurologic examination.
- List the items in a neurologist's "toolkit."
- Discuss the difference between decorticate and decerebrate postures and what those postures indicate.
- Discuss what is meant by "primitive" reflexes in children and adults.
- Discuss the differences between dementia, delirium, and depression.
- Describe how ICU delirium is evaluated.
- Describe some common evaluation scales used in coma evaluation and cognitive recovery from head trauma.
- List several of the major types of dementing diseases.
- List common neurologic tests and procedures and what they are intended to evaluate.

- Explain the significance of asymmetric EEG findings.
- Discuss how the DSM-IV classification codes are applied in psychiatric diagnoses.

IX. REFERENCES AND RESOURCES CONSULTED

American Psychiatric Association. (1994). *Quick reference to the diagnostic criteria from DSM-IV.* Washington, DC: Author.

American Speech-Language-Hearing Association. (1997). *National outcomes measure system.* Rockville, MD: Author.

Anderson, D. (Ed.). (2003). *Dorland's illustrated medical dictionary* (30th ed.). Philadelphia: W. B. Saunders.

Bonner, J. S., & Bonner, J. J. (Eds.). (1991). *The little black book of neurology: A manual for neurologic house officers* (2nd ed.). St. Louis, MO: Mosby Yearbook.

Chenitz, W. C., Stone, J. T., & Salisbury, S. A. (1991). *Clinical gerontological nursing.* Philadelphia: W. B. Saunders.

Daniels, R., Nosek, L., & Nicoll, L. (2007). *Contemporary medical-surgical nursing.* Clifton Park, NY: Delmar Cengage Learning.

Ely, W. D. (2002). *Confusion assessment method for the ICU (CAM-ICU): Training manual.* Nashville, TN: Vanderbilt University.

Flaherty, A. W. (2000). *The Massachusetts General Hospital handbook of neurology.* Philadelphia: Lippincott Williams & Wilkins.

Folstein, M., & Folstein, S. E. (2001). *Mini Mental State Examination.* Lutz, FL: Psychological Assessment Resources, Inc.

Folstein, M., Folstein, S.E., & McHugh, P., (1975). Minimental state, a practical method for grading the cognitive status of patients for the clinician. Journal of Psychiatric Research, 12, 189–198.

Gelb, D. J. (Ed.). (2005). *Introduction to clinical neurology* (3rd ed.). Philadelphia: Elsevier Butterworth Heinemann.

Gilroy, J. (1990). *Basic neurology.* New York: Pergamon.

Hagen, C. (2008). Personal communication.

Hagen, C., & Malkmus, D. (1977, November). *Rancho Los Amigos scale for head injury.* Paper presented at the American Speech-Language-Hearing Association Annual Convention, Atlanta, GA.

Hagen, C., & Malkmus, D. (1979, November). *Intervention strategies for language disorders secondary to head injuries.* Paper presented at the American Speech-Language-Hearing Association Annual Convention, Atlanta, GA.

Heilman, K. M., Watson, R. T., & Greer, M. (1977). *Handbook of neurologic signs and symptoms.* New York: Appleton-Century-Crofts.

House, J. W., & Brackmann, D. E. (1985). Facial nerve grading system. *Otolaryngology—Head and Neck Surgery, 93,* 146–147.

Jacobs, J. W., Bernard, M. R., & Delgado, A. (1977). Screening for organic mental syndromes in the medically ill. *Annals of Internal Medicine, 86,* 40–46.

Levin, H. S., O'Donnell, V. M., & Grossman, R. G. (1979). The Galveston orientation and amnesia test: A practical scale to assess cognition after head injury. *Journal of Nervous System and Mental Disorders, 167,* 675–684.

Nichols, D. G., Lappe, D. G., Haller, J. A., & Yaster, M. (Eds.). (1996). *Golden hour: The handbook of advanced pediatric life support.* St. Louis, MO: Mosby Yearbook.

Pfeiffer, E. (1975). A short portable mental status questionnaire for the assessment of organic brain deficits in elderly patients. *Journal of the American Geriatric Society, 23,* 433–441.

Plum, F. (1985). Neuro-ophthalmology. In J. B. Wyngaarden & L. H. Smith (Eds.), *Cecil textbook of medicine* (17th ed.). Philadelphia: W. B. Saunders.

Plum, F., & Posner, J. B. (1980). *The diagnosis of stupor and coma* (3rd ed.). Philadelphia: F. A. Davis.

Ross, B. G., Fradet, G., & Nedzelski, J. M. (1996). Development of a sensitive facial grading system. *Otolaryngology—Head and Neck Surgery, 114*(3), 380–386.

Samuels, M. A. (Ed.). (1978). *Manual of neurologic therapeutics.* Boston: Little, Brown.

Schwamm, L. H., Van Dyke, C., & Kiernan, R. J. (1987). The neurobehavioral cognitive status examination: Comparison of the cognitive capacity screening and MMSE in neurologic populations. *Annals of Internal Medicine, 107,* 486–491.

Scott, T. F. (1999). The neurologic examination. In S. M. Shah & K. M. Kelly (Eds.), *Emergency neurology: Principles and practice* (pp. 3–13). Cambridge: The Cambridge Press.

Sessler, C. N., Gosnell, M., Grap, M. J., Brophy, G. T., O'Neal, P. V., Keane, K. A., et al. (2002). The Richmond agitation-sedation scale: Validity and reliability in adult intensive care patients. *American Journal of Critical Care Medicine, 166,* 1338–1344.

Strub, R. L., & Black, F. W. (1993). *The mental status examination in neurology* (3rd ed.). Philadelphia: F. A. Davis.

Teasdale, M. J., & Jennett, B. (1974). Assessment of coma and impaired consciousness: A practical scale. *Lancet, 11,* 81–84.

Weiner, W. J., & Goetz, C. G. (1999). *Neurology for the nonneurologist.* Philadelphia: Lippincott Williams & Wilkins.

Weisberg, L. A., Strub, R. L., & Garcia, C. A. (1983). *Essentials of clinical neurology.* Baltimore: University Park Press.

CHAPTER 5

Nutrition, Hydration, and Swallowing

Speech-language pathologists (SLPs) are frequently consulted when patients have dysphagia or oral feeding problems. SLPs are asked to determine if any behavioral therapy, oral exercises or nonnutritive stimulation, texture or diet style adjustment, feeding assistance or technique, positioning, oral prosthesis, or adaptive equipment would decrease a risk for aspiration or benefit oral intake. SLPs are asked to participate in the management plan if a risk for aspiration prevents consideration of oral intake or if a food aversion complicates adequate nutrition. All members of the care team generally understand that dysphagic and malnourished patients have delayed recoveries and more frequent complications, leading to increased lengths of stay in the hospital and, correspondingly, increased costs. In children, dysphagia and feeding problems present a number of special concerns. Preterm neonates and newborns with congenital disorders often have upper airway problems, gastrointestinal disorders, neurologic disorders, and metabolic or systemic conditions requiring special nutritional management. Malnourished children are more susceptible to infection. Malnutrition can compromise neurologic development, growth, and learning. Allergic responses and specific food allergies are increasingly being identified in children. These food allergies may prevent adequate nutrition and can be life threatening. In settings where adults are treated, clinicians must be particularly mindful of the unique concerns in dietary management for safe and adequate nutrition and hydration of elderly patients and individuals with cognitive impairments.

Dysphagia is a medically related condition; thus, SLPs working with individuals with dysphagia need to understand its causes and medical management. Involvement with the assessment and treatment of patients at any age who are nutritionally compromised or fluid deficient necessitates a basic understanding of normal nutrition and hydration requirements; the procedures that are used to diagnose nutrition, hydration, and swallowing disorders; and the medical management of nutrition and fluid and electrolyte balance. The ideal management of dysphagia and feeding disorders in children involves multidisciplinary team collaboration with a nutrition specialist (registered dietitian), gastroenterologist, pediatrician, SLP, and, when indicated, a pediatric allergist, lactation specialist, psychologist, and other specialists.

I. CHAPTER FOCUS

This chapter reviews medical terminology and abbreviations commonly encountered in discussions of disorders of nutrition and hydration. Conditions associated with dysphagia and feeding disorders across the age span are described. Procedures, tests, and therapies for the medical management of dysphagia and nutrition and hydration deficits in adults and children are discussed. Illustrations of diagnostic and management procedures also are provided. Special attention is given to *pediatric dysphagia* and feeding disorders in children and to issues in nutrition and dietary and swallowing management of elders. Further discussion of nutrition in the elderly is found in Chapter 14. Reference tables and figures related to adult and pediatric nutrition and hydration management are included.

II. TERMINOLOGY AND ABBREVIATIONS

A. Anatomic Terminology

See Figure 5–1 for an illustration of the structures of the digestive tract and Figure 5–2 for an illustration of the anatomy of the urinary tract.

Adrenal glands. Small, triangular glands located on top of both kidneys. An adrenal gland is made of two parts: The outer region is called the *adrenal cortex* and the inner region is called the *adrenal medulla*; these glands secrete *hormones* (hydrocortisone, corticosterone, aldosterone, and androgen) and *epinephrine* and *norepinephrine* to regulate metabolic functions in the body, heart rate, and blood pressure.

Bile duct. Duct formed by the union of the common hepatic duct and the cystic duct; carries bile into the duodenum.

Bladder (urinary). Hollow, muscular, sac-like cavity for the storage of urine prior to elimination.

Cardia. Small area of the stomach near the esophagastric junction.

Cardiac valve, cardiac orifice, cardiac sphincter. Opening into the stomach at the junction of the esophagus.

Cecum. First part of the large intestine.

Celiac. Pertaining to the abdomen.

Cervical esophagus. Upper portion of the esophagus.

Chief salivary glands. Three pairs of glands with ducts opening into the oral cavity, including the **parotid glands** (with *Stensen's duct*, see Figure 5–1) located below the ear; **sublingual glands** with 10 to 30 ducts located on the floor of the mouth; and the **submandibular glands** (*Wharton's duct*) located below the mandible.

Colon. Large intestine from the cecum to the rectum, including the *ascending colon*; *transverse colon*; *descending colon*; and *sigmoid*, or pelvic, *colon*.

Common hepatic duct. Duct formed by the union of the right and left hepatic ducts, which receive bile from the liver.

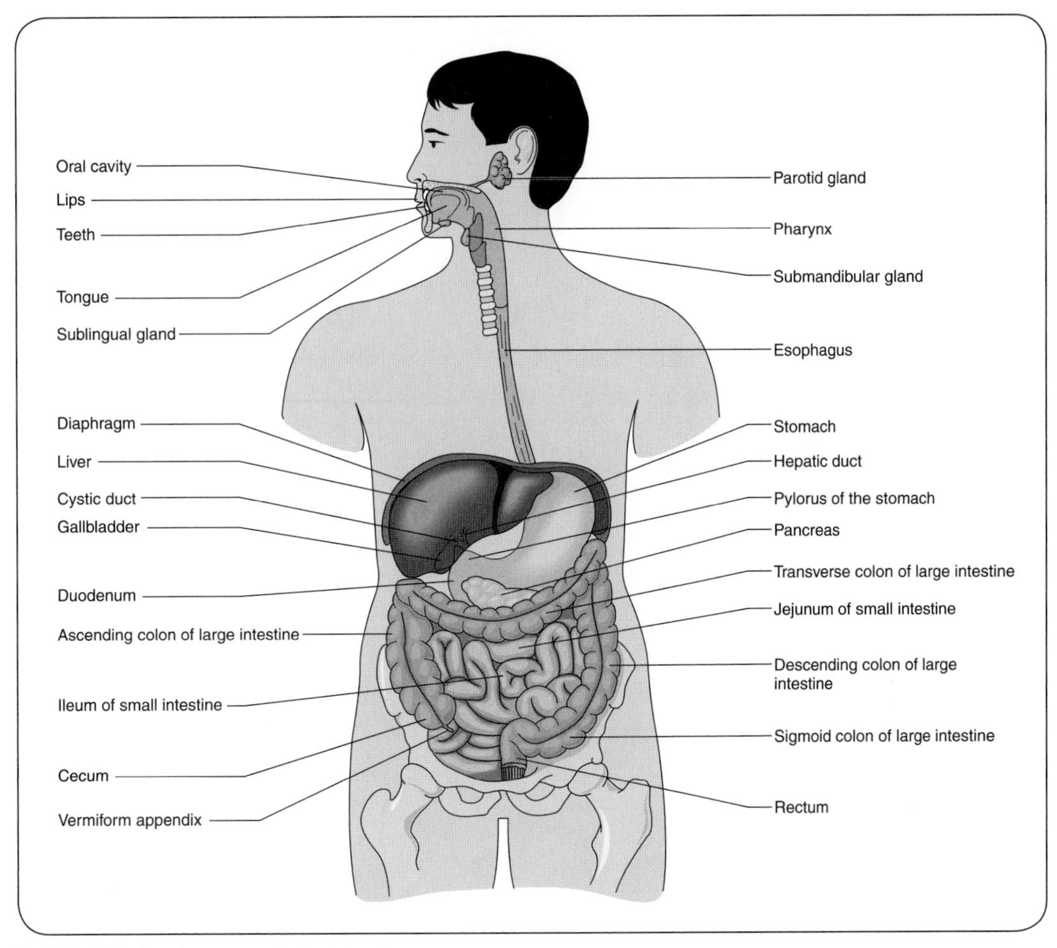

FIGURE 5–1 Anatomy of the digestive tract. Source: Delmar/Cengage Learning

Duodenum. First part of the small intestine extending from the *pyloric valve* to the *jejunum.*

Enteric. Pertaining to the intestine.

Epigastric. Pertaining to the region above the stomach.

Epiglottis. The cartilaginous flap at the base of the tongue that serves to protect the *glottis,* which is the opening between the vocal folds into the airway, during swallowing.

Fundus. Enlarged upper portion of the stomach extending to the left of the *cardiac valve* (stomach orifice).

Gallbladder. A small, pear-shaped organ located next to the liver; stores and concentrates bile for release in digestion.

Ileum. Third part of the small intestine extending from the jejunum to the *cecum.*

Jejunum. Second part of the small intestine extending from the *duodenum* to the *ileum.*

Kidneys. Two bean-shaped organs located behind the abdominal cavity on either side of the spinal cord in the lumbar region. The kidneys filter wastes (*urea, creatinine,* and *uric acid*) from the blood and reabsorb materials that the body needs to retain in the

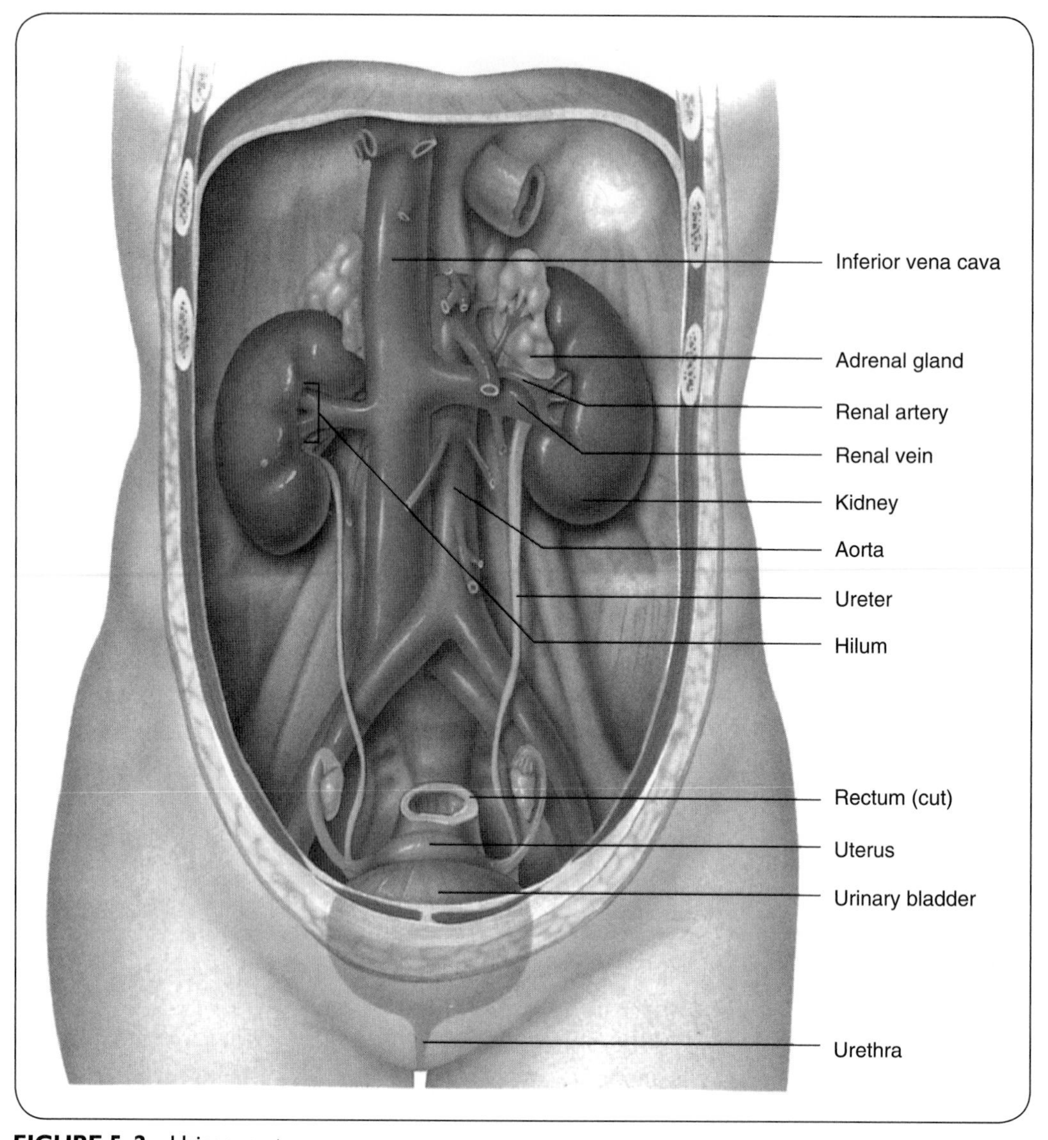

FIGURE 5–2 Urinary system. Source: Delmar/Cengage Learning

bloodstream before producing urine. The kidneys produce a substance called *renin*, which controls blood pressure, and *erythropoietin*, which regulates red blood cell production in the bone marrow.

Liver. Organ that manufactures a thick greenish or yellowish-brown fluid called **bile**. Bile contains a fatty substance (*cholesterol*), bile acids, and pigments. One of the pigments manufactured by the liver is called *bilirubin*, which is produced when red cells are destroyed in the liver. The liver helps to keep the amount of sugar (*glucose*) in the blood in a normal balance through a process called **glycogenesis**. It can also convert glycogen to glucose when blood sugar levels are low. The liver manufactures blood proteins, removes old erythrocytes, releases bilirubin, and removes poisons from the bloodstream. Bile released by the liver travels down the *hepatic duct* into the *cystic duct* and into the gallbladder where it is concentrated and then mixed with pancreatic juices for digestion. The term **portal system** refers to the blood vessels passing to and from the liver. The *hepatic vein* goes from the liver to the vena cava.

Mesentery. Peritoneal fold that carries the blood supply and attaches the jejunum and ileum to the posterior abdominal wall.

Mesocolon. Mesentery attaching the colon to the posterior abdominal wall.

Nares. Openings into the nose, pronounced "nar-eez"; a single nasal opening is called a **naris**.

Omenta. Peritoneal sheets connecting the stomach with other visceral organs (liver, spleen, and transverse colon).

Pancreas. Organ located next to the duodenum leading out of the stomach. The pancreas is both an **exocrine gland** (excreting amylase and lipase outward into the duodenum through the pancreatic duct to aid in digestion) and an **endocrine gland** (secreting insulin and glucagon into the bloodstream). Insulin is essential for the metabolism of blood sugar and for maintenance of the proper blood sugar level.

Peritoneum. A serous membrane sac composed of the parietal peritoneum lining the abdominal wall and visceral peritoneum containing the viscera in position.

Pylorus, pyloric sphincter, pyloric valve. Valved opening between the stomach and the duodenum.

Pyriform space, sinus. Recess area between the larynx and hypopharyngeal wall.

Small intestine. Proximal portion of the intestine from the *pylorus* to the *ileocecal junction*.

Small salivary glands. Salivary glands distributed throughout the tongue, cheeks, and lips.

Stomach. Organ that prepares food both chemically and mechanically for transport into the small intestine for further digestion.

Thoracic esophagus, distal esophagus. Lower esophagus that passes through the thorax.

Trigone of the bladder. A triangular space at the base of the bladder where the ureters enter and the urethra drains out.

Ureters. Membranous tubes leading from each kidney for urinary passage to the bladder.

Urethra. Membranous tube leading from the bladder for urinary drainage.

Vallecula. Recess on either side of juncture of the base of the tongue and the epiglottis; the plural form is **valleculae.**

B. Descriptive, Diagnostic, and Syndrome Terminology

Achalasia. A common disorder characterized by dilation of the esophagus caused by failure of the cardiac sphincter to relax. This condition can produce aspiration tendencies when the patient is supine (lying on the back). Patients with achalasia typically complain of chest pain, regurgitation, or nocturnal cough. An **epiphrenic diverticulum** occurring just above the diaphragm can be associated with achalasia and other esophageal motility disorders.

Achlorohydria. Lack of hydrochloric acid in the stomach juices.

Acidosis. A condition in which the pH level of the blood falls *below* 7.35.

Acoria. A lack of satisfaction after eating not due to hunger.

Adenotonsillar hyperplasia. Enlarged tonsils or adenoids, potentially leading to airway obstruction.

Ageusia. A loss of taste sensation.

Albumin. A plasma protein considered a good indicator of nutritional status; normal levels in adults should be between 4 and 6 g/dL.

Alkalosis. A condition in which the pH level of the blood is *above* 7.45.

Alliaceous. Tasting like onions or garlic.

Allotriogeusia. Referring to a perverted appetite or sense of taste.

Amblygeusia. Reduced taste sense.

Amino acids. Small substances that are the chief structure of proteins and are produced when proteins are digested and broken down.

Amylase. An enzyme produced by the pancreas that breaks down starch. Lipase, also produced by the pancreas, breaks down triglycerides and lipids.

Anabolism. Constructive phase of metabolism in which the body cells synthesize protoplasm for growth and repair.

Anaphylaxis. An acute reaction to an allergen, for example, a bee sting or certain foods, usually beginning with a tingling sensation, *urticaria* (itching), or a metallic taste in the mouth. Other symptoms can include hives, a sensation of warmth, difficulty breathing or swallowing, vomiting, diarrhea, cramping, a drop in blood pressure, and loss of consciousness. These symptoms may begin within several minutes to 2 hours after exposure to the allergen, but life-threatening reactions may get worse over a period of several hours. Some patients experience what is called a *biphasic reaction*. Often these second-phase symptoms occur in the respiratory tract and may be more severe than the first-phase symptoms. Studies suggest that biphasic reactions occur in about 20% of anaphylactic reactions.

Angioedema. An allergic form of edema, rapid in onset and potentially life threatening, often involving the upper airways, mucous membranes, and bowels.

Ankyloglossia. Tongue tied.

Anorexia. Loss of appetite or desire for food.

Anthropometric assessment. Measures of body size, weight, and proportion as a part of the nutritional assessment.

Aphagia. A complete inability to swallow.

Aphthous stomatitis. Small ulceration of the mucous membrane of the mouth.

Aposia. Lack of thirst.

Aptyalism. Lack of saliva secretion.

Ascites. An accumulation of fluid in the peritoneal cavity.

Aspiration. The entry of secretions, fluids, food, or any foreign substance into the airway.

Asterixis. A motor condition usually associated with hepatic coma and other metabolic conditions in which there are intermittent sustained contractions of muscle postures of the extremities; "liver flap."

Atresia of the esophagus. A congenital absence of the esophageal opening or a congenital esophageal stricture.

Azotemia. Excessive urea or other nitrogenous substances in the blood. *Prerenal azotemia* refers to decreased renal perfusion secondary to congestive heart failure (CHF), shock, or volume depletion.

Barrett's esophagus, Barrett's metaplasia. Referring to a condition characterized by metaplastic epithelium occurring in the lower esophagus following chronic peptic esophagitis.

Basal energy expenditure (BEE), basal metabolic rate (BMR). An individual's energy needs for basic tissue metabolism can be calculated by a mathematical equation that determines caloric requirements depending on the *age*, *sex*, *weight*, and *height* of the patient. The *BEE equation* is sometimes referred to as the **Harris-Benedict** equation or formula (see Table 5–9, Dietitian's Nutritional Assessment).

Bile. Digestive substances produced in the liver and stored in the gallbladder.

Biliary. Carrying or containing bile.

Bilirubin. Pigment produced from the destruction of hemoglobin in the liver and released into bile.

Body mass index (BMI). Calculation of the BMI is the preferred method for determining obesity. The formula is the same for children and adults. Calculate BMI by dividing the person's weight in pounds (lb) by the height in inches (in.) squared and multiplying by a conversion factor of 703; thus the formula is: weight (lb)/[height (in.)]$^2 \times 703$. With the metric system, the formula for BMI is the weight in kilograms divided by the height in meters squared. Because height is commonly measured in centimeters, divide the height in centimeters by 100 to obtain the height in meters. In general, a BMI of less than 22 in adults indicates malnutrition and greater than 27 is considered obese.

Borborygmi. Rumbling or splashing bowel sounds.

Bougie. Tapered, flexible, sausage-shaped tubes of varying diameters used to dilate an orifice.

Buccal. Pertaining to the cheek.

Bulimia. A voracious appetite.

Cachexia. A general wasting away of body tissue; state of malnutrition, emaciation, debilitation, and anemia.

Cacogeusia. A bad taste.

Calorie. The amount of heat necessary to raise the temperature of 1 gram of water 1°C; a **kilocalorie**, kcal, is sometimes called a "large calorie" or "food calorie."

Candidiasis (moniliasis, thrush). Curdlike creamy patches of fungal growth. *Candida albicans* in the mouth or upper gastrointestinal tract may be found in association with antibiotic therapy, diabetes, immune suppression therapy, or immunodeficiency diseases.

Catabolism. Destructive phase of metabolism in which body stores are broken down to maintain basal energy requirements.

Cathartics. Drugs that induce movement of digested material through the bowels (laxatives).

Celiac disease. A genetically determined chronic immunologic intolerance to gluten, causing damage to the villi of the small intestine and resulting in malabsorption of nutrients. This condition is diagnosed by small bowel biopsy and genetic screening for DQ2 and DQ8 markers. Individuals with this condition are required to follow a **gluten-free diet (GFD)**. Celiac disease is thought to be variable, with some individuals having symptomatic conditions and others having silent or latent conditions. Celiac disease is most frequently characterized by diarrhea, abdominal pain or distention, constipation, failure to thrive, and, less frequently, *dermatitis herpetiformis*, *aphthous* (mouth) *ulcers*, and vomiting. It can present at any time but it is most typically found in toddlers and in populations at known risk for the condition, such as individuals with **type 1 diabetes mellitus (T1 DM)** and **Down syndrome**.

Cerebral palsy (CP). Referring to several forms of congenital (present at birth) **static encephalopathies**, resulting from intrauterine or perinatal brain damage, or metabolic, genetic, or systemic factors. The degree and types of speech, language, cognitive, sensorimotor, and swallowing disorders found in children with CP vary depending on the area(s) of the brain that is (are) involved. Movements or postures are characterized as *spastic*, *athetotic* (writhing), *dystonic*, *ataxic*, or *tremorous*.

Cheilosis. An abnormal condition of the lip characterized by reddening and fissures at the corners seen in riboflavin and other B-complex vitamin deficiencies.

Cholecystitis. Inflammation of the gallbladder.

Chyle. The milkylike fluid secreted during intestinal digestion made up of lymph and emulsified fats.

Cirrhosis. A degenerative liver disease characterized by changes in the lobes of the liver and in fat infiltration of the liver's cells.

***Clostridium difficile* (C-diff).** An "overgrowth" organism that causes colitis or enteritis, characterized by watery diarrhea usually brought on by repeated enemas, prolonged nasogastric tube insertion, or gastrointestinal tract surgery. The overuse of antibiotics, especially penicillin (ampicillin), clindamycin, and cephalosporins may also alter the normal intestinal flora and increase the risk of developing this disease. C-diff is a common and difficult to manage complication in children who have had prolonged enteral feedings.

Cleft lip/palate, bifid uvula. Incomplete fusion (unilateral or bilateral) of the tissues of the lip, maxillary processes, or hard or soft palate during fetal development.

Colostrum. The first milk secreted by mothers after delivery.

Congenital cardiac anomalies. Cardiac defects in neonates can include a number of conditions, such as *atrial septal defect* (ASD), *ventricular septal defect* (VSD), *tetrology of Fallot* (TOF), *truncus arteriosus*, *transposition of the great arteries* (TGA), and *hypoplastic left heart syndrome* (HLHS).

Congenital intestinal obstruction. Disorders in neonates that can include *atresia* and *stenosis* of the bowel, *meconium ileus*, *meconium plug syndrome*, *small left colon syndrome* (SLCS), and *hypertrophic pyloric stenosis.*

Continence. The ability to control bowel or bladder elimination.

Creatinine. One of the nonprotein constituents of blood and a component of renal products (urine) formed as the end product of *creatine* metabolism by muscle.

Creatinine height (production) index (CHI). A urine test used to determine lean body mass and degrees of protein depletion.

Deglutition. Swallowing.

Deglutition therapist. An individual trained to provide therapy for swallowing disorders. Deglutition therapy may be a subspecialty of nursing, SLP, or other health professions.

Dehydration. A condition that results from a low volume of body water.

Dentalgia. Pain in a tooth.

Dermatomyositis. A collagen disease characterized by edema; muscular weakness; skin rash; and, in some cases, mucosal lesions.

Diabetes insipidus. A rare form of diabetes characterized by excessive thirst and the passage of large volumes of dilute urine caused by the inability of the kidney tubules to reabsorb water; also called **nephrogenic diabetes insipidus (DI)**. **Central DI** is associated with hypothalamic damage affecting mechanisms associated with an *antidiuretic hormone* (ADH) *deficiency*.

Diabetes mellitus. The most common form of diabetes, commonly referred to as "sugar" diabetes, in which there is a disorder in the metabolism of insulin (hormone produced by the pancreas) and of carbohydrate, protein, and fat, with associated disorders of the structures or functions of the blood vessels. **Type 1 insulin-dependent diabetes mellitus (IDDM)**, formally referred to as juvenile diabetes, is characterized by little or no endogenous insulin secretion. **Type 2 non-insulin-dependent diabetes mellitus (NIDDM)**, the more common form of diabetes mellitus, is characterized by abnormalities in insulin secretion and resistance to the action of insulin, contributing to hyperglycemia. Secondary diabetes can be drug induced or occur as a consequence of other conditions, such as pancreatic disease, hormonal dysfunction, pregnancy, medications, and genetic defects. The term *brittle diabetes* refers to diabetes that is difficult to control with both medication and diet.

Diarrhea. The passage of watery, unformed stools accompanied by abdominal cramping.

Diverticula. Abnormal pouches in the walls of a hollow structure, such as the esophagus or the intestines.

Diverticulitis. Inflammation of the diverticula.

Dumping syndrome. Condition, frequently occurring after a gastrectomy and sometimes following a fundoplication, in which the stomach empties too rapidly and the patient experiences sweating, faintness, flushing, and diarrhea.

Duodenal atresia. Total obstruction of the intestinal lumen (duodenum); often seen in conjunction with Down syndrome.

Dysphagia. An impaired ability to chew or swallow solid or liquid substances often associated with discomfort and aspiration.

Dysphagia management team. A group of health care professionals who collaborate on the evaluation and management of dysphagic persons. At a minimum, these teams usually include a dietitian, an SLP or occupational therapist, a nurse, and a physician.

Edema. An excess of water in the interstitial space within body tissues.

Edentulous. Lacking teeth.

Electrolytes. Chemical compounds that dissolve and separate molecules that carry either a positive or a negative electrical charge.

Emesis. Vomited stomach contents.

Enteritis. Inflammation of the intestine.

Enterostomal therapist. A nurse who has been certified or trained in the care of patients' ostomies.

Eosinophilic esophagitis. A condition in which the cellular structure of the walls of the esophagus have a much higher than normal number of eosinophils. These cells increase in response to allergens and bacteria; thus, eosinophilic esophagitis is felt to be related to an allergic response to certain foods and exposure to other environmental irritants.

Eructation. The discharge of gas from the stomach through the mouth (belching).

Esophageal atresia. An abnormality in which the esophagus terminates prematurely, before extending to the stomach.

Failure to thrive (FTT). In children, FTT is typically defined by one or more of the following factors: a two or greater percentile drop on the growth charts within a 3- to 6-month period; weight to age below the third percentile; or the weight to length ratio below the third percentile.

Fick equation. Formula to determine directly the amount of oxygen consumed in which cardiac output = oxygen consumed (mL/minute × 100) divided by arterial oxygen content minus venous oxygen content. A *reverse Fick equation* refers to an indirect oxygen consumption computation in which resting energy expenditure (REE) = VO_2 1/minute × 5 kcal × 60 minutes × 24 hours.

Flatus. Intestinal gas released from the rectum.

Fluid balance. The state in which water remains in normal amounts and percentages in the body's tissues.

Fluid intake. All sources of fluid consumed or introduced into the body.

Fluid output. All fluid eliminated from the body (through drainage tubes, catheters, wounds, sweating, exhalation, vomiting, defecation, or urination).

Food allergies. A wide array of foods may bring on allergic responses, but the most common problem foods are peanuts, nuts, and shellfish, followed by fish, eggs, wheat, soy, and milk. An allergy to cow's milk is referred to as *cow's milk protein allergy*, or CMPA.

Food jags. Referring to a selective preference in children for an extremely limited variety of foods (e.g., a child who eats only bagels and American cheese).

Free water. Sodium-free water contained in solid foods, enteral feedings, and humidified air.

Gastralgia. Pertaining to pain in the stomach.

Gastric paresis, gastroplegia. Paralysis of part or all of the stomach that is sometimes associated with diabetes.

Gastric ulcers, peptic ulcers. Erosions of gastric mucosa. Acute gastric ulcer can be caused by trauma, major surgery, alcohol abuse, or increased steroid secretions. *Chronic gastric ulcer* can be caused by *chronic peptic disease* usually involving the nonacid secreting antral area of the stomach (antrum). Chronic peptic disease can also produce *peptic strictures* of the esophagus.

Gastrocele. A hernia of the stomach.

Gastrodynia. Pain in the stomach.

Gastromegaly. Abnormally large stomach.

Gastroschisis. Antenatal herniation of the abdominal contents through a paraumbilical (around the umbilicus) defect in the abdominal wall.

Glossodynia. Painful tongue due to a chronic inflammatory process or nutritional deficiency.

Glucose. An odorless, clear or yellowish, thick syrup made up of dextrose (with dextrins, maltose, and water) that results from incomplete hydrolysis of starch; glucose is not normally found in urine, so its presence is indicative of **diabetes mellitus**. An abnormal increase of glucose in the blood is referred to as **hyperglycemia**, and an abnormally low glucose content in the blood is referred to as **hypoglycemia.**

Halitosis. Offensive mouth odor.

Hematemesis. Vomiting blood.

Hemoptysis. Expectoration of blood.

Hiatus hernia, hiatal hernia. A protrusion of part of the stomach through the esophageal opening of the diaphragm.

Hirschsprung's disease. A congenital aganglionosis (absence of nerve cells) causing disruption of the normal colonic transport.

Hypercalcemia. An excessive amount of calcium in the blood. ***Hypo*calcemia** is a deficit of calcium in the blood.

Hyperchloremia. An excessive amount of chloride in the blood. ***Hypo*chloremia** is a deficit of chloride in the blood.

Hyperemesis. Excessive vomiting.

Hyperkalemia. An excessive amount of potassium in the blood. ***Hypo*kalemia** is a deficit of potassium in the blood.

Hypermagnesemia. An excessive amount of magnesium in the blood. ***Hypo*magnesemia** is a deficit of magnesium in the blood.

Hypernatremia. An excessive amount of sodium in the blood. ***Hypo*natremia** is a deficit of sodium in the blood.

Hyperphosphatemia. An excessive amount of phosphate in the blood. ***Hypo*phosphatemia** is a deficit of phosphate in the blood.

Hypertonic solution. A mixture of water with a higher amount of dissolved ionic substances than normally found in the blood.

Hypervolemia. Excessive amount of fluid (water) in the blood. ***Hypo*volemia** is below average amount of fluid (water) in the blood.

Iatrogenic malnutrition. Malnutrition inadvertently produced by medical treatment.

Icterus. Jaundice; yellowish discoloration of the skin, sclera membranes (whites of the eyes), and secretions due to high levels of bilirubin in the blood.

Ileus. Obstruction of the small intestine.

Imperforate anus. A group of congenital anorectal anomalies often associated with infants who have **tracheoesophageal fistulae (TEF)** or **VATER** (*v*ertebral, *a*nal, *t*racheal, *e*sophageal, and *r*enal congenital abnormalities) syndromes. In most cases of imperforate anus, the rectum terminates with a fistula into either the urethra in the male or into the vagina in the female.

Intraventricular hemorrhage. Bleeding within the ventricles.

Intussusception. The common cause of acute intestinal obstruction in infants between 3 and 24 months of age characterized by a telescoping of one segment of the bowel into the more distal segment, usually at the junction of the terminal ileum and the ileocecal valve.

Kwashiorkor syndrome. A malnutrition syndrome associated with a severe protein deficiency.

Low birth weight (LBW). Any child, regardless of gestational age, born with a birth weight of less than 2500 g (5 pounds, 8 ounces).

Malabsorption syndromes. Syndromes resulting in impaired absorption of nutrients by the small bowel.

Malacia. Softening; examples pertinent to SLP include: **laryngomalacia**, softening of the laryngeal tissues; **tracheomalacia**, softening of the tracheal tissues; **bronchomalacia**, softening of the lung tissues.

Mallory-Weiss syndrome. Laceration of the distal esophagus and proximal stomach caused by retching, vomiting, or hiccups. This disorder is seen frequently in chronic alcoholism but may be found in association with other conditions affecting the upper gastrointestinal tract.

Malnutrition. A condition resulting from a lack of proper or adequate nutrients in the diet or from malabsorption.

Marasmus. Malnutrition associated with chronic illness, especially when patients have been maintained on inadequate diets.

Megadose. Ingesting more of a substance than the amount recommended to sustain health (e.g., a megadose of some vitamins can be harmful).

Melena. Black stool or black vomit due to the presence of blood in the gastrointestinal tract.

Metabolic rate, basal metabolic rate (BMR). The rate at which the body burns calories.

Mic-Key. Brand name (rather than nickname) for a pediatric gastrostomy feeding tube opening.

Micturition. Urination; the act of voiding.

Mild alkali syndrome. A disorder that, if unrecognized, can cause irreversible kidney disease; brought on by excessive use of antacids and dehydration.

Milliequivalent. The unit used to measure electrolytes (mEq/liter).

Nausea. Feeling unwell with a desire to vomit.

Necrotizing enterocolitis. A severe, often fatal, disease occurring most frequently in premature infants, characterized by temperature instability, abdominal distention, residual aspirates, bloody stools, bilious vomiting, *acidosis*, **disseminated intravascular**

coagulation (DIC), and *pneumotosis intestinalis*. Necrotizing enterocolitis is associated with conditions such as *asphyxia, hyaline membrane disease, patent ductus arteriosus*, sepsis, and *polycythemia*.

Nitrogen balance. The state of the body relative to ingestion and excretion of protein. A *positive nitrogen balance* indicates adequate protein ingestion. A *negative nitrogen balance* indicates protein depletion and malnutrition; **nitrogenous waste** refers to substances containing nitrogen that are mostly excreted in urine, including **uric acid** and **urea.**

Obesity. A condition in which there is an excessive amount of body fat; clinically, obesity is diagnosed when patients have a BMI of 30 or greater.

Occlusal. In dentistry, pertaining to the contacting (biting) surfaces of the teeth; referring generally to closure.

Odynophagia. Pain associated with swallowing.

Omphalocele. A congenital defect that can vary from a small bulge at the base of the umbilicus to a sac containing the intestines.

Patent. A tube or vessel that is open and unobstructed.

Perinatal asphyxia. A state of decreased oxygenation to the newborn at the time of delivery sufficient to cause neurologic damage.

Periodontal disease. Disease of the gums, leading to tooth decay and tooth loss related to aging, inadequate oral hygiene, or diseases and conditions producing poor oral hygiene such as deficient salivation.

Peristalsis. The rhythmic muscular contractions within hollow organs, for example, the movement of contents through the alimentary (gastrointestinal) tract.

Periventricular leukomalacia (PVL). Damage to the white matter of the brain.

pH. The expression of hydrogen ion concentration in fluids.

Phenylketonuria (PKU). A congenital disorder in which infants are born lacking the enzyme to break down phenylalanine, which could potentially lead to mental retardation. PKU screening tests are performed to detect phenylketonuria or phenylalanine following delivery on all infants in U.S. hospitals, and if PKU is detected, a low-protein, phenylalanine restricted diet is implemented through adulthood.

Pica. A craving to eat unusual or nonnutritive substances.

Piecemeal swallow. An inability to clear the entire bolus with one swallow.

Pierre-Robin sequence. A congenital craniofacial anomaly with micrognathia, glossoptosis, and a U-shaped posterior cleft palate.

Pitting edema. A condition in which a "pit" or impression is left after pressure is applied to edematous skin tissue.

Plasma. The fluid component of blood.

Polydipsia. Excessive thirst.

Polyphagia. Excessive eating.

Polyuria. Excessive urination.

Presbyphagia, presbyesophagus. Swallowing and esophageal dysmotility problems related to normal physiological changes in aging and associated pathologic conditions.

Proctalgia. Pertaining to pain in or around the rectum.

Projectile vomiting. Vomiting with great force.

Protein-calorie malnutrition (PCM) syndrome. Two overlapping syndromes of malnourishment in children (diagnoses are sometimes used with adults) are included as forms of PCM, ***kwashiorkor syndrome***, and **marasmus**. Kwashiorkor syndrome refers to the severe protein deficiency with edema and ascites and stunted growth found in poorly nourished children; marasmus refers to the severe cachexia with growth deficiencies in children with inadequate diets (and a history of early weaning or lack of breastfeeding). Children with PCM are frequently found to have mental retardation, possibly as a result of decreased myelination.

Pseudodiverticula. Esophageal glands that have become dilated, appearing to be diverticula.

Ptyalism. Excessive secretion of saliva.

Pyloric stenosis. A congenital condition seen in newborns characterized by an overgrowth of muscle fibers, diminishing the lumen of the pylorus.

Pyrosis. Heartburn.

Recommended daily (dietary) allowance (RDA). The daily amount of nutrients that the body needs (varies by age, weight, and activity level).

Reflux. The expulsion of stomach contents into the esophagus or hypopharynx.

Renin. A substance produced by the kidney that controls the narrowing of blood vessels all over the body, thus controlling blood pressure.

Respiratory distress syndrome, hyaline membrane disease. A condition seen in premature newborns who lack sufficient surfactant in the lungs to allow them to breathe adequately.

Retropulsion, reverse peristalsis. Esophageal or intestinal dysmotility causing contents to be pushed upward through the esophagus or gastrointestinal tract.

Rhabdomyolysis. Disintegration or breakdown of muscle characterized by myoglobin in the urine.

Riley-Day syndrome. Familial dysautonomia in which there is a delay in the cricopharyngeal sphincter relaxation, resulting in aspiration tendencies.

Rokitansky's diverticulum. A traction diverticulum in the esophagus.

Rumination. Rechewing food regurgitated from the stomach; more often seen in infants.

Saliva. The secretions that contain *amylase* and serve to moisten, dissolve, and transport food for digestion.

Sandifer's syndrome. A dystonic torticollis posture seen in children in response to GER, hiatal hernia, or esophagitis.

Schatski's ring. Lower esophageal stricture in the region of the squamocolumnar junction.

Scleroderma, progressive systemic sclerosis. A systemic disease characterized by skin tightening and fibrosis of smooth muscles with which there may be an associated dysphagia.

Seatorrhea. Excessive fat in the stool.

Serum albumin and transferrin. A measure of visceral protein stores and malnutrition.

Short bowel syndrome. State of malabsorption caused by resection of a large part of the small intestine to correct colitis, atresia, volvulus, and other GI abnormalities.

Sialoadenitis, sialadentitis. Inflammation of a salivary gland usually characterized by painful swelling of the gland.

Sjögren's syndrome. Inflammation of the lacrimal glands and salivary glands sometimes affecting swallowing.

Skin turgor. The fullness of the skin in relationship to the underlying tissue; an indicator of fluid balances in the body.

Stasis. Not moving.

Stomatitis. Inflammation of the mucosa of the mouth.

Strangury. Painful urination due to spasmodic muscle contraction.

Subglottic stenosis. Narrowing of the airway below the level of the vocal folds usually characterized by stridor and uncoordinated **suck-swallow-breath (SSB)** patterns.

Swallow control center. An area of the medulla oblongata on the floor of the fourth ventricle where the central nervous system nuclei that control swallowing are located.

Third spacing. A condition in which body fluids become trapped in interstitial areas usually due to a loss of plasma proteins. Third spacing can occur suddenly when a patient is *burned,* suffers a *crushing injury*, goes through *surgical manipulation*, or has an *allergic reaction*; or it can occur slowly in certain types of liver or kidney diseases.

Tracheoesophageal fistula (TEF). Abnormal opening between the trachea and esophagus.

Trench mouth (Vincent's infection). An inflammatory condition of the gums associated with pain, ulcerations, fever, bleeding, and lymphadenopathy.

Trismus. An inability to open the mouth fully; it can occur in patients who have undergone surgery or radiation treatment to the mouth.

Turgor. The fullness of the skin relative to the underlying tissue.

Tympanites. A condition that results when intestinal gas accumulates and is not expelled (intestinal distention); *meteorism.*

Urgency. A sensation of needing to urinate immediately.

Very low birth weight (VLBW). Any child, regardless of gestational age, who weighs less than 1500 grams (3 pounds, 3 ounces); birth weight less than 1000 grams (2 pounds, 2 ounces) is described as an **extremely low birth weight (ELBW).**

Volvulus. A twisting of the bowel (or other organ) on itself, causing an obstruction.

Waterbrash. Stomach contents that are regurgitated into the mouth.

Wilms' tumor. A malignant tumor occurring in childhood that is curable if treated early with surgery, radiation, or chemotherapy.

Xerostomia. Insufficient secretion of saliva; dry mouth.

Zenker's diverticulum. A posterior diverticulum of the esophagus usually in the cervical esophagus.

Zollinger-Ellison syndrome. A syndrome of extreme gastritis marked by hypergastrinemia, gastric hypersecretion, and peptic ulceration.

C. Abbreviations

AA. Age adjusted
a.c. Before meals (*ante cibum*)
ACBE. Air contrast barium enema
ADH. Antidiuretic hormone
A/G. Albumin globulin (ratio)
AKI. Acute kidney injury
Alb. Albumin
ALP. Alkaline phosphatase
AODM. Adult-onset diabetes mellitus
Aq. Water (*aqua*)
ASD. Atrial septal defect
ATC. Around the clock
ATP. Adenosine triphosphate
Ba. Barium
BaE. Barium enema
BAO. Basal acid output
BEE. Basal Energy Expenditure
b.i.d. Two times a day (*bis in die*)
BM. Bowel movement
BMI. Body mass index
BMR. Basal metabolic rate
BPD. Bronchopulmonary dysphagia
BRP. Bathroom privileges
B.S. Blood sugar
BUN. Blood urea nitrogen
BW. Body weight
Ca. Calcium
Cal. Calorie
CCK-PZ. Cholecystokinin-pancreotzymin
C & DB. Cough and deep breaths
CDCA. Chenodeoxycholic acid
C-diff. *Clostridium difficile*
CHO. Carbohydrate
Cho. Cholesterol
cib. Food (*cibus*)
Cl. Chloride
CLD. Chronic lung disease
CMPA. Cow's milk protein allergy
CRF. Chronic renal failure
CUC. Chronic ulcerative colitis
DAT. Diet as tolerated
D5W. 5% dextrose in water
D5RL. 5% dextrose in Ringer's lactate
D5S. 5% dextrose in saline
DHFT. Dobbhoff (enteric) feeding tube
EBM. Expressed breast milk
E. coli. *Escherichia coli*
EE. eosinophilic esophagitis
EGD. Endoscopic gastroduodenoscopy
EIP. Esophageal intraluminal pseudodiverticulosis
ERCP. Endoscopic retrograde cholangiopancreatography
ESRD. End-stage renal disease
FB. Foreign body
FBS. Fasting blood sugar
Fe. Iron
F/F. Removable full denture
FN. Fully nourished
FOS, FOF. Full of stool, full of feces
FTT. Failure to thrive
GB. Gallbladder
GEJ. Gastroesophageal juncture
GER. Gastroesophageal reflux
GERD. Gastroesophageal reflux disease
GGT. Gamma-glutamyl transferase, gamma-glutamyl transpeptidase
GI. Gastrointestinal, gastroenterology
GIP. Gastric inhibitory peptide

GNB, GNR. Gram-negative bacillus, gram-negative rod

GTT. Glucose tolerance test

GU. Genitourinary

HAA. Hepatitis-associated antigen

HAV. Hepatitis A virus

HBIG. Hepatitis B immune globulin

HBV. Hepatitis B virus

HCl. Hydrochloric acid

HCV. Hepatitis C virus

Hyper al. Hyperalimentation

I & O. intake and output

IBS. Irritable bowel syndrome

IBW. Ideal body weight

ICG. Indocyanine green

IDDM. Insulin-dependent diabetes mellitus

INF. Intravenous nutritional fluid

IRDM. Insulin-resistant diabetes mellitus

IUGR. Intrauterine growth restriction

IV. Intravenous

IVC. Intravenous cholangiography

IVF. Intravent hemorrhage

IVP. Intravenous pyelogram

JJT/JT. Jejunostomy tube

K. Potassium

kcal. Kilocalorie

kg. Kilogram

KUB. Kidneys, ureters, and bladder

LB. Large bowel

LDH. Lactic dehydrogenase

LES. Lower esophageal sphincter

LFT. Liver function test

LGI. Lower gastrointestinal (tract)

LS scan. Liver spleen scan

L/W. Length to weight ratio

MN. Midnight

MOM. Milk of magnesia

M & R. Measure and record

MVit. Multivitamin

Na. Sodium

NCS. No concentrated sweets

NDD. National Dysphagia Diet

NEC. Necrotizing enterocolitis

NG. Nasogastric tube

NH_3, NH_4. Ammonia, ammonium

NIDDM. Non-insulin-dependent diabetes mellitus

NIT. Nasointestinal tube

NN. Negative for sugar and acetone

NPO. Nothing by mouth (*non per os*)

NPO $\bar{p}$ MN. Nothing by mouth after midnight

NSS. Nonnutritive stimulation, nonnutritive sucks

N&V. Nausea and vomiting

Nx. Nourishment

OCG. Oral cholecystography

O&P. Ova and parasites

P. Phosphorus

PAB. Prealbumin

p.c. After meals (*post cibum*)

PCM. Protein caloric malnutrition

PEM. Protein energy malnutrition

PDA. Patent ductus arteriosus

PEG. Percutaneous endoscopic gastrostomy

PEJ. Percutaneous endoscopic jejunostomy

PKU. Phenylketonuria

p.o. By mouth (*per os*)

PP. After meals (*postprandial*)

PROM. Premature rupture of membranes

PTC. Percutaneous transhepatic cholangiography

PUD. Peptic ulcer disease

q. Every (*quaque*)

***q.* a.m.** Every morning

q.h. Every hour (*quaque hora*)

q.i.d. Four times a day (*quarter in die*)

***q.* s.** Every shift

***q.* 2h.** Every 2 hours

RDA. Recommended daily allowance

SB. Small bowel

SBS. Short bowel syndrome

S-G. Swan-Ganz (catheter)

SSB. Suck-swallow-breathe

T & A. Tonsillectomy and adenoidectomy

TEF. Tracheoesophageal fistula

t.i.d. Three times a day (*ter in die*)

TOF. Tetralogy of Fallot

TPN. Total parenteral nutrition

U/A. Urinalysis

UDCA. Ursodeoxycholic acid

UES. Upper esophageal sphincter

UGI. Upper gastrointestinal

UTI. Urinary tract infection

VCU. Voiding cystourethrogram

VFSS. Videofluoroscopic swallow study

VLBW, ELBW. Very low birth weight; extremely low birth weight

Wt. Weight

III. PROCEDURES, TESTS, AND THERAPIES

Also see "Commonly Ordered Tests and Procedures" in Chapter 3; Chapter 7 for more elaborated descriptions of radiologic studies; Chapter 4 for descriptions of neurologic studies; and "Gastrointestinal and Other Abdominal Surgeries and Procedures" in Chapter 13.

Abbott-Rawson tube. A type of double-channel tube for injecting or aspirating fluid from the stomach.

Acid perfusion test. A test comparing subjective responses to saline versus decinormal hydrochloric acid perfused into the esophagus through a nasogastric tube; used to differentiate cardiovascular midchest pain from painful esophageal reflux.

Artificial saliva. Oral wetting agent prepared with properties similar to saliva and used to diminish "dry mouth," or xerostomia, and to assist with digestion of foods.

Auscultation of swallowing. Listening by means of a stethoscope to swallowing sounds (*cervical auscultation*) to determine the presence of aspiration; or listening to stomach sounds (*stomach auscultation*, or *left upper quadrant* [LUQ] *auscultation*) to determine if a nasogastric tube is properly placed. In the latter procedure, an air bolus is injected through the nasogastric tube after placement, and LUQ auscultation is used to listen for the air released ("whoosh" sound) into the stomach.

Balloon tamponade. An emergency procedure using a balloon catheter to control bleeding from esophageal varices.

Barium fluoroscopy; upper GI study; upper esophageal series; barium fluorogram; cinesophagram. Radiologic studies of oral, pharyngeal, hypopharyngeal, and esophageal structures and dynamic functions through the use of x-ray with barium (or barium with air).

Depending on its purpose, the study may utilize fluoroscopy, rapid series films, videofluoroscopy (videotapes or digital image recordings), or cinefluoroscopy (motion picture films).

Barium swallow (BaS); modified barium swallow (MBS), videofluoroscopic swallow study. Radiologic study using thin and thick liquid barium, paste barium, barium pills, barium-coated cookies, or barium mixed with soft solid food substances (e.g., pudding, marshmallows, applesauce) for the purpose of examining swallowing structures and dynamic swallowing functions with particular attention to the oral and pharyngeal phases of swallow and aspiration risks.

Celestin tube. Latex tube used to bypass tumors in the esophagus.

Cholecystography. X-ray examination of the gallbladder using radiopaque dye.

Colonoscopy. Examination of the *upper and lower portions* of the colon. A **sigmoidoscopy** refers to an examination of the rectosigmoid, or *lower portion*, of the large bowel.

Dialysis. A procedure that removes water and toxic chemicals from the body and is used when the kidneys can no longer perform that function. **Hemodialysis** is a procedure using an artificial kidney machine to filter wastes from the bloodstream. **Peritoneal dialysis** is a procedure in which fluid is introduced through a peritoneal catheter into the abdominal cavity, causing highly concentrated wastes circulating in the peritoneum to diffuse out of the bloodstream and into the fluid for removal. **Continuous arteriovenous hemofiltration (CAVH)** is a method similar to dialysis in which blood is removed from the body and waste is filtered out. This procedure is amenable for use in intensive care units with critically ill patients.

Dilation, dilatation. Expansion of an organ, orifice, or stricture in a tube, such as the esophagus, usually with an instrument such as specially gauged dilators, or "bougies," referred to as *bouginage dilation*.

Electroglottography (EGG). Technique used to examine laryngeal displacement and glottal motions during speech and swallowing through the use of a two-channel oscilloscope, a pressure transducer (with electrodes placed on each side of the thyroid cartilage), and an amplifier.

Elemental diet. Specially prepared formulas in which the protein chains are broken down, or "predigested," to allow for absorption in individuals who have food allergies or malabsorption syndromes.

Enteral hyperalimentation. Nutrition and hydration support through feeding tubes introduced into the gastrointestinal tract (see Figure 5–6 for illustrations of various routes of enteral [tube] feeding).

Enterostomy. The creation of an opening into the intestine.

Entriflex tube, En-tube Plus. Types of feeding tubes.

Epinephrine pens. Self-injectable doses of epinephrine prescribed for emergency use for individuals who have a known severe cardiovascular collapse in response to foods and other allergens.

Esophageal gastric tube airway, esophageal obturator airway. Tube with an inflatable balloon cuff obturator inserted into the esophagus to occlude the esophagus and prevent aspiration of stomach contents during endotracheal intubation and ventilation (Figure 5–3).

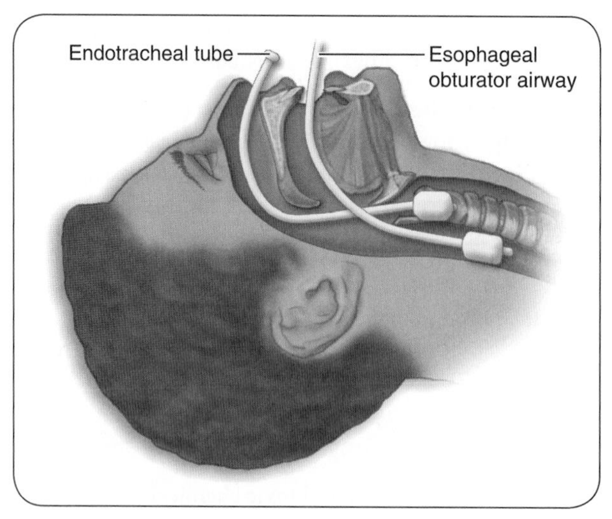

FIGURE 5–3 Esophageal obturator airway. Source: Delmar/Cengage Learning

E-Stim. In dysphagia treatment, E-Stim is used for the purpose of enhancing a motor response of the swallowing musculature to improve swallowing functions by applying **neuromuscular electrical stimulation** (NMES), which is a low-voltage current delivered through the skin to excite motor nerves, causing muscle contraction.

Extracorporeal hemoperfusion. A procedure utilizing sorbents to remove potential toxins, for treatment of drug overdoses that are not removed by dialysis, or for the removal of ammonia and other toxins from the patient in hepatic coma.

Fiberoptic endoscopic examination of swallowing safety (FEESS). Endoscopic examination of oropharyngeal functions during swallowing. FEESS studies may be videotaped.

Fiberoptic endoscopy. Visualization and, in some cases, biopsy tissue sampling through the use of a fiberoptic, flexible endoscope inserted into a hollow organ (*nasendoscopy, colonoscopy, duodenoscopy, gastroduodenoscopy, esophagastroscopy, gastroscopy, peritoneoscopy, laryngoscopy, proctosigmoidoscopy*, etc.). Figure 5–4 illustrates an endoscopic examination of the upper gastrointestinal (GI) tract.

Frazier Free Water Protocol. A hydration protocol that originated with the Frazier Rehabilitation Center in Louisville, Kentucky, which essentially allows most individuals to have access to water despite having a diagnosis of dysphagia.

Fundoplication, Nissen fundoplication. Procedure in which the upper portion of the stomach wall is wrapped around the stomach opening to prevent chronic, severe gastric reflux, as illustrated in Figure 5–5.

Gamma-glutamyl transferase (GGT). A test performed on blood serum to determine the level of an enzyme found in the liver, kidney, prostate, heart, and spleen. Increased levels of GGT can indicate a number of conditions, including cirrhosis, liver necrosis, hepatitis, alcoholism, neoplasm, acute pancreatitis, acute myocardial infarction, nephrosis, and acute cholecystitis.

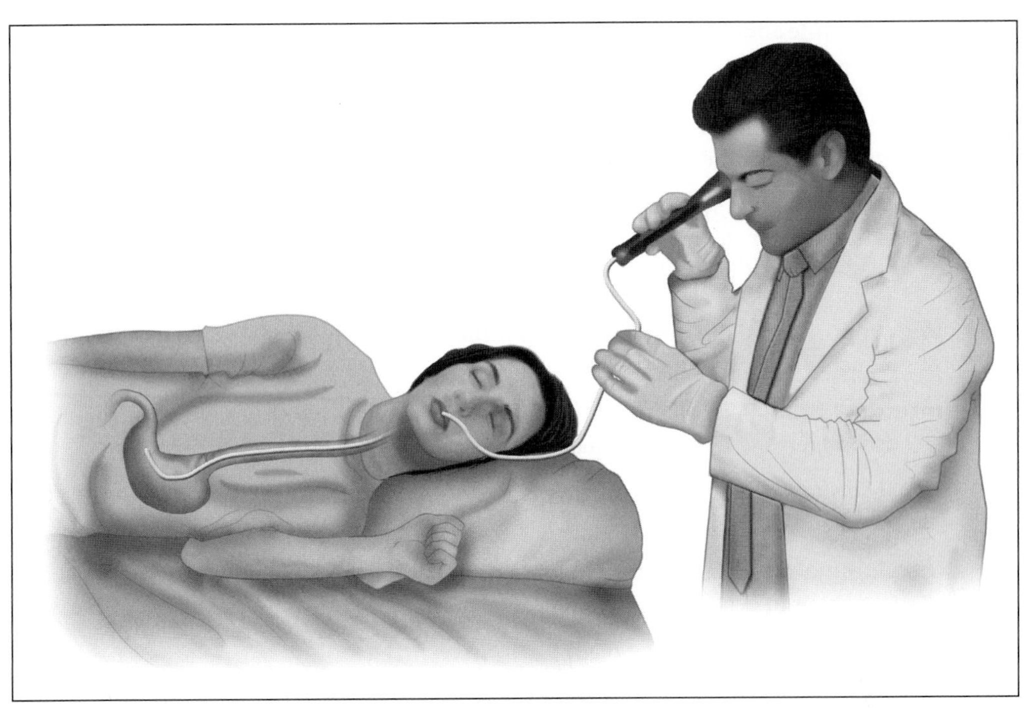

FIGURE 5–4 Gastrointestinal endoscopy. Source: Delmar/Cengage Learning

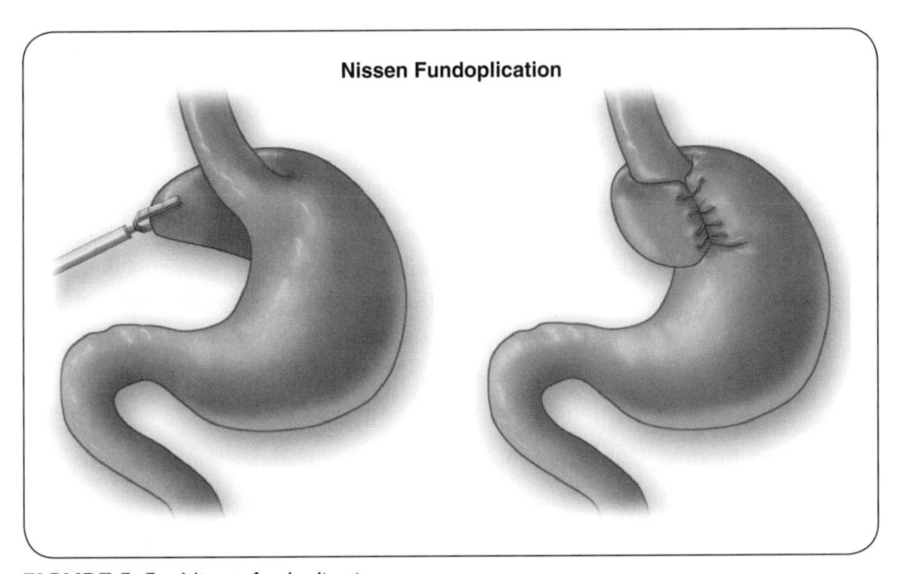

FIGURE 5–5 Nissen fundoplication. Source: Delmar/Cengage Learning

Gastraview, Gastragrafin study. Trademarked names for contrast preparations used in radiologic studies. Gastraview studies are usually ordered to examine for fistulae in the GI tract prior to abdominal surgeries when barium residues would be problematic.

Gavage. Feeding directly into the stomach by way of a tube.

Haberman feeder, Dr. Brown Bottle. Two examples from several types of nipple devices and bottle shapes used to feed infants with structural (e.g., cleft palate) or oral motor weakness (CP with low tone) and a related difficulty with intraoral pressure, sucking, and swallowing. These and similar devices are used when a slower flow rate with bottle feeding is found (usually during the videofluoroscopic swallow study) to facilitate oral intake.

Heme Quant test. A quantitative assay to detect a heme-positive reaction (presence of blood) in the patient's stool (feces).

Hepatic antigen. A test to determine the presence of the hepatitis B virus.

H_2 receptor blockers, protein pump inhibitors. Drugs administered for the purpose of reducing or eliminating gastric acid secretion.

Intestinal tube. Referring to any type of tube used to provide an access for nutrition, to decompress the stomach or small bowel, or to obtain fluids from the intestine.

Intraesophageal pH monitoring, pH probe. Procedure for monitoring gastric reflux across a 24-hour sampling period.

Intraluminal multiple electrical impedance. Measure of electrical resistance in the esophagus to determine the volume of material passing through and clearing the esophagus.

Ketonic diet. Special high-fat diet.

Lavage. To wash out a cavity. *Gastric lavage* is used to remove stomach contents by aspiration and flushing out contents with a stomach tube ("stomach pump"). *Diagnostic peritoneal lavage* (DPL) is a procedure used to examine for a ruptured bowel or bleeding into the peritoneum.

Manometry. An intraluminal measure of pressures used to determine the force and velocity of peristalsis of the upper and lower esophageal sphincters. *Manofluoroscopy* combines computerized manography with barium fluoroscopy to examine for pressure gradients relative to bolus flow actions.

Mecholyl test. A test using a cholinergic drug, mecholyl, to evaluate esophageal achalasia.

Methylene blue test. Use of a blue-colored dye (0.5 mL in 30 mL of water) mixed with food in a clinical evaluation of swallow; any evidence of blue coloring detected in the aspirate from tracheostomy suctioning indicates aspiration of the swallowed material. Food coloring may also be used to assess aspiration in the same manner.

Minnesota tube. A multiple balloon tube apparatus similar to the Stengstaken-Blakemore tube used to treat esophageal or stomach varices.

Murphy drip. Continuous bladder irrigation through a triple-lumen urinary catheter (Foley catheter).

Nasendoscopy, nasopharyngoscopy. Procedures for directly visualizing the nasal, palatal, pharyngeal, laryngeal, and esophageal structures usually with a fiberoptic endoscope.

Nasogastric (NG) feedings. Enteral nutrition and hydration support through the use of a tube passed into the nasal passages through the pharynx and esophagus into the upper GI tract.

Nasojejunal (NJ) feedings. Feedings by way of a tube inserted through the nose and into the stomach for passage through the pyloric sphincter and duodenum into the jejunum (Figure 5–6).

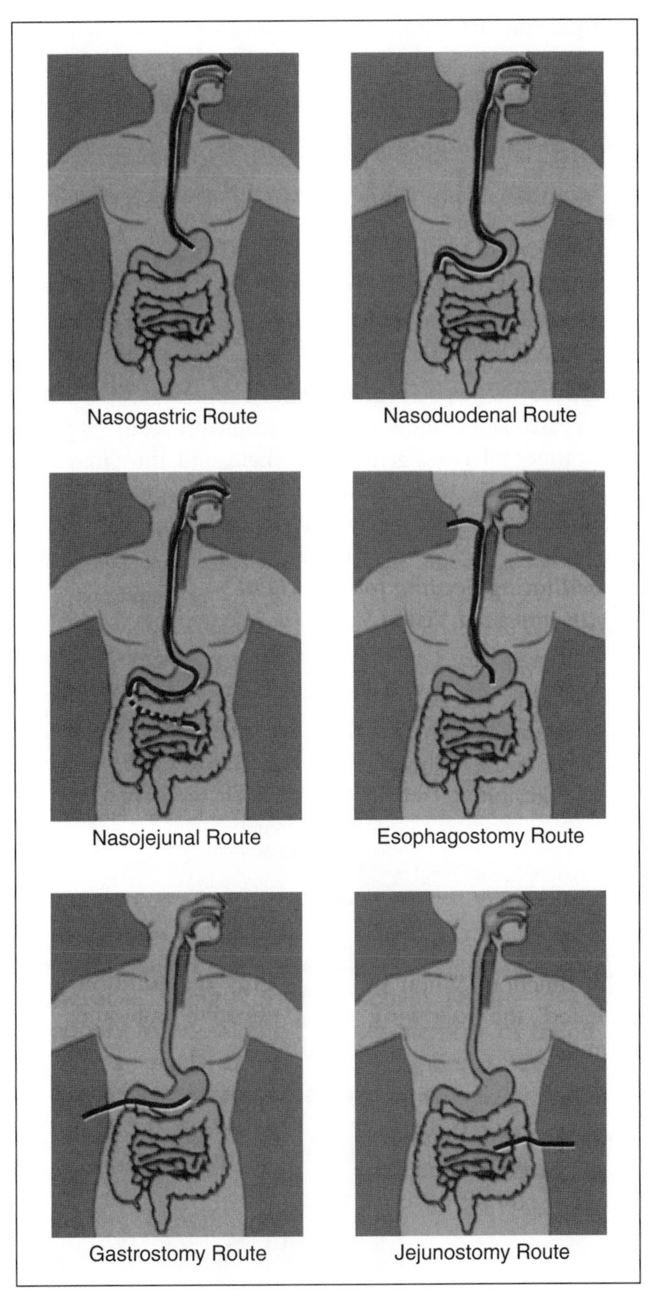

FIGURE 5–6 Enteral feeding routes. Source: Delmar/Cengage Learning

Nonnutritive suck. Inserting a gloved little finger or pacifier in a newborn's or infant's mouth for the purpose of assessing the sucking ability of the child or to provide oral stimulation.

Oral glucose tolerance test (OGTT). Test for excessive levels of glucose in the blood following the oral administration of a volume of glucose.

Orogastric feedings. Enteral feedings preferred for infants in which oral tubes rather than nasogastric tubes are used. Newborns are "nose breathers" and the nasogastric tube may partially occlude the airway and compromise the infants' respiration.

Panorex. Trademarked name of a radiologic procedure using two axes of rotation to obtain a panoramic radiograph of the dentition and the dental arches.

Parenteral hyperalimentation. A method used to supply the necessary nutrients directly into the bloodstream usually by means of a catheter inserted through a **central venous catheter placement**, or cannulation, which is referred to as a **"central line."** The subclavian vein or a right atrial catheter placement is most often used for parenteral hyperalimentation (Figure 5–7). The term **total parenteral nutrition (TPN)** is a synonym (see definition).

Percutaneous endoscopic gastrostomy (PEG). An endoscopic procedure performed for insertion of a gastrostomy tube. This endoscopic procedure is preferred in cases where a patient cannot tolerate a general anesthetic and, thus, may be performed by a gastroenterologist with only local anesthesia and mild sedation. See Figure 5–6 for illustrations of methods for direct feeding tube placement in the GI tract and Figures 13–2 and 13–3 in Chapter 13, illustrating related gastric surgeries and other procedures.

Pharyngotomy. Creation of an opening into the pharynx usually for the purpose of providing a feeding method.

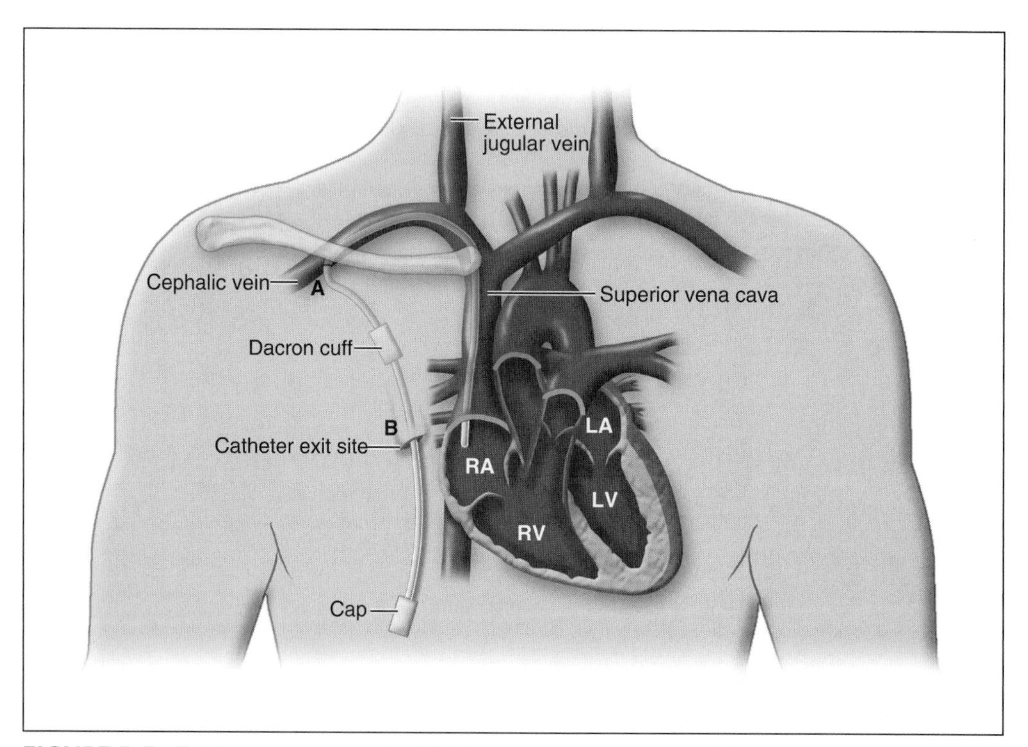

FIGURE 5–7 Total parenteral nutrition (TPN). (A) Vascular access site. (B) Cutaneous exit site of the catheter. Source: Delmar/Cengage Learning

Prealbumin (PAB) assessment. A blood test used to determine the adequacy of nutritional support. A PAB level of ≤15 mg/dL indicates **protein energy (caloric) malnutrition (PEM)**.

Renal biopsy. A percutaneous technique used to extract and examine kidney tissue.

Scintigraphy. A radionuclide study used to detect gastroesophageal reflux, esophageal motility, and aspiration.

Small bowel biopsy and duodenal aspiration. To achieve this small bowel study, a lubricated, mercury-filled Rubin-Quinton tube or Carey capsule is placed in the oropharynx and swallowed by the patient, allowing the tube to enter the stomach. It is then manipulated under fluoroscopic guidance through the pylorus into the duodenum. With negative pressure (suction), contents and mucosa can be aspirated from the tip of the tube.

Small bowel studies, lower GI studies, large bowel studies, barium enemas. Radiologic examinations of the small and large intestines.

Stool culture. A test performed on feces to determine the presence of organisms.

Surface electromyography (sEMG). In dysphagia treatment, sEMG is used to monitor the surface activity of the muscles involved in swallowing as a biofeedback tool for training swallowing maneuvers in rehabilitation.

Sweat chloride. Test for cystic fibrosis.

Total parenteral nutrition (TPN), parenteral hyperalimentation (hyper al). Long-term intravenous nutrition, or TPN, is a nutritional support method in which an *amino acid-glucose-lipid infusate* is introduced directly into a central vein (usually the subclavian vein) by means of disposable tubing and an *infusion pump* to maintain a constant infusion rate through a large intravenous catheter. TPN is used with patients who have severe digestive abnormalities and is prescribed to provide an amount of nitrogen that meets or exceeds the amount required to maintain nutritional equilibrium to allow protein synthesis and weight maintenance or gain. Patients who are likely to receive TPN include those who are in a *mild catabolic state* following surgery or are severely malnourished and require nutritional therapy prior to surgery; those in *a hypermetabolic state* (as found after bodily trauma, severe burns, head injury, cancer, and sepsis); those with pancreatitis; those *without a functioning gut;* and those with a *gastrointestinal obstruction*, or *short bowel syndrome.*

Tube feedings. Introducing nourishment through an enteral tube directly into the GI tract. The term *gastric gavage* is synonymous.

Ultrasonographic examinations of dysphagia. Use of ultrasound for detecting soft tissue movements during swallow and determining any aspiration tendencies. This technique is felt to be useful with infants or other patients who are not easily studied with fluoroscopy.

Umbilical catheter. A central catheter inserted directly into the umbilical vessels (artery or vein) in neonates.

Urinary catheter. A small-bore tube usually placed into the bladder to drain urine. Indwelling catheters, such as the triple-lumen Foley catheters, have small inflatable balloons to secure the tube for an extended period. Condoms attached to tubing ("condom catheters") and external urinary devices with adhesive bags may be used for the collection of urine from males and infants.

Videofluoroscopic swallow study (VFSS). A modified barium swallow study conducted under fluoroscopy and recorded (videotaped or with digitized images) to examine dynamic swallowing functions and risk for aspiration from the oral phase, pharyngeal phase, and upper esophageal phase of swallow.

IV. ENTERAL AND PARENTERAL NUTRITION

When oral intake is not possible, safe, or sufficient to meet a patient's nutritional needs, then **enteral hyperalimentation** (nutrition by way of tubes placed in the *GI tract*) or **TPN** (nutrition by way of solutions infused directly into the *bloodstream*) are necessary (see Figure 5–7). Enteral hyperalimentation is usually achieved through a lubricated, small-bore, weighted feeding tube (such as a **Dobbhoff feeding tube**) that is passed through a nostril into the nasopharynx and esophagus into the stomach or directed through the stomach for transpyloric passage into the duodenum or jejunum. Enteral feeding may be temporary, through the use of nasogastric, nasoduodenal, or nasojejunal tubes, or long term, through the use of *gastrointestinal tubes* (G-tubes). G-tubes are placed *percutaneously* (through the skin) directly into the stomach, duodenum, or *jejunum* (JJTs) or directly into the esophagus. Feeding tubes sometimes have both a gastric and a jejunal port for bolus feedings directly into the stomach via the gastric access and continuous (pump) feedings into the small bowel via the jejunal port. Percutaneous feeding tubes can be removed or "taken down" once the patient achieves the ability to maintain nutrition and hydration needs safely by oral intake (see Figure 5–6). In small children, the button opening into a G-tube is sometimes called a Mic-Key, referring to the brand name for a low-profile feeding tube (see Figure 13–3).

When enteral feeding tubes are inserted, placement is confirmed through LUQ auscultation or x-ray. The hospital's dietitians select the formulas, methods, and rates for the enteric feeding solutions. Feedings may be bolus feedings that are intermittent (at particular times of day) or continuous, depending on the type of solution required and the patient's medical and nutritional status. Volumes and feeding rates will be calculated according to the individual factors for adults and children. Table 5–1 lists generally recommended fluid requirements for infants and children.

An **infusion pump**, or gravity infusion, specifically designed for prescribed infusion rates with enteral feeding may be selected, depending on the patient's needs and tolerances. Enteral feeding products commonly used include *Dobbhoff feeding tubes* with Dobbhoff enteric feeding bags and pump

TABLE 5–1 Generally recommended fluid requirements for children

WEIGHT OF CHILD	TARGET
1–10 kg	100 mL/kg
11–20 kg	1,000 mL + 50 mL/kg > 10 kg
>20 kg	1,500 mL + 20 mL/kg > 20 kg

Source: Adapted from Klint, A., & Scott, L. (2008). *Collaboration between the clinical dietitian and speech-language pathologist in the treatment of children with feeding difficulties.* Guidelines presented at the Pediatric Feeding and Swallowing Training Module, Vanderbilt University, Nashville, TN, January 2008, with permission.

(Biosearch Medical Products, Inc.); *Corpak feeding tubes*; *Flexiflo Flexitainer* feeding bag and enteral feeding formula (Ross Laboratories); *Kangaroo tube-feeding set* with a Kangaroo 220 enteral feeding pump (Chesebrough-Ponds, Inc.); *Life Care Pump* (Abbott Laboratories); *IVAC Enteral feeding pump* (IVAC Corporation); and *Moss compression feeding catheters* designed for surgical patients.

TPN, described earlier, is used with nutritionally depleted patients for whom enteral (GI tract) hyperalimentation is not an option (see definition of TPN). TPN solutions consist of a *nitrogen source* (protein), *hypertonic dextrose* and *lipids*, and *supplementary vitamins* and *minerals*, which are infused into a central vein, typically the subclavian vein, or the internal jugular. *Right atrial catheters* are placed for long-term TPN, and the most commonly used catheters are Hickman, Broviac, and Centracil catheters (see Figure 5–7). Other intravenous solutions are not recommended to be "piggybacked" onto a TPN line; however, a Hickman catheter has a double lumen, which allows for continuous TPN infusion and intermittent infusion of medications and additional therapies. TPN can be infused through a **peripherally inserted central venous catheter (PICC) line**. These lines are preferred in the home setting, because they have a lower infection rate. Peripheral parenteral support utilizes a moderate osmolality formula and lipids.

V. NUTRITION, HYDRATION, AND ORAL FEEDING IN INFANTS AND CHILDREN

A. Nutrition and Hydration

The GI tract of the *premature* infant often does not tolerate adequate fluid volumes to meet the infant's fluid or caloric demands. Additionally, prior to reaching a gestational age of approximately 32 to 34 weeks, the infant lacks a coordinated suck-swallow-breathe (SSB) pattern and, thus, has not adequately developed the oral motor ability to allow for adequate intake from a breast or bottle. Consequently, enteral feeding is typically used until the infant reaches a gestational age of 32 to 34 weeks and has no evidence of respiratory distress. Table 5–1 provides a summary of the fluid needs of neonates and children. Table 5–2 provides a summary of the recommended dietary allowances for infants and children.

TABLE 5–2 Generally recommended daily allowance (RDA) for caloric needs in children

AGE RANGE	TARGET
Birth to 6 months	108 kcal/kg
6–12 months	98 kcal/kg
1–3 years	102 kcal/kg
4–6 years	90 kcal/kg
7–10 years	70 kcal/kg

Source: Adapted from Klint, A., & Scott, L. (2008). *Collaboration between the clinical dietitian and speech-language pathologist in the treatment of children with feeding difficulties.* Guidelines presented at the Pediatric Feeding and Swallowing Training Module, Vanderbilt University, Nashville, TN, January 2008, with permission.

Food Aversions

Children who are born prematurely or with severe medical conditions (e.g., VATER syndrome) often experience long-term (months to years) periods of nonoral, enteral feeding and little, if any, positive oral nutritive experiences. Additionally, children who have had gastrointestinal allergic responses (e.g., eosinophilic esophagitis) or have undergone surgeries of the gastrointestinal tract (e.g., Nissen fundoplications [see Figure 5–5] for severe reflux) are likely to develop negative responses to oral intake. These negative experiences coupled with a lack of normal physiologic, sensory, and motor experiences associated with oral intake may cause the child to develop a severe adverse response (retching, vomiting, food refusals) to food or oral contact of any sort. These negative reactions complicate efforts to wean the child from tube feeding to the bottle, cup, and spoon. These children are described to have food aversions, or "sensory issues" with oral nutritional and hydration, and orally related activities such as oral hygiene and may benefit from a progressive, behavioral program of desensitization therapy to slowly introduce food items.

VI. ADULT NUTRITION AND HYDRATION

Nutrition is the process by which the body uses food and fluid to reach and maintain health. To maintain proper nutrition the body needs *calories, water, carbohydrates, proteins, fats, vitamins*, and *minerals*. **Vitamins** are the chemical substances necessary for normal tissue growth and maintenance of health. The functions of various vitamins are outlined in Table 5–3.

Severe nutritional deficiencies can accompany debilitating diseases, such as *metastatic cancer, infections, thyrotoxicosis, impaired intestinal absorption disorders, connective tissue diseases, chronic behavioral disorders*, and *conditions associated with alcoholism*. Nutritional deficiencies can result from the lack of a single vitamin or deficiencies in multiple nutrients. Lack of vitamin B_1, **thiamine**, is commonly associated with neurologic nutritional deficiencies, especially alcoholic neuropathies. **Alcoholic-nutritional peripheral neuropathies** are found in advanced stages of alcoholism. This disorder is characterized by axonal degeneration mainly involving the small pain- and temperature-mediating fibers in the lower distal extremities. Elders are particularly at risk for nutritional deficiencies due to medical disorders, cognitive disorders, and medication effects as well as behavioral, social (isolation), emotional (depression), economic (e.g., lack of funds to purchase protein-rich, nutritious foods) conditions, and other factors (e.g., ill-fitting dentures). Chapter 14 provides additional description of nutrition and hydration in elders.

The signs of nutritional deficiencies include:

- *Apathy* and *listlessness*
- *Darkening of the skin*
- Red, *sore mouth* with fissuring at the corners
- Red, *sore tongue*
- *Burning feet*
- *Anemia*
- *Muscle wasting*
- *Weight loss*

TABLE 5–3 Vitamins and their functions

VITAMIN	FUNCTION
A (Retinol)	Growth of cells; promotion of skin, hair, and epithelial cells
B_1 (Thiamine)	Normal digestion, carbohydrate metabolism, nervous system functions
B_2 (Riboflavin)	Normal growth, light accommodation, formation of certain enzymes
B_3 (Niacin)	Carbohydrate, fat, and protein metabolism; prevents loss of appetite
B_6 (Pyridoxine)	Healthy gums and teeth; red cell formation; carbohydrate, fat, and protein metabolism
B_9 (Folic acid)	Red cell formation, protein metabolism, normal intestinal tract functioning
B_{12} (Cyanocobalamin)	Protein metabolism, red cell formation, healthy nerve cells
C (Ascorbic acid)	Healthy bones, teeth, and gums; formation of blood vessels and capillary walls; proper healing; facilitation of iron and folic acid absorption
D (Calciferol)	Absorption of calcium and phosphorus
E (Alpha-tocopheral)	Red cell formation, protection of essential fatty acids
Pantothenic acid	Metabolism
H (Biotin)	Enzyme activity; metabolism of carbohydrates, fats, and proteins
K (Menadione)	Production of prothrombin (for blood clotting)

Based on: Lewis, L. W., & Timby, B. K. (1988). *Fundamental skills and concepts in patient care* (4th ed.). Philadelphia, PA: J. B. Lippincott.

Caloric needs of children (see Table 5–2), young adults, adults, and elders vary by body size, level of activity, and other factors. Elders have a lower resting metabolic rate than younger individuals, and fat stores tend to be increased while protein stores are decreased in advanced age. Most active adults require between 2000 and 3000 calories per day. To achieve, or maintain, *ideal body weight* (IBW), dietitians generally recommend a daily intake of 25 calories per kilogram of body weight. Plant and animal sources provide the amino acids that the body refashions into the protein it requires. The term "protein complementation" refers to a process by which two or more *plant sources* are ingested together at the same meal to provide the same total protein found in a single animal source.

Carbohydrates provide an easily metabolized source of energy, and many carbohydrate sources (e.g., grains, cereals, fruits, vegetables) have undigestible fiber, which promotes elimination of solids. Fats have a higher energy value than carbohydrates and protein sources (two and one-half times the amount of either). Alcohol is also high in calories, providing 7 calories per gram.

Water is an essential part of wellness, and fluid intake must be maintained at a fairly constant level (Tables 5–4 and 5–5). Minerals, such as potassium, calcium, phosphorus, and so on, are the substances that, when dissolved in the body, help to regulate the body's processes—such as conduction of nerve impulses. The healthy body maintains regulatory processes to ensure that fluid reserves and electrolytes are in proper balance. Following neurologic damage to the hypothalamus, water balance disorders can arise from disturbances in the neuromechanisms affecting the

TABLE 5–4 Average water balances (70 kg male)

Intake	2,500 mL/day (about 35 mL/kg/day baselitne)
Oral Liquids	1,500 mL
Oral Solids	700 mL
Metabolic	250 mL (through internal metabolic resources)
Output	1,400–2,300 mL/day
Urine	800–1,200 mL
Stool	250 mL
Insensible losses	600–900 mL (through lungs and skin)

Based on: Gomella, L. G. (Ed.). (1989). *Clinician's pocket handbook* (6th ed.). East Norwalk, CT: Appleton &Lange.

TABLE 5–5 Indicators of fluid imbalances

Changes in weight
Changes in blood pressure
Elevated body temperature (fluid deficit)
Weak, rapid, thready pulse (fluid deficit)
Full, bounding pulse (fluid excess)
Shallow respiration (fluid deficit)
Moist and labored respiration (fluid excess)

release of the **antidiuretic hormone (ADH)**, causing conditions such as *diabetes insipidus* and *hypo-* and *hypernatremia.* Hypothalamic damage can also lead to temperature regulation disorders. Tables 5–5 and 5–6 summarize the conditions indicative of fluid or electrolyte imbalances. To calculate volume equivalents from standard volume referents in the U.S. to metric measurements, see Table 5–7. When considering fluid intake measures it is also important to remember that solid food also contains variable amounts of fluid. For further discussion of specific metabolic disorders in critically ill patients, see Chapter 11.

TABLE 5–6 Indicators of electrolyte imbalances

CONDITION	INDICATORS
Hypernatremia	Confusion, stupor, coma, muscle tremors, seizures, pulmonary, and peripheral edema.
Hyponatremia	Lethargy, confusion, coma, muscle twitches, irritability, seizures, nausea, vomiting, ileus.
Hyperkalemia	Weakness, flaccid paralysis, hyperactivity, deep tendon reflexes, confusion, EKG changes.
Hypokalemia	Weakness, flaccid paralysis, hyperactivity, deep tendon reflexes, confusion, EKC changes.
Hypercalcemia	Anorexia, nausea, vomiting, polyuria, polydipsia, abdominal pain, kidney stones, fatigue, hypotonia, lethargy, coma.
Hypocalcemia	Peripheral and perioral paresthesia, hyperactive deep tendon reflexes, carpopedal spasm, abdominal cramps, Chvostek's sign (facial twitches), lethargy and irritability (in infants), EKG changes, generalized seizures, tetany, laryngospasm.
Hypermagnesemia	Nausea, vomiting, hypotension, hyporeflexia, weakness, drowsiness, coma, bradyrhythmias, respiratory failure.
Hypomagnesemia	Weakness, muscle twitches, asterixis, tremors, vertigo, convulsions, tachycardia.
Hyperphosphatemia	Renal failure.
Hypophosphatemia	Weakness, rhabdomyolysis, cardiac and respiratory failure, impaired leukocyte and platelet function, paresthesia, hemolysis.

Based on: Gomella, L. G. (Ed.). (1989). *Clinician's pocket handbook* (6th ed.). East Norwalk, CT: Appleton & Lange; and from Lewis, L. W., & Timby, B. K. (1988). *Fundamental skills and concepts in patient care* (4th ed.). Philadelphia: J. B. Lippincott.

Table 5–7 Volume equivalents

1 Teaspoon	=	5 mL*
1 Tablespoon	=	15 mL
1 Ounce	=	30 mL
Juice glass	=	120 mL (4 oz)
Average drinking glass	=	240 mL (8 oz)
Coffee cup	=	210 mL
Milk carton	=	240 mL
1 Quart	=	946 mL

* 1 mL equals 1 cc; however, it has become more acceptable in medicine to use **mL** as the preferred volume measurement.

VII. IATROGENIC MALNUTRITION IN THE ELDERLY

Malnutrition and dehydration caused by improper management or inadvertent errors in nutrition and hydration management are serious problems with the elderly. Malnutrition and dehydration can be caused by **polypharmacy**, which means using combinations of drugs that affect the body's management of fluid stores, metabolism, or appetite. *Diuretic drugs* need to be monitored to ensure that proper fluid balance is maintained.

Other factors potentially leading to malnutrition include:

- *Pain*, affecting appetite
- *Poor oral hygiene*
- Improper *dietary restrictions*
- *Lack of* or *poorly fitting dentures*
- *Improperly packaged* food items (difficult to open)
- *Decreased mobility* (inability to obtain food or water independently when needed)

Environmental factors, including unpleasant surroundings or odors, the lack of sensory aids (e.g., hearing aids, glasses) during meals, and neurologic deficits (e.g., hemianopsia or neglect of one side of the food tray) can also affect the older person's appetite, ability to eat independently, and, consequently, nutritional status.

VIII. PRESCRIBED DIETS

A. Diet Styles

In hospitals, diet orders are written by the physician, and the nurse or ward clerk is responsible for communicating the orders to the dietary service or department (see Chapter 2). Hospitals

TABLE 5–8 Prescribed diet styles

DIET STYLE	DESCRIPTION
Prescribed therapeutic diets	Diets for special needs such as sodium restricted, low residue, or diabetic diet therapies.
Clear liquid diet	A diet consisting of water, clear fruit juice, clear broth, gelatin, tea, or coffee.
Full liquid diet	A diet of liquid and strained fruit juices, soups, vegetable juice, milk, ice cream, gelatin, tea, and coffee.
Pureed diet	A diet similar to a full liquid diet but including pureed fruits, vegetables, and meats.
Mechanical soft diet	A diet style that includes ground meats and in which fruits and vegetables are well-cooked and soft enough to be easily chewed by edentulous persons.
Light or convalescent diet	A diet in which fried, rich, or raw foods are eliminated; and foods are generally prepared by steaming or boiling for easier digestion.
Dysphagia diet	Diet style usually ordered for patients with dysphagia related to oropharyngeal weakness and/or dyscoordination who have some risk of aspiration or other swallowing difficulties.
Regular diet	Standard diet served from the kitchen for patients who do not require any dietary therapies.

vary somewhat as to the diet styles that can be ordered for the patient, and the characteristics of a particular diet style (e.g., "mechanical soft" diet) may differ among institutions. Table 5–7 provides a volume equivalent reference for metric measurements of dietary intake. Table 5–8 lists diet styles that are commonly found in medical facilities.

B. National Dysphagia Diet

The National Dysphagia Diet (NDD), published in 2002 by the American Dietetic Association, aims to establish standard terminology and practice applications of dietary texture modification in dysphagia management. The NDD's diet levels were developed through consensus by a panel of dietitians, SLPs, and a food scientist. It proposes the classification of foods according to eight textural properties across four levels of semisolid/solid foods to represent points along continua for each property (McCullough, Pelletier, & Steele, 2003). A hierarchy of diet levels was proposed: **Level 1**: Dysphagia-Pureed (homogenous, very cohesive, pudding-like, requiring very little chewing ability); **Level 2**: Dysphagia-Mechanical Altered (cohesive, moist, semisolid foods, requiring some chewing); **Level 3**: Dysphagia-Advanced (soft foods that require more chewing ability); and **Level 4**: Regular (all foods allowed).

TABLE 5–9 Dietitian's nutritional assessment

ASSESSMENT	PURPOSE
Nutrition History	Examines the patient's food habits, preferences, weight, and any weight changes.
Somatic Protein	Includes a height-to-weight ratio and mid-arm circumference measure to indicate skeletal muscle stores.
Triceps Skinfold	Indicates fat stores.
Visceral Proteins	Examines serum albumin, serum transferrin or total iron binding capacity (TIBC) and total lymphocyte count.
Nitrogen Balance	Indicates the adequacy of nutritional support.
Basal Energy Expenditure (BEE) Requirement	Requirements for energy and protein will vary depending upon the nutritional status of the patient, stresses, and activity factors. The Harris-Benedict formula for computing BEE is: Male = 66 + (13.7 × weight, in kg) + (5 × height, in cm) − (6.8 × age, in years) Female = 665 + (9.6 × weight, in kg) + (1.8 × height, in cm) − (4.7 × age, in years).

C. Nutritional Requirements and Restrictions

Determination of the need for nutritional supplements or restrictions, the timing and type of enteral feeding, and other specific dietary needs require a **nutritional assessment** by a dietitian, as described in Table 5–9.

IX. NUTRITION AND HYDRATION NOTES

A. Fluid and Electrolyte Management

The "Doctor's Orders" section of the patient's medical chart will contain the stated **dietary orders**, any **IV fluid orders**, and orders for **fluid replacement** or any **electrolyte imbalance correction therapies**. These orders are based on findings from the admitting physical examinations, daily vital signs, laboratory findings, I & O records, nutritional assessment, and related studies such as those pertaining to dysphagia. Certain prescribed diets, such as those restricting *potassium* (**K**) and *sodium* (**Na**), are intended to correct electrolyte and fluid imbalances.

TABLE 5–10 Infant formula guidelines

AGE	FORMULA VOLUME PER FEEDING	FEEDINGS PER DAY
1 month	126 mL (4.1 oz)	6
2 months	142 mL (4.6 oz)	5
3 months	161 mL (5.2 oz)	5
4 months	168 mL (5.4 oz)	5
5 months	191 mL (6.2 oz)	4
6 months	179 mL (5.8 oz)	5
7–9 months	131 mL (4.2 oz)	5
10 months	136 mL (4.4 oz)	5
11 months	125 mL (4.0 oz)	5
12 months	141 mL (4.5 oz)	4

Source: From Kenner, C. A. (1998). *Nurse's clinical guide: Neonatal care,* 2nd ed. Reprinted with permission from Lippincott Williams and Wilkins.

B. Bedside Charting

Usually, at the end of the bed or in a rack near the patient's bed, there will be a chart for daily recording of vital signs and, when ordered, all **intake and output**, or **ins and outs (I & O)**. Nurses are responsible for recording all measurable daily food and liquid ingestion and excretion. Certain medical conditions, such as dehydration, necessitate more frequent monitoring. Infants require especially careful monitoring of nutrition/hydration intake during illness to ensure that they take the recommended volume (Table 5–10). Additional information about fluid and nutritional needs of neonates and children is provided in Tables 5–1 and 5–2.

C. Feeding Orders

The SLP's findings regarding indications for special dietary orders, feeding precautions, and feeding guidelines or therapies should be clearly and concisely written in the *consultation report* or *progress notes* and a place where the information is readily accessible to nurses or others who are feeding the patient. Warning "stickers," armbands, and posters are commercially available to alert nurses to special feeding precautions; and feeding guidelines can be posted above the patient's bed or on the bed stand, as long as the information does not convey protected health information. Information that states or indicates the medical condition *should not be posted* in a manner that would allow visitors and others to read it. For example, posting something like "John's Cancer Diet" is not allowable. When special dietary adjustments, such as a dysphagia diet style, are recommended by the SLP's assessment, it may be best to communicate these recommendations directly to the physician, following the reporting guidelines outlined in Chapter 2, and to the dietitian or in a conference with the **dysphagia management team**.

Typically, dysphagia diet styles for aspirating patients restrict thin liquids and solid foods and are prepared for easier movement through the oral and pharyngeal phases of swallow. Thickening agents are usually added to liquids. There are complications to thickeners, especially with children, so careful consideration must be given to any dietary style recommendation and, when indicated, consultation with gastroenterology should be considered.

Dysphagia diet style consistencies can range from solids, prepared similarly to the mechanical soft diet, to thickened paste/pureed solid foods. Patients with an esophageal stricture or obstruction who are not at risk of thin liquid aspiration may benefit from a pureed or full liquid diet style. Dysphagia diets need to be tailored to the individual needs and problems of the patient, taking into account any food allergies and other precautions.

X. CLINICAL COMPETENCIES

The learner outcomes, skills, and competencies gained from information contained in this chapter include the ability to:

- Read, interpret, and use anatomic terminology related to nutrition, hydration, and swallowing in adults and children.
- Read, interpret, and use descriptive, diagnostic, and syndrome terminology related to nutrition, hydration, and swallowing in adults and children.
- List commonly ordered laboratory tests for evaluation of nutrition, hydration, and swallowing in adults and children.
- Describe the essential features and differences between enteral and parenteral methods of nutritional support.
- Discuss factors taken into account in the management of nutrition and hydration in neonates, infants, and young children.
- Discuss factors taken into account in the evaluation and management of nutrition and hydration in adults.
- List the reasons why a special bottle might be employed with a child who has a cleft palate.
- List the signs of malnutrition.
- Describe the importance of adequate hydration in adults and children.
- Explain why children who are born prematurely might develop aversions to oral intake.
- Discuss factors that can impair adequate nutrition in the elderly.
- Discuss methods to determine caloric and nutrition needs in adults and children.

XI. REFERENCES AND RESOURCES CONSULTED

Anderson, D. (Ed.). (2003). *Dorland's illustrated medical dictionary* (30th ed.). Philadelphia: W. B. Saunders.

Andreoli, T. A., Carpenter, C., & Grigg, R. C. (Eds.). (2007). *Cecil essentials of medicine* (7th ed.). Philadelphia: W. B. Saunders.

Arvedson, J. C., & Brodsky, L. (Eds.). (2002). *Pediatric swallowing and feeding: Assessment and management* (2nd ed.). San Diego, CA: Singular.

Ayres, S. M., Schlichdrig, R., & Sterling, M. J. (1988). *Care of the critically ill* (3rd ed.). Chicago: Yearbook Medical.

Barrocas, A., Belcher, D., Champagne, C., & Jastram, C. (1995). Nutrition assessment practical approaches. *Clinics in Geriatric Medicine, 11*, 675–713.

Bender, A. (1982). *Dictionary of nutrition and food technology* (5th ed.). London: Butterworth.

Chenitz, W. C., Stone, J. T., & Salisbury, S. A. (1991). *Clinical gerontological nursing*. Philadelphia: W. B. Saunders.

Daniels, R., Nosek, L., & Nicoll, L. (2007). *Contemporary medical-surgical nursing*. Clifton Park, NY: Delmar Cengage Learning.

Davis, M. A., Gruskin, K. D., Chiang, V. W., & Manzi, S. (Eds.). (2005). *Signs and symptoms in pediatrics: Urgent and emergent care*. Philadelphia: Elsevier Mosby.

Gomella, L. G. (Ed.). (1989). *Clinician's pocket handbook* (6th ed.). East Norwalk, CT: Appleton & Lange.

Gomella, L. G. (Ed.). (1993). *Clinician's pocket reference* (7th ed.). East Norwalk, CT: Appleton & Lange.

Groher, M. E. (Ed.). (1984). *Dysphagia: Diagnosis and management*. Stoneham, MA: Butterworth.

Hendricks, K. M., & Duggan, C. (Eds.). (2005). *Manual of pediatric nutrition* (4th ed.). Hamilton, Ontario: BC Decker.

Hunter, T. B., & Taljanovic, M. S. (2003). Glossary of medical devices and procedures: Abbreviations, acronyms, and definitions. *Radiographics, 23*, 195–213.

Jablonski, S. (2005). *Dictionary of medical acronyms and abbreviations* (5th ed.). Philadelphia: Elsevier Saunders.

Johnson, A. F., & Jacobson, B. H. (Eds.). (2007). *Medical speech-language pathology: A practitioner's guide* (2nd ed.). New York: Thieme.

Karnell, M. P. (1994). *Videoendoscopy: From velopharynx to larynx*. San Diego, CA: Singular.

Keir, L., Wise, B., Krebs, C., & Kelley-Arney, C. (2008). *Medical assisting: Administrative and clinical competencies* (6th ed.). Clifton Park, NY: Delmar Cengage Learning.

Kenner, C. A. (1992). *Nurse's clinical guide: Neonatal care*. Springhouse, PA: Springhouse.

Klint, A., & Scott, L. (2008). *Collaboration between the clinical dietitian and speech-language pathologist in the treatment of children with feeding difficulties*. Guidelines presented at the Pediatric Feeding and Swallowing Training Module, Vanderbilt University, Nashville, TN, January 2008.

Langmore, S., Schatz, K., & Olsen, N. (1988). Fiberoptic endoscopic examination of swallowing safety: A new procedure. *Dysphagia, 2*, 216–219.

Lewis, C. M. (1986). *Nutrition and nutritional therapy*. East Norwalk, CT: Appleton-Century-Crofts.

Lewis, L. W., & Timby, B. K. (1988). *Fundamental skills and concepts in patient care* (4th ed.). Philadelphia: J. B. Lippincott.

Logemann, J. A. (1983). *Evaluation and treatment of swallowing disorders.* San Diego, CA: College-Hill Press.

McCullough, G., Pelletier, C., & Steele, C. (2003, November 4). National dysphagia diet: What to swallow? *The ASHA Leader*, pp. 16, 27.

Morris, S. E., & Klein, M. D. (2000). *Pre-feeding skills: A comprehensive resource for mealtime development* (2nd ed.). Austin, TX: Pro-Ed.

Perlman, A. L. (1991). Neurology of swallowing. *Seminars in Speech and Language, 12*, 171–184.

Persons, C. G. (1987). *Critical care procedures and protocols.* Philadelphia: J. B. Lippincott.

Rizzo, D. C. (2007). *Fundamentals of anatomy & physiology* (2nd ed.). Clifton Park, NY: Delmar Cengage Learning.

Robinson, C. H., Lawler, M. R., Chenoweth, W. L., & Garwick, A. E. (1986). *Normal and therapeutic nutrition* (17th ed.). New York: Macmillan.

Rosenthal, S. R., Sheppard, J. J., & Lotze, M. (1995). *Dysphagia and the child with developmental disabilities.* San Diego, CA: Singular.

Seikel, J. A., King, D. W., & Drumright, D. G. (2005). *Anatomy and physiology of speech, language, and hearing* (3rd ed.). Clifton Park, NY: Delmar Cengage Learning.

Willett, M. J., Patterson, M., & Steinbock, B. (1986). *Manual of neonatal intensive care nursing.* Boston: Little, Brown.

CHAPTER 6

Medical Genetics

One of the most exciting areas of current medical science is the application of research in human genetics to a vast array of medical conditions. Genetic research is unfolding rapidly and having a profound influence on clinical medical practices with patients of all ages and across a wide range of disorders. The field of medical genetics has been advanced by the completion of the **Human Genome Project** in 2003. This project was initially coordinated by the National Institutes of Health (2008) and the Department of Energy in the United States, and it was ultimately completed with the help of international partners within the Human Genome Organization (HUGO). Although there were several goals, the primary aim of the project was mapping the complete content and sequence of the human genome. Attaining that goal has resulted in revolutionary insights into diseases and their prevention and treatment. With an increased understanding of genetics in human development and disease, there has been a growing interest in **developmental biology**—the study of the processes involved in the development of complex organisms from a one-cell embryo. Developmental biology is an outgrowth of **embryology** that integrates embryologic research into the genetic, biochemical, physiologic, and cellular factors that contribute to normal and abnormal human development. These areas of medical science are increasingly suggesting or providing genetic and other biologic evidence for the basis of many of the conditions encountered in medical speech-language pathology with which causal factors were previously not known.

I. CHAPTER FOCUS

This chapter highlights fundamental concepts and terminology that may be encountered in readings and patient care discussions related to genetically related conditions. The full gamut of genetically based conditions and diseases and congenital anomalies one might encounter in clinical practice cannot be listed or reviewed here, but certain disorders that provide an illustration or example are mentioned. Discussions related to specific genetic conditions, congenital and perinatally acquired disorders, teratogenic factors, and the related communication and swallowing disorders are discussed in other chapters. Several inherited neurologic syndromes are listed in

Chapter 10, Neurologic and Psychiatric Disorders, and disorders with associated feeding, swallowing, and nutrition disorders are discussed in Chapter 5.

A comprehensive review of the basic sciences underlying medical genetics, inborn errors in metabolism, genetic mapping, and gene therapies exceeds the scope of this chapter. Readers should consult the references cited at the end of this chapter. Texts on medical genetics are highly recommended reading for students interested in inherited speech, language, hearing, cognitive, and developmental disabilities. Genetics texts are an essential addition to the libraries of medical speech-language pathologists (SLPs), particularly those working in settings where individuals with genetic syndromes are commonly seen. The intent of this chapter is to provide a general overview of medical genetics, including some of the terminology and basic concepts that will be encountered in readings, medical records, and patient care discussions related to genetically and nongenetically based congenital conditions and diseases. SLPs who work with children who have velopharyngeal insufficiency (VPI), usually due palatal clefting, need to have a heightened sensitivity to genetic abnormalities. Occasionally, it is the speech-language pathologist who is the first to recognize that a child's facial, dental, oral-pharyngeal structural features might be characteristic (phenotypic) of a genetic disorder.

II. TERMINOLOGY AND ABBREVIATIONS

A. Terminology

Abortion. Referring to any terminated pregnancy prior to fetal viability (before 24 weeks); abortions may be *spontaneous* (accidental or due to natural causes) or *planned* (elective). In medical terminology, a *miscarriage* is referred to as an abortion.

Affected pedigree member method. A method of genetic analysis of the extent to which relatives share alleles of a given disease at a location that would be more frequent than by chance alone.

Allele. Variant form of a gene found at the same locus of homologous chromosomes. A diploid organism gets one set of their alleles (genes) from one parent and another set of alleles from the other parent; thus, variations from the combination of these genes determine the inherited characteristics (e.g., hair color, height, blood type, and risk for diseases).

Allogenic. Tissues in transplantation that are from the same species but have different antigens.

Allograft, homograft. Transplanted tissue graft between individuals who are not identical twins and have different genotypes; an **isograft** is a tissue graft from an identical twin; an **autograft** is a graft from the patient's own tissue; and a **xenograph** is a graft from another species.

Amniocentesis. A prenatal procedure involving the removal of amniotic fluid to examine fetal cells.

Aneuploidy. A chromosome number that is not the exact multiple of the **haploid**; for example, **trisomy** indicates the presence of an extra chromosome and **monosomy** indicates the absence of a chromosome.

Anomaly. Any deviation from normal physical form or function.

Apoptosis. Programmed cell death, as compared to cell death caused by disease or injury.

Autoimmune disorder. An abnormal immune system response in which the body reacts adversely to its own tissues.

Autosomal. The 22 non-sex-determining chromosomes in humans; that is, chromosomes other than the Y and X chromosomes.

Autosomal dominant inheritance. Phenotypic inheritance determined by mutant alleles on both of the paired autosomes.

Autosomal recessive inheritance. Phenotypic inheritance determined by only one mutant allele in the paired autosomes.

Banding. Referring to one of the staining techniques for elucidating chromosomal characteristics and structural abnormalities, which are described as C bands, G bands, Q bands, and R bands.

Benign neoplasm. A tumor that does not invade surrounding tissues or metastasize (spread) to another location.

Benign trait. Genetically based variant that is not clinically significant; for example, the blood group ABO is considered to be a *benign polymorphism*, or benign trait.

Birth defect. An abnormal condition present at birth but not necessarily a genetic disorder.

Blood group. Blood type, a phenotype classification based on the presence or absence of inherited antigenic substances on the surface of red blood cells.

Branchial cleft cyst. A common congenital mass typically presenting as a lateral neck mass or a fistula that drains into the skin.

Cancer-related genes. Genes that are associated with the development of cancers categorized as **oncogenes**, which are genes known to be associated with unregulated cell growth and responsible for tumor development; **tumor suppressor genes**, such as gatekeeper genes, or p53; and **deoxyribonucleic acid (DNA)-repair genes**, which repair the damage to a cell's DNA before cell proliferation has occurred.

Carrier. Referring to a person who has a *recessive,* mutated gene along with its corresponding normal allele, which masks the development of a disease in that individual, but the disease can be transmitted to his or her offspring.

Chiasma. Anatomically referring to a decussation or crossing; in genetics *chiasmata* are the intersections, or crossovers, of chromosomal material between chromosome pairs.

Chimera. An organism formed by two different zygotes; transplantation results in chimerism.

Chorionic villus sampling. A prenatal test performed under ultrasonic guidance at 8–10 weeks' gestation in which cells are taken from the primitive placenta (chorion) to identify genetic disorders. Other forms of prenatal testing may involve cells taken from amniotic fluid or the umbilical cord for biochemical and chromosomal analysis.

Chromosomal disorder. Birth defect caused by errors in part of or in an entire chromosome.

Chromosome. Organized threadlike structure contained within the nucleus of cells of the body consisting of the protein chromatin and a single (double-helix) strand of DNA, which contains genes, regulatory elements, and nucleotide sequences. A normal human cell has 46 chromosomes, with 22 pairs of *autosomes* and 2 *sex chromosomes.*

Clone. In molecular biology, cloning refers to a method for making multiple copies of a defined DNA sequence in vivo through repeated mitosis to produce genetically identical cells or organisms from a single ancestor.

Codon. The triplet combination of DNA units, or bases (adenine (A), thymine (T), guanine (G), and cytosine (C), that provides the code for a specific amino acid or the "stop" message of a gene.

Complex inheritance. A non-Mendelian pattern of trait inheritance, usually the result of two or more alleles interacting with environmental factors.

Congenital. Present at birth, not necessarily due to a genetic disorder.

Cytogenetics. The genetic study of cells and chromosomes.

Deformation syndrome. Dysmorphic features caused by intrauteral factors (e.g., **intrauterine growth restriction**).

de novo. From the Latin "from the beginning;" in genetics, a de novo finding indicates neither parent apparently possesses or has transmitted the genetic mutation.

Deoxyribonucleic acid (DNA). Our hereditary material, a large molecule contained in nearly every cell of the body in humans carrying the genetic information needed to replicate and produce proteins.

Disruption. Birth defect caused by factors such as *teratogenic* agents, disruption of blood flow to the fetus, or a rupture of the amniotic sac with entrapment.

Dizygotic (DZ) twins. Fraternal (not identical) twins.

Dominant. A trait that is expressed phenotypically in heterozygotes.

Dysmorphism. Any morphologic or developmental abnormality.

Ecogenetic disorder. A genetic predisposition to a particular disease that is triggered by an environmental factor.

Ectoderm. One of the three primary layers of the developing embryo giving rise to the skin; nervous system; and neural crest structures, including craniofacial structures.

Embryonic stem (ES) cells. Cells that are derived from eggs that are fertilized outside a woman's body in vitro. Embryonic cells are **pluripotent**, as compared to adult stem cells, which are **multipotent** (see later); however, researchers have found that pluripotent embryonic stem cells can be generated from adult skin cells (fibroblast cultures).

Empiric risk. The risk probability, based on observation, for a particular genetic factor to occur in a given family.

Enzyme. A protein that facilitates, enhances, or accelerates a particular chemical reaction in the body.

Epistasis. A double mutation where one mutation blocks the phenotype of another mutation but not due to dominance factors.

Eugenics. Selective breeding; the opposite of **dysgenics**.

Expressivity. The degree, from mild to severe, to which a particular genotype is expressed. This term is sometimes confused with **penetrance**, which refers to the extent to which the signs or symptoms of a particular disease are expressed within a population or fraction of individuals who actually have the genotype for that disease.

Failure to thrive. Growth failure in neonates, infants, and children; adults, particularly elders, may be diagnosed with the condition *failure to thrive* when there is a lack of a positive response to nutritional and other therapies.

Familial. A trait that is present in several family members and more common among relatives than in the general population.

Fate. The predictable genetic lineage of a particular embryologic cell as determined by developmental biology through "*fate mapping.*"

Fetoscopy. Endoscopic visualization of a fetus.

Fetus. The unborn, developing infant during the time frame from 12 weeks' gestation through term or delivery.

Fragile X. A genetic mutation characterized by a mutation of the FMR 1 gene on the long arm of the X chromosome. Currently fragile X is implicated in a number of disorders, including *fragile X mental retardation protein* (FMRP) syndrome and *fragile X associated tremor/ataxia syndrome* (FXTAS). It is suspected to be associated with other disorders, including some types of autism spectrum disorder (ASD), epilepsy, anxiety disorders, and attention-deficit hyperactivity disorder (ADHD).

Functional gene test. An assay to test for the presence of specific proteins to determine if a target gene is present and active.

Gamete. One-half of a chromosome pair; the reproductive cell, either an ovum or sperm, that contains a *haploid* number of chromosomes (23).

Gatekeeper genes. Genes that regulate cell proliferation and serve to suppress tumors.

Gene. An organism's unit of inheritance and a subunit of DNA. The human body has 20,000–25,000 genes, each containing the code for a specific, functional product, which is typically a protein such as an enzyme. A gene's coded information is *expressed* through its translation into proteins or ribonucleic acid (RNA).

Gene map. The arrangement of genes on each chromosome. Gene mapping is one of the main purposes of the Human Genome Project.

Gene pool. All of the alleles within a population. A large gene pool indicates genetic diversity, whereas inbreeding produces a small gene pool and less robust populations with fewer "adaptive" traits (traits that help to ensure survival).

Gene product. The protein produced from the code of a specific gene (e.g., human growth hormone).

Gene therapy. Treatment of diseases through the transfer of selected DNA sequences.

Genetic map, genome map. The relative order and arrangement of the position of genes and other DNA markers within chromosomes as determined by *linkage analysis.*

Genetic marker. Any unique characteristic of DNA that allows for differentiation of the locus and tracing of classifiable alleles through a family.

Genetics. The study of the inheritance of traits from parents to offspring.

Genetic screening. Testing to identify risk factors for a particular trait or condition.

Genome. The complete genetic material (DNA) in an individual's chromosomes; the internal "blueprint" for building and maintaining a living organism.

Genotype. An individual's actual genes, as compared to **phenotype** (defined later).

Germ cells. Either an egg or sperm cell, the reproductive cells of the body; compare to *somatic cells* (defined later).

Germline mutation. Cancers arise from mutations in genes that can be inherited, referred to as a *germline mutation*, or develop over a person's lifetime due to environmental factors (exposure to carcinogens) or mutagens.

Haploid. The number of chromosomes in each gamete (one of a pair of chromosomes), which in humans is 23.

Hemolytic disease of the newborn. Referring to Rh incapability (see the definition in Abbreviations) between a mother who is Rh^- and a fetus that is Rh^+. When small amounts of blood pass between the placenta and the mother's bloodstream, the mother will form antibodies to the fetus' Rh^+ blood, and those antibodies can damage fetal red blood cells. Preventive measures with Rh^- mothers to protect the fetus are now routine.

Heritability. The extent to which a disease is determined by genetic factors.

Heterozygous. Individuals with two different alleles at the same location.

Homozygous. Individuals with the same alleles at a given location.

Host. In molecular biology, a host organism, such as *Escherichia coli* (a bacterium), is introduced to yeast to isolate and grow recombinant DNA.

Inborn error of metabolism. Referring to the cause of a large class of inherited (genetic) diseases such as *phenylketonuria* (PKU) and *maple syrup urine disease* that are known to be related to genetic alterations in the code for specific enzymes. These alterations cause a specific protein defect that blocks normal metabolic functions and leads to pathologic, metabolic conditions. Infant screening is used to identify many of these conditions and prevent adverse consequences.

Inbreeding, consanguinity. Mating with close relatives.

Index case. The first case in a family to be identified to have a familial trait in the pedigree.

***In situ* hybridization.** Mapping a gene by hybridizing a DNA molecule that has been radioactively labeled.

***In vitro* fertilization.** The process of fertilizing an egg outside the body and then introducing the fertilized egg(s) back into the uterus.

Karyotype. Referring to an individual's chromosomal composition. In cytogenetics, karyotypes are the organized profile of a person's chromosomes, arranged, and presented graphically as a **photomicrogram**, from largest to smallest, to allow for easier identification of genetic abnormalities.

Kindred. Extended family members.

Linkage analysis. Tracing patterns of heredity in large, at-risk families.

Locus. A particular place in a DNA sequence.

Male-to-male transmission. Genetic inheritance limited to fathers and sons.

Malignant neoplasm. A tumor that is capable of invading surrounding tissues or *metastasizing* (spreading) to another location.

Maternal inheritance. Genetic inheritance limited to the mother and to her offspring.

Maternal serum screening. Prenatal tests that examine for certain proteins and other substances in the blood of the mother to identify fetal abnormalities; for example, neural tube defects and certain trisomies.

Mendelian. Referring to the predictions of autosomal dominant, autosomal recessive, and X-linked inheritance patterns, as initially described by Gregor Mendel in his classic study of the inheritance of seven traits in peas, which he demonstrated to be determined by a single gene.

Mitochondrial inheritance. Single gene disorders where the locus for the mutation is in the mitochondria of the chromosome.

Monozygotic (MZ) twins. Twins coming from a single zygote, or identical twins.

Mosaic. An individual with two or more genotypes coming from two different cell types; a *mosaic* refers to the occurrence of different genotypes in an individual developed from a single zygote (fertilized egg).

Multipotent. Referring to progenitor cells that are capable of differentiating into a limited number of cell fates as compared to *pluripotent* cells (see later).

Mutagen. An agent that causes a change in the molecular sequence, number, or arrangement of a given gene.

Mutation. A spontaneous, permanent, inheritable change in a chromosome structure or DNA sequence; a mutation can be harmful, beneficial, or of no consequence.

Neoplasm. Abnormal cell growth; neoplasms may be benign or malignant.

Neural tube defects. These defects include *spina bifida* (meningomyelocele) and *anencephaly* (see Chapter 4), which are thought to be caused by a combination of genetic and environmental factors.

Odds ratio. A statistical comparison of the probability of individuals who share a given inherited trait to ultimately develop a particular disease.

Oligonucleotide array. An array of microscopic spots of DNA features arranged on a silicone or glass chip (**gene chip**) used for the purpose of identifying genotypes, gene expression profiling, or for resequencing mutant genes.

Ontogeny. The biological developmental history of an organism.

p53. Tumor-suppressing gene; mutations in the gene are found in about half of all cancers.

Pedigree. A standard method of graphing the family tree of inherited conditions (discussed in greater detail later).

Penetrance. The likelihood that a gene will have any phenotypic expression and cause a particular disease, such as cancer.

Pharmacogenetics. The pharmacological application of research in biochemical genetics, which is concerned with genetically determined variations among individuals in their responses to drugs.

Pharmacokinetics. The study of the body's absorption, distribution, metabolism, and excretion of drugs.

Phenotype. The manifestation (structure, function, or behavior) of our genetic inheritance and its interaction with environmental factors; the physical expression of a genetic trait.

Pluripotent. Referring to a stem cell that could potentially give rise to either fetal or adult cell types and any of the three germ layers (endodermal, mesodermal, and epidermal). Pluripotent cells in immunology are discussed in Chapter 12.

Polygenic. Trait inheritance that is multifactorial and determined by different genes.

Polymorphism. In molecular biology, referring to certain points of mutation in a genotype; when a locus has more than one allele with a frequency of greater than 1%, it is said to be polymorphic. Because humans have a large number of polymorphisms, with the exception of identical twins, each of us is genetically unique. This genetic uniqueness is the basis of **DNA profiling** in forensics.

Prevalence. At a given point in time, the number of persons with a particular trait or disease within a given population.

Prion. An infectious protein implicated in the transfer of several rare neurodegenerative diseases.

Proband. The *index case*; in pedigree graphs, the proband denotes the individual of interest with a given trait.

Prophylactic surgery. Surgery performed for the purpose of avoiding the development of a cancerous tumor; for example, prophylactic breast surgery in women who have been identified to have a mutated version of the ***BRCA1*** or ***BRCA2*** **genes**, which are the genes known to restrain cell growth. Women who inherit a mutated version of *BRCA1* are also at higher risk for ovarian cancer.

Qualitative trait. An observation that an individual has or does not have a trait.

Quantitative trait. A measurement of the difference of occurrence of a trait within a population.

Recessive gene. A gene that is expressed only in the presence of a counterpart (recessive) allele on the matching chromosome.

Recombinant DNA technology. Reconstructing a DNA molecule *in vivo* from segments of two or more DNA molecules.

Regulation. Decreasing (*down-regulation*) or increasing (*up-regulation*) the rate of a gene expression.

Retrovirus. A virus that is capable of propagating DNA from its RNA through *enzyme reverse transcriptase,* in which the virus uses an enzyme to "reverse-transcribe" its RNA genomes into DNA, which is then integrated into the host genome and replicated along with it. The human immunodeficiency virus (HIV) is a retrovirus.

Ribonucleic acid (RNA). The genetic material in cellular organisms that directs the transfer of information from the DNA. RNA is required to determine the protein structure and protein production needed by a cell for its development.

Sex chromosomes. The X and Y chromosomes; normal females carry two X chromosomes and normal males carry one X and one Y chromosome.

Simplex. A familial pedigree where only one member is affected by a genetic disorder.

Somatic cells. Cells of the body (derived from *soma,* which is Greek for "body"); somatic cells are all the body's cells other than germline (sex-determining) cells (see earlier).

Sporadic. Referring to a new mutation.

Stem cell. A type of cell that is capable of reinvigoration and differentiation into diverse types of specialized cells.

Syndrome. A pattern of abnormalities.

Teratogen. Any environmental agent (e.g., a medication or an infectious agent) that causes a congenital malformation in a fetus.

Trait. A feature or characteristic.

Triple test. A test that determines the risk to a mother of having a child with Down syndrome.

Trisomy. Referring to three representations of a given chromosome instead of the normal two.

Two hit model. In medical genetics, the theory that cancer can develop when both alleles of a tumor-suppressing gene in a given cell have become inactivated.

Universal donor. A person with type O Rh^- blood who can donate blood to any recipient.

Universal recipient. A person with AB Rh^+ blood who can receive blood from any donor.

Variable expression. A genotype that may produce phenotypes of varying severity.

Vector. In molecular genetics, referring to the use of a host molecule to clone a gene or DNA fragment.

Velopharyngeal incompetence (VPI). Referring to various congenital abnormalities of the hard and soft palates and oropharyngeal structures, resulting from a lack of normal embryologic development for midline fusion of oral structures (between 4 and 8 weeks' gestation), or the *result of surgical removal of palatal and velopharyngeal tissues,* causing an open port between the oropharyngeal cavity and the nasal cavity. VPI can be associated with a *complete cleft lip and palate, cleft palate,* or *submucous cleft* (which is typically associated with a **bifid uvula**). Recently, the gene *IRF6* has been identified as a contributor to about 12% of cleft lip and palate cases.

X linkage. Inheritance patterns found on the X chromosome but not the Y chromosome.

Y linkage. Inheritance patterns found on the Y chromosome but not the X chromosome.

Zygote. The union of two gametes; a fertilized cell (ovum).

B. Abbreviations

ABO. Blood groups, blood types

DNA. Deoxyribonucleic acid

DZ. Dizygotic

FISH. Fluorescence *in situ* hybridization (test)

FLK. Funny looking kid

MZ. Monozygotic

p. For *petit*, referring to the short arm of a chromosome

PCR. Polymerase chain reaction

q. The long arm of a chromosome

Rh. The initial reference comes from *Rh*esus monkeys that were used in experiments that led to the discovery of the Rh system in which Rh positive individuals have a polypeptide, Rh-D, encoded by a gene on chromosome 1, whereas Rh negative individuals lack this antigen.

RNA. Ribonucleic acid

sib. Sibling (brother or sister)

SKY. Spectral karyotyping

SNP. Single nucleotide polymorphism

STRP. Short tandem repeat polymorphism

tDNA. Transfer DNA

VNTR. Variable number of tandem repeats

X. Referring to the X chromosome

Y. Referring to the Y chromosome

III. BASIC CONCEPTS IN HUMAN GENETICS

Genetically based diseases and normal variations in human traits are typically divided into four categories: **single gene disorders**, **multifactorial inheritance**, **chromosomal defects**, **mitochondrial defects**, and disorders occurring in families but of **unknown etiology**.

A. Single Gene Disorders

Most of us will recall from a high school science class, single gene disorders are often called **Mendelian traits**, or diseases, and include those rare conditions that can be linked to a *single mutation* at an individual locus. The frequency of occurrence of these disorders can often be linked to ethnic origin or regional descent. Certain disorders occur more frequently in one particular ethnic group or regional origin than another. For example, Jews from Eastern European origin have offspring with a higher frequency of *Tay-Sachs disease* than is found in the general population. Single gene disorders can be due to **autosomal recessive** or **autosomal dominant inheritance**, or **X-linked recessive** or **X-linked dominant inheritance**, or **mitochondrial inheritance** (see Terminology). In autosomal dominant inheritance, every affected individual has an affected parent and will pass on the *trait* to the next generation. Both males and females have an equal (50%) likelihood of inheriting the trait, and there is a 50-50 chance of passing the trait with each pregnancy. In autosomal recessive inheritance, the affected individual *may* have parents with normal phenotypes; that is, their physical appearance, intelligence, behavior, or medical status is apparently "normal." Although male and female offspring are also equally (25%) likely to inherit the trait, the trait is more likely to be seen in the siblings of the affected individual than in the parents. Medical geneticists caution that single gene inheritance is not "simple" and that "dominant" and "recessive" are not rigid categories. Jorde, Carey, Bamshad, and White (1999) suggest that the distinctions between dominant and recessive traits become blurred as we learn more about them. Some dominant traits have a more severe expression in homozygotes than in heterozygotes (e.g., anchondroplasia) (Jorde et al., 1999). It is important to recall that genetic inheritance refers to inherited **traits**, which may or may not be expressed as a disease. Heterozygotes can inherit a recessive trait without having the clinical expression (phenotype) of a disease. Although these individuals are "clinically normal," they may be found to have enzymatic abnormalities or other features that indicate the presence of the trait. In some individuals, the *disease* may be recessive but the *trait* is dominant (Jorde et al., 1999).

B. Multifactorial Inheritance

A large number of diseases and deformities, such as cleft lip and palate and spina bifida, are known to result from a combination of small variations and influences coming from more than one mutant allele at multiple locations, rather than a single error in genetic information. Environmental factors may also have a role in neural tube defects like spina bifida. In multifactorial inheritance, genetic influences can add or detract characteristics from the phenotype. Although cleft lip and palate is considered a multifactorial condition, genetic counselors can predict certain factors that will increase the potential for inheritability, including *consanguinity* (mating with a close relative); *severity of the disorder* in the affected parent (the more severely the expression of the disease in the parent the more likely he or she is to have a child with the disorder); *sex of the child*; and the *number of other children affected* with some variant of the phenotype in the family. These factors are taken into account when conducting genetic counseling. The phenotypes for cleft lip and palate are listed in Chapter 13, Surgeries and Other Procedures.

Diseases in which the phenotype presents later in life may also be multifactorial. Alzheimer's disease (AD), for example, has variable expressivity and genetic heterogeneity. There appears to be a familial autosomal dominant form of AD that accounts for about 10% of cases. About 1% of individuals with Down syndrome (trisomy 21) have AD. But in the majority of individuals with this diagnosis, the origin is believed to be multifactorial. Several genetic mutations (*PSEN1, PSEN2, APP, APOE)* have been described to be fully or partially *penetrant* and vary with regard to the age of onset or rapidity of progression. The phenotype of a patient with AD principally includes a progressive loss of global cognitive functions.

C. Chromosomal Defects

Chromosomal defects include diseases where the phenotype is determined by mutations, or physical changes, which alter the number or structure of a chromosome. This can include *deletions*, *additions*, *inversions*, *translocations*, *insertions*, and "*rings*," occurring during chromosomal paring and creating abnormalities in the chromosomal origin, number, or function. For example, the presence of an extra copy of chromosome 21 produces **Down syndrome**, or trisomy 21. Chromosomal abnormalities are also found on the sex chromosomes, as is the case with **Turner's syndrome** (45X), which is one of the more frequent chromosomal abnormalities. As in other chromosomal defects involving the sex chromosomes (*Klinefelter's syndrome*, XYY and XXX syndromes), a *nondisjunction* occurs during one of the stages of meiotic division in spermatogenesis, which results in abnormal pairings of the chromosomes. In the case of Turner's syndrome an end-to-end, rather than longitudinal, pairing results, and this chromosomal abnormality causes a number of physical abnormalities in the developing fetus. Another type of chromosomal abnormality is called **uniparental disomy**, where offspring inherit two copies of a given chromosome from one parent, instead of one from each parent. Two conditions that are most often discussed in this category are *Prader-Willi syndrome* and *Angelman syndrome.* In these disorders, the child has inherited an extra copy of chromosome 15. Children with Prader-Willi syndrome have two copies of chromosome 15 from their mother, due to an inheritance of a deletion from the father. In Angelman syndrome, both chromosomes 15 come from the father due to an inherited deletion from the mother. The phenotype for Prader-Willi includes difficulty feeding as an infant, with overeating later leading to obesity; characteristic facial features; small hands and feet; short stature; hypogonadism; speech delay; and mental retardation. In Angelman syndrome, the newborns may have a normal phenotype (appear to be normal), but by about 6 months, developmental delays may be apparent. Eventually, the phenotype includes severe mental retardation; speech impairment; hand flapping; frequent laughing and excitability; and wide-based gait with a balance disorder, including ataxia. These children are described to have seizures that involve unusual laughter pattern called **gelastic seizures**. Another rarer uniparental disomy is **Beckwith-Wiedemann syndrome**, due to disomy of chromosome 11. The phenotype with these children includes a large tongue, protrusion of the umbilicus, severe hypoglycemia with related morbidities, and other severe complications, including malignancies of the kidney, adrenal glands, and liver.

An X-related chromosomal disorder receiving considerable attention by geneticists recently is **fragile X** (see definition). Like other genetic conditions inherited through the

X chromosome, males are more likely to have phenotypical expressions of the disorder than females. The carrier females have two X chromosomes, whereas males have only one; thus, the normal chromosome can compensate for the defective one. As discussed earlier, the defect has been identified to be abnormal repetitions of the nucleotide CGG on the long arm of an X chromosome. The greater the number of abnormal repetitions, the more likely a full blown syndrome will result. Several childhood and adult-onset disorders are now known or suspected to be associated with this genetic abnormality, including **fragile X associated tremor, ataxia syndrome (FXTA); fragile X mental retardation protein (FMRP) syndrome**; and other disorders, such as variants of autism spectrum disorders (ASD), epilepsy, and hyperactivity disorders.

In some cases, the culprit chromosomal mutation or deletion disorder is not clear. For example, **CHARGE syndrome** is an autosomal dominant condition with genotypic heterogeneity. Most individuals are found to have the chromodomain helicase DNA-binding protein-7 (*CHD7*) gene; however, there have been case reports of individuals who meet the phenotypic clinical criteria for CHARGE syndrome but who have a variety of underlying cytogenetic abnormalities (including 22q11.2 deletions) and single gene mutations (including *SEMA3E* gene mutations). The phenotype of children with CHARGE syndrome includes multiple congenital abnormalities, such as characteristic face and hand dysmorphology, hypotonia, urinary tract anomalies, orofacial clefting, deafness, and dysphagia and tracheoesophageal anomalies (Thelin & Swanson, 2006). The acronym "CHARGE" refers to **c**oloboma of the eye, **h**eart defects, **a**tresia of the choanae, **r**etardation of growth and/or development, **g**enital and/or urinary abnormalities, and **e**ar abnormalities and deafness. This list of abnormalities is no longer strictly applied in the diagnosis, but "CHARGE" continues to be used to refer to this syndrome.

D. Mitochondrial Defects

Mitochondria are specialized structures in cells that contain genes and also play a crucial role in metabolism. Mitochondrial inheritance is non-Mendelian in that it comes exclusively from the mother. Thus, defects associated with these disorders are traced through the maternal lineage. There are several diseases occurring later in life that are now thought to be related to mitochondial defects, including forms of AD, osteoporosis, Parkinson's disease, stroke, and diabetes mellitus. Mitochondrial defects and environmental factors are also potentially implicated in certain forms of deafness. For example, some individuals may be genetically predisposed to acquire inner ear, hair cell damage that is triggered by toxicity from the aminoglycoside class of antibiotics. This condition is referred to as **mitochondrial deafness**.

E. Teratogens

Environmental agents that lead to birth defects are called **teratogens**. A prime example is **fetal alcohol syndrome (FAS)**, caused by an excessive exposure of the fetus to alcohol intake by the mother during a critical period of development (less than the first 12 weeks). These children typically have low birth weight, developmental delays, characteristic craniofacial dysmorphology, and central nervous system (CNS) and cardiac abnormalities. There are many suspected teratogenic factors potentially affecting fetal development; several of the verified teratogens are listed in Table 6–1.

TABLE 6–1 Teratogenic factors

TYPE OF TERATOGEN	DEFECTS (varies by the amount and timing of exposure)
Maternal Infections	
Rubella	Profound hearing loss, cardiac and central nervous system (CNS) abnormalities, cataracts
Cytomegalovirus (CMV)	Severe sensorineural hearing loss, CNS abnormalities, and developmental delays
Toxoplasmosis	Seizures, low tone, feeding difficulties, developmental delays
Syphilis	Skin rashes, sores, jaundice, anemia, seizures, swollen liver and spleen, developmental delays
Varicella zoster	Low birth weight (LBW) due to abnormal growth during fetal development (intrauterine growth retardation), distinctive skin abnormalities, incomplete development (hypoplasia) of certain fingers and/or toes or rudimentary digits
Maternal Diseases	
Diabetes	Cardiac abnormalities, neural tube defects
Systemic lupus erythematosus	Congenital heart block
Phenylketonuria (PKU)	Cardiac abnormalities, microcephaly, developmental delays
Graves' disease	Small for gestational age, congenital hyperthyroidism, developmental delays
Maternal Radiation	Cataracts, microcephaly, small for gestational age, cancer, developmental disabilities
Maternal Drug Use	
Angiotensin-converting enzyme (ACE) inhibitors	Orthopedic defect, renal dysgenesis
Alcohol	Craniofacial dysmorphology, cardiac and CNS abnormalities, LBW, developmental delay
Aminopterin	Craniofacial dysmorphology, limb defects neural tube defects, LBW
Carbamazepine	Spina bifida
Carbinazole/methimazole	Hypothyroidism, goiter
Cocaine	Intracranial hemorrhage
Fluconazole (high doses)	Limb and craniofacial defects

continues

TABLE 6–1 Teratogenic factors *(continued)*

TYPE OF TERATOGEN	DEFECTS (varies by the amount and timing of exposure)
Isotretinoin	Hydrocephalus, CNS defects, micrognathia, cardiac defects
Methotrexate	Craniosynostosis, craniofacial dysmorphology, limb defects
Phenytoin	Craniofacial dysmorphology, hypoplastic phalanges and nails
Solvent abuse	Small for gestational age, developmental delay
Streptomycin	Hearing loss
Tetracycline	Stained teeth
Thalidomide	Limb reduction and abnormalities, ear abnormalities
Valproic acid	Spina bifida, craniofacial abnormalities
Warfarin	Nasal hypoplasia, CNS defects due to hemorrhage

Based on: Jorde, L. G., Carey, J. C., Bamshad, M. J., & White, R. L. (1999). *Medical genetics* (2nd ed., p. 301). St. Louis, MO: Mosby.

F. Pedigree Construction

The study of trait inheritance of genetic conditions often involves the construction of a pedigree. A pedigree is the genetic family tree, or the scientific genealogy of a family. The symbols for constructing a pedigree are conventional and are provided in Figure 6–1. Females are represented with a circle and males with a square. A diagonal cross through the symbol denotes "deceased." A filled circle or square refers to an affected individual. A large dot in the center of a circle or square refers to a carrier. Connecting lines between symbols differ depending on relationships; for example, a line connecting a circle and square denotes "marriage," a cross through that line denotes "divorce," a double line denotes "consanguinity" (mating with a close relative), and a connecting dotted line denotes a nonmarriage "union." Pedigree symbols denote the family generations using Roman numerals (I, II, III) and birth order within generations (numbers next to squares or circles), or number of females and males (numbers within the squares or circles). An arrow pointing to a particular square or circle denotes the **proband**, or the person of interest.

IV. CLINICAL COMPETENCIES

The learner outcomes, skills, and competencies gained from information contained in this chapter include the ability to:

- Read, interpret, and use basic terminology and abbreviations related to medical genetics.
- Define what is meant by "cancer-related genes."
- Differentiate between a "genotype" and a "phenotype."
- Describe the difference between single gene inheritance patterns and multifactorial abnormalities.

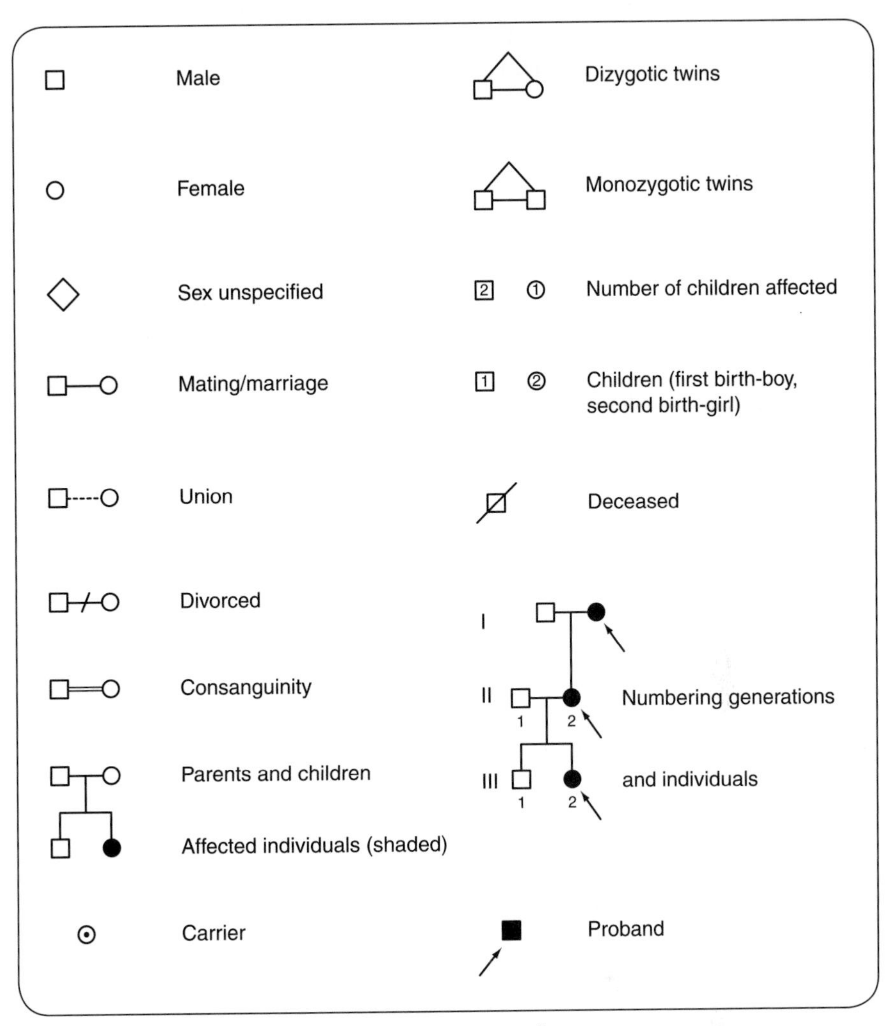

FIGURE 6–1 Symbols for constructing a genetic pedigree. Source: Delmar/Cengage Learning

- Define a "karyotype."
- Describe conditions that are the result of chromosomal deletion or addition defects.
- List known teratogenic agents and the disorders they cause.
- Describe the symbol system used in construction of a genetic pedigree.

V. REFERENCES AND RESOURCES CONSULTED

Boys Town Research Hospital. (2008). *Areas of research—Hereditary communication disorders.* Retrieved April 2008, from

http://www.boystownhospital.org/research/Areas/Hereditary/index.asp

Crow, J. F. (2000). Origins, patterns, and implications of human spontaneous mutation. *National Review of Genetics, 1*, 40–47.

Dale, J. W., & von Shantz, M. (2003). *From genes to genomes: Concepts and applications of DNA technology.* Chichester, West Sussex: John Wiley & Sons.

Jablonski, S. (2005). *Dictionary of medical acronyms and abbreviations* (5th ed.). Philadelphia: Elsevier Saunders.

Jorde, L. G., Carey, J. C., Bamshad, M. J., & White, R. L. (1999). *Medical genetics* (2nd ed.). St. Louis, MO: Mosby.

Keats, B. J. B., Popper, A. N., & Fay, R. R. (Eds.). (2002). *Genetics and auditory disorders.* New York: Springer-Verlag.

King, R. A., Rotter, J. I., & Motulsky, A. G. (Eds.). (2004). *The genetic basis of common diseases* (2nd ed.). Oxford: Oxford Press.

Lengauer, C., Kinzler, K. W., & Volgelstein, B. (1998). Genetic instabilities in human cancers. *Nature, 396*, 643–649.

Meuller, R. F., & Young, I. D. (2001). *Emery's elements of medical genetics* (11th ed.). Edinburgh: Churchill Livingstone.

National Institutes of Health. (2008). *Human Genome Project.*

Retrieved August 2008, from http://www.ornl.gov/sci/techresources/Human_Genome/home.shtml

Nussbaum, R. L., McInnes, R. R., Willard, H. F., & Boerkoel, C. F. (2004). *Thompson and Thompson genetics in medicine* (6th ed., Rev. reprint). Philadelphia: Elsevier Saunders.

Shelton, B. K., Ziegfeld, C. R., & Olsen, M. M. (2004). *Manual of cancer nursing* (2nd ed.). Philadelphia: Lippincott Williams & Wilkins.

Speechville Express. (2007). *Speechville Express syndromes.* Retrieved April 2008, from http://www.speechville.com/associated-disabilities/syndromes.html

Thelin, J. W., & Swanson, L. A. (2006). CHARGE syndrome. *The ASHA Leader, 11*(14), 6–7.

Wilson, G. N. (2000). *Clinical genetics: A short course.* New York: Wiley-Liss.

CHAPTER 7

Imaging Studies and Radiologic Oncology

In most hospital-based settings, speech-language pathologists (SLPs) are directly involved in the radiologic evaluation of swallowing. They may assist or receive assistance from the radiologist or radiology technician in conducting the **videofluoroscopic swallow studies (VFSS)**, or **modified barium swallows (MBS)**. The SLPs' diagnostic and management plan decisions are often informed by radiologic imaging studies. Findings from radiologic studies of the nervous system, particularly by studies of brain structures are also factors considered in the evaluation and treatment planning of individuals referred with communication disorders secondary to neurologic causes. Patients with traumatic brain injuries frequently have orthopedic injuries that may complicate communication or swallowing therapies. The extent and nature of these injuries are evaluated with radiologic studies. Radiation therapies may be a part of the history or treatment plan for individuals with brain tumors or head and neck cancer. It is essential that SLPs have fundamental knowledge of radiologic therapies and studies and the various imaging procedures as well as their purposes and be familiar with the related terminology and abbreviations encountered in medical records and reports.

I. CHAPTER FOCUS

This chapter reviews terminology and abbreviations encountered in radiologic studies, diagnostic imaging procedures, and radiologic therapies in oncology that are frequently encountered in medical SLP practice. Fundamental concepts in radiologic and imaging procedures and methods for administration of radiation oncology are reviewed. Related discussions and descriptions are found elsewhere in this text, especially in Chapters 3, 4, 5, 13, and 14.

II. TERMINOLOGY AND ABBREVIATIONS

A. Terminology (see also Chapters 3, 4, and 5)

Abdominal decubitus (position). Position in which patients are examined lying flat.

Acute abdominal series (AAS). Includes a kidneys, ureters, and bladder (KUB) study and x-rays for acute (sudden) abdominal disorders.

Adhesions. Abnormal fibrous bands between structures.

Adynamic. Not moving.

Aerated. Filled with air.

Aerophagia. Swallowing air.

Air-barium double contrast (ABDC), air contrast barium enema (ACBE). Techniques used when examining the gastrointestinal (GI) tract that involve giving the patient both barium and effervescent (gas-producing) crystals to swallow or by enema, allowing for better examination of the mucosa than is possible with barium alone.

Air-space disease. Lung disease involving the alveolar sacs.

Alopecia. Hair loss.

Alpha ray. Least penetrating form of radiation; positively charged helium nuclei.

Analog. In PET scanning, a radiopharmaceutical agent that is biochemically equivalent to a natural body compound.

Anechoic. Structures that fail to respond to echoes, as with sonography.

Anger camera. Instrument used for recording the distribution of gamma-emitting radioactivity, named for its inventor, Hal Anger.

Angiocardiogram. An x-ray study using radiopaque contrast medium to examine the heart and its vascularities as well as its great vessels.

Angiogram. An x-ray study using a bolus of radiopaque contrast medium to examine blood vessels. Various *rapid series studies* are used for cardiac, pulmonary, and cerebral angiography. *Digital subtraction angiography* (DSA) uses a minimal contrast load.

Anterior cervical plates. Plates and screws fixed to the anterior cervical spine for stabilization.

Aortogram. An x-ray study using radiopaque contrast medium to examine the aorta.

Aplasia of the lung. Incomplete development of the lung.

Aplastic anemia. A type of anemia caused by bone marrow destruction, for example, resulting from chemotherapy or radiation therapy effects.

Arteriogram. An x-ray study using radiopaque contrast media to study arteries.

Arthrogram. An x-ray study using radiopaque contrast media to study joints.

Artifact. An artificially produced image, as in "movement artifact."

Ascites. An accumulation of fluid in the abdominal (peritoneal) spaces.

Atelectasis. Collapsed, airless portion of the lung.

Austen-Moore. A type of hip prosthesis, sometimes used to refer to any hip replacement implant.

Barium swallow, esophagram. Fluoroscopic study used to examine the swallowing mechanism, esophagus, and esophageal peristalsis. (Also see Chapter 5.)

Barrett's esophagus, Barrett's metaplasia. A condition characterized by metaplastic epithelium occurring in the lower esophagus following peptic ulcer disease.

Basilar skull fracture. Fracture at the base of the cranium.

Beta rays. Radiation capable of penetrating body tissues for a few millimeters.

Betatron. A machine used to deliver high-energy radiation for megavoltage radiation therapy.

Bezoar. A collection of foreign bodies in the GI tract; for example, hair mass/ball.

Bilbao-Dotter tube. Tube used to conduct an enteroclysis (high enema) or duodenography.

Blowout fracture. Fracture of the floor of the orbit with possible entrapment of the orbital contents; hemorrhage into the maxillary sinuses is usually present.

Bone scan. Radioactive isotope study of bony structures (stress fractures, abscess, metastases).

Brachytherapy. Radiation therapy where a source of radiation is inserted near the area of the body being treated.

Bronchogram. An x-ray study using radiopaque contrast medium for examination of the bronchi.

Bucky grid. A grid placed between the x-ray machine and the patient to absorb ambient radiation and to reduce blurs on the film.

C-spine. X-ray study of all seven cervical vertebrae for trauma, neck pain, and neurologic disorders involving the upper spine.

Calcification. Deposits of calcium salts in tissues.

Calculus. Abnormal accumulation of mineral salts usually forming a stone-like body.

Carrier. Nonradioactive element or compound with the same chemical properties as a radioactive molecule.

Cassette. The covering of x-ray film providing protection from light exposure and containing a grid to enable the use of a lesser amount of radiation to obtain a desired result.

Cavitary lesions. Lung cavities seen with abscesses, cancer, or tuberculosis.

Cesium-137. Radionuclide used to study vaginal cancer.

Cholangiogram. An x-ray study using contrast medium to examine the bile ducts.

Cholecystogram. An x-ray study using contrast medium to examine the gallbladder and its contents (i.e., gallstones).

Cineradiography. Radiologic studies using motion picture film for recording; this term may be applied to videotape recording.

Cisternogram. An x-ray study of the base of the brain.

CM line, OM line. Canthomeatal, or orbitomeatal, line defined by an imaginary line from the lateral canthus of the eye to the meatus of the ear.

Cobalt-60. Radionuclide used in radiation therapy.

Coin lesion. Circular-shaped pulmonary lesions seen with granulomas and some carcinomas.

Collimator. The device in an x-ray machine that restricts diffusion of x-ray beams and focuses the beam at the desired area.

Communicating hydrocephalus. A condition where there is increased cerebrospinal fluid (CSF) in the brain despite the existence of a normal egress between the CSF and ventricles; communicating hydrocephalus is due to a problem with the resorption of CSF. (See Chapter 10 for additional discussion of hydrocephalus.)

Consolidation (pulmonary). Solidification of the lung, as found with pneumonia.

Contra coup. Referring to an injury to the brain occurring on the side opposite to the traumatic blow.

Contrast media. Compounds, usually having iodinated organic molecules, that are injected or imbibed for the purpose of obtaining better delineation of structures during x-ray.

Curie. A unit of radioactivity.

Cyclotron. A machine capable of producing megavoltage external radiation by creating accelerated, charged particles electromagnetically.

Decubitus. Lying down.

Degenerative joint disease (DJD). Osteoarthritis.

Density. Compactness.

Depressed skull fracture. Fracture of the cranial bones with depressed fragments of bone.

Diaphanogram. Infrared photographic examination.

Diffuse esophageal spasm. An esophageal contraction that occurs in response to thermal stimulants (hot or cold) and/or gastroesophageal reflux.

Digital subtraction. The use of a computer to subtract x-ray images instantaneously from low doses of contrast medium within a vessel.

Discrete. Well-defined.

Disseminated idiopathic skeletal hyperostosis (DISH). Extensive anterior hypertrophic spurs of the cervicothoracic spine.

Dosimetrist. Technical specialist in calculating radiation dosage.

Dry CT. A computed tomogram taken without contrast medium.

Dysmotility. An impairment in the normal peristaltic activity of the esophagus or intestines.

Echoencephalogram. An ultrasound study of the brain used to examine for tumors and other masses.

Electrokymogram. An x-ray study of the dynamic movements of the heart or other organs.

Enhanced CT. A computed tomogram taken after introduction of a contrast agent.

Epiphysis. The articulated end of bone where growth occurs.

Extrinsic masses. Growths that are outside the bowel but exert pressure on the GI tract.

Fibrosis. Where normal tissue has been replaced with fibrous tissue.

Film. A light-sensitive, thin cellulose sheet used for recording x-ray images.

Film badge. A badge containing a strip of material sensitive to ionizing radiation used to detect exposure to beta and gamma radiation.

Fluoroscopy. An x-ray study using a fluorescent surface to view the shadows of structures of the body after they are exposed to an x-ray beam.

Fractionation. Administration of radiation therapy in measured doses over a period of time to diminish radiation effects on normal tissues.

Gamma rays. Electromagnetic waves emitted from the atoms of radioactive elements. Gamma rays may be used in diagnostic scanning or radioactive implant therapies.

Gantry. The frame of the MRI scanner.

Gastraview, Gastragrafin study. Referring to the trade names for contrast agents used most often in radiologic studies prior to abdominal surgery when barium residues are not desired.

Gray units. Preferred units for quantifying radiation dosage. One unit of gray (Gy) equals 100 rads; thus 1 cGy = 1 rad.

Half-life. The time required for half of the radioactivity in a radioactive substance to disintegrate.

Hiatus hernia; hiatal hernia. Protrusion of the wall of the stomach through the hiatus (esophageal opening) of the diaphragm.

Hilum. The triangular depression on the medial surface of each lung that contains the hilar lymph nodes and through which blood and lymph vessels, nerves, and bronchi pass (the left should be 2–3 cm higher than the right).

Infiltrates. Radiodensities in the lungs indicating permeation of substances into the lung spaces.

Inflammatory joint disease (IJD). Referring to rheumatoid arthritis, gout, and pseudogout.

Interstitial pulmonary disease. Pulmonary disease of the tissues between the air (alveolar) spaces.

Intrathecal, thecal space. Within a sheath; usually pertaining to the space within the covering of the brain or spinal cord.

Intravenous pyelogram. An x-ray study using an injected contrast agent excreted from the bladder for examination of the urinary tract.

Intrinsic mucosal mass. Benign or malignant growths within the mucosa.

Intrinsic nonmucosal mass. Mural, or wall, tumors; benign or malignant growths covered by normal mucosa.

Ionization. Separating stable molecules into their charged particles called *ions*.

Ionmeter. A device used to measure radiation.

Iridium-192. A radionuclide used in internal radiation therapy.

Irradiation treatment. Therapeutic use of radiation beams and radionuclides.

Kilovolt. One thousand volts.

Kilowatt. One thousand watts.

Kyphosis, cervicothoracic kyphoscoliosis. Humpback; an abnormal anterior convexity of the cervicothoracic spine.

Linear accelerator. A device capable of generating megavoltage radiation dosage.

Linear skull fracture. Fracture line across the skull.

Luxury perfusion. Increased blood flow around the margins of a brain lesion.

Lymphangiogram. An x-ray study using a contrast medium to examine the lymph glands and lymphatic ducts.

Magnetic resonance angiography (MRA). An imaging study used principally to examine diseases involving the cerebrovascular system, such as aneurysms or other vascular malformations.

Magnetic resonance imaging (MRI). An imaging technique that uses magnetic movements of atomic nuclei to delineate tissues. Radio waves are directed toward a body area contained in an external magnetic field. When the radio waves are turned off, the hydrogen nuclei emit microwaves and weak radio waves that are detected and interpreted by a computer to construct transsectional images.

Mammogram. An x-ray or xeroradiographic study of the breast tissue for early detection of tumors.

Megavolt. One million volts.

Myelitis. Inflammation of the bone marrow.

Noncontrast computed tomogram (nc CT). Computed tomogram taken without a contrast agent; *dry CT*.

Oblique. Positioning at approximately a 45° lateral angle from the x-ray beam.

Obstruction hydrocephalus. A condition where there is an excessive accumulation of CSF in the brain owing to a blockage of the egress of CSF from the ventricular system, usually due to stenosis or obstruction of the Sylvian aqueduct.

Orthovoltage. Low to medium voltage energy used in radiation therapy (140–450 kV) as palliative treatment for cancer.

Osteoma. Tumor arising from bone tissue.

Osteomalacia. Softening of bone tissue due to calcium depletion associated with pain, tenderness, and muscle weakness; usually the result of a vitamin D deficiency.

Osteopenia. Lack of bone tissue.

Osteoporosis. Abnormal demineralization of bone tissue.

PACS. Picture Archiving and Communication System.

Panorex™. Trademarked name for a radiologic procedure using two axes of rotation to obtain a panoramic radiograph of the dentition and dental arches.

Portable chest film. Use of a portable x-ray machine to examine a patient unable to be transported to the radiology suite.

Positron emission tomography (PET) and single proton emission computed tomography (SPECT). Two types of emission computed tomography that permit imaging of metabolic activity from measurements of radioactivity within body sections.

Radiodermatitis. Skin inflammation due to radiation exposure.

Radiolucent. Structures or substances that permit the passage of radiation beams (appearing dark on an x-ray film).

Radionecrosis. Tissue death caused by radiation exposure.

Radiopaque. Structures or substances that restrict the passage of radiation beams (appearing white on an x-ray film).

Rarefaction. Decreased density.

Reticular infiltrates. Interstitial lung infiltrate pattern.

Roentgen. The international term for a unit of exposure to x-ray doses. This eponym refers to Wilhelm Roentgen, the German physicist who discovered x-rays.

Scan. General term for methods of visualizing organs, structures, and transverse body sections obtained through computed tomography, ultrasonography, scintigraphy, and other forms of diagnostic imaging.

Scintilligraphy. Studies that involve producing two-dimensional images from the scintillations emitted by radionuclide material administered internally.

Scintiscan. Radionuclide study used to detect scintillations produced when a radioactive substance is introduced into the body. In dysphagia evaluation, scintiscans are used to examine gastric reflux, esophageal motility, and aspiration.

Scoliosis. Curvature of the spine.

Sella, sella turcica. A shallow depression in the sphenoid bone at the base of the brain.

Shield. In radiology, a protective structure or garment containing lead used to prevent the passage of radiation.

Sialogram. An x-ray study of the salivary ducts and the secreting portion of the gland feeding the duct.

Spondylitis. An inflammation of the vertebrae.

Sternal wires. Surgical staples closing a suture in the sternum that are left in place following chest surgeries.

Tertiary waves, tertiary peristalsis. A condition usually found in the elderly in which there are multiple regions of dilation and narrowing of the esophagus during swallow; also called **corkscrew esophagus** and **presbyesophagus**.

Thermography. Recording of heat patterns within body structures; used to detect breast cancer and other inflammatory conditions.

Thyroid scan. Technetium-99 scan to evaluate thyroid function.

Tics. In radiology, referring to diverticula.

Tomography. Diagnostic radiographic studies in which images of single planes across tissues are produced in a series at different depths of an organ or area of the body.

Ultrasonography. Diagnostic studies using high-frequency sound waves that are projected and detected as they strike tissues of varying densities. These data are analyzed by a computer to create a series of images of the structure.

Valsalva maneuver. Procedure for increasing oral, pharyngeal, and nasal cavity pressures by holding the nose and mouth closed during forced exhalation against a closed glottis.

Venogram. An x-ray study of the veins, using a radionuclide contrast agent.

Wedge angle. In Doppler flow ultrasonography, the scanner is usually held at a "wedge" angle, rather than perpendicular, to the vessel being studied.

Xenon-127. Radioactive gas inhaled in ventilation x-ray studies of the lungs.

Xeroradiography. Dry radiologic techniques in which the x-ray image is made on a powdered surface and transferred photographically to specially treated paper.

B. Abbreviations

AAS. Acute abdominal series

Abd. CT. Abdominal computed tomogram

ACDF. Anterior cervical (spine) diskectomy with fusion

AM. Auditory meatus

AP. Anteroposterior

AU-198. Radioactive gold

AXR. Abdominal x-ray

Ba. Barium

B/K. Bladder/kidney (scan)

CAT, CT. Computed or computerized axial tomogram/tomography, computed or computerized tomogram/tomography

C CT. Contrast computed tomography

cGy. Centi-grays

CHIPES. Potentially poisonous compounds that are radiopaque (mnemonic stands for **c**hloral hydrate, **h**eavy metals, **i**odides, **p**henothiazines, **e**nteric coated, and **s**olvents)

Ci. Curie; mCi millicurie; μCi, microcurie; nCi, nanocurie; pCi, picacurie

CM. Costal margin, canthomeatal (line)

CPB. Competitive protein binding

CR. Computerized radiography

C-spine. Cervical spine (study)

CT. Computed tomogram

CXR. Chest x-ray

DR. Digital radiography

DWI. Diffuse-weighted magnetic resonance imaging

EMI. Electronic Musical Instruments (British company that built the first computed tomographic scanner, then called an "EMI scanner")

ERCP. Endoscopic retrograde cholangiopancreatogram

ERT. External radiation therapy

ESR. Electron spin resonance

F, Fr. French scale, a method for denoting the size of catheters and tubes based on units of 0.33 mm in diameter; for example, an 18 F tube is approximately 6 mm in diameter

fMRI. Functional magnetic resonance imaging

G. Glabella

GA-167. Gallium-167; radioactive gallium (used in whole body scanning studies)

I-131. Iodine-131; radioactive iodine (used in liver, kidney, and thyroid studies)

IC. Iliac crest

IRT. Internal radiation therapy

IVC. Intravenous cholangiogram

IVP. Intravenous pyelogram

KUB. Kidneys, ureters, bladder (study)

kV. Kilovolt

kW. Kilowatt

LCBF. Local cerebral blood flow

LL. Left lateral

MAMA™. Trademark name of a videofluoroscopic positioning chair used with children under 60 pounds

MFG. Manofluorogram

MRA. Magnetic resonance angiogram

MRI. Magnetic resonance imaging

MRS. Magnetic resonance spectrography/ spectragram

MRV. Magnetic resonance venogram

MUGA. Multigated acquisition (heart scan)

nc CT. Noncontrast computed tomogram

NMR. Nuclear magnetic resonance

OCG. Oral cholecystogram

OM. Orbitomeatal (line)

P-32. Phosphorus-32; radioactive phosphorus (used for palliative treatment of hematologic disorders)

PA. Posterior-anterior

PACS. Picture Archiving and Communication System

PET. Positron emission tomography/tomogram

PTHC. Percutaneous transhepatic cholangiogram

PWI. Perfusion-weighted magnetic resonance imaging

Ra. Radium

Rads. Radiation absorbed doses

rCBF. Regional cerebral blood flow

RISA. Radioiodinated human serum albumin

RL. Right lateral

ROI. Region of interest

RPG. Retrograde pyelogram

SBFT. Small bowel follow-through

SN. Sternal notch

SP. Symphysis pubis

SPECT. Single photon emission computed tomography/ tomogram

TBI. Thyroxine binding index

TC. Thyroid cartilage

Tc-99m. Technetium-99m; radioactive technetium (used in tracer studies of the brain, skull, lungs, spleen, liver, thyroid, and bony structures)

TEE. Transesophageal echocardiogram

TRF. Thyrotropin releasing factor

TRH. Thyrotropin-releasing hormone

TSH. Thyroid-stimulating hormone

2-D echo. Two-dimensional echocardiogram

U. Umbilicus

UGI. Upper GI

VCUG. Voiding cystourethrogram

V/Q. Ventilation-perfusion (lung) scan

XP. Xiphoid process

III. FUNDAMENTAL CONCEPTS

A. Contrast Agents and Barium Sulfate

It is sometimes desirable to change the radiodensity of the tissues being examined by injecting drugs containing iodine, called *contrast media*, or *contrast agents.* Barium sulfate is also introduced to delineate hollow structures better. Other non-barium contrast agents, such as "Gastraview" or "Gastragrafin," may be used to examine for fistulae prior to abdominal surgery. These latter agents are used when barium residues are not desirable.

During special studies, such as **cerebral angiography**, a water-soluble radioactive contrast agent is introduced percutaneously through catheterization of the femoral artery up to the major brachiocephalic arteries of the brain to enhance blood vessels prior to radiography. Sometimes the contrast agent is injected directly into the internal carotid arteries.

Some patients have a mild to severe adverse response to contrast media. These allergic reactions include feeling hot and itchy (**urticaria**); having a metallic taste in the mouth; and developing hives, angina, bronchospasm, and nausea and vomiting. In severe cases, irreversible shock can occur, resulting in death.

B. Plain (Still) Film Studies (Radiographs)

Plain film studies are used for a variety of purposes, including examination of orthopedic injuries and of nasogastric feeding tube placement; for screening purposes in chest, cardiac, abdominal, GI, renal, and skeletal examination; and in lymphangiography, cisternography, venography, sialography, and vascular studies, including cerebral angiography. Radiography uses x-ray produced images recorded on film. X-ray photons directed toward body structures are either absorbed or deflected as they pass through the electrons of the structures in their path. A radiographic image is a reflection of the electron density differences within the tissues that the x-ray has encountered in its path. The factors that affect electron density are the thickness of the structure and its physical state (gas, liquid, or solid).

C. Fluoroscopic Studies

Fluoroscopy permits immediate and continuous viewing of the x-ray image by using a phosphor screen. The resulting image is then magnified and transferred to a monitor for viewing and, in some cases, video-recorded for review. Rapid series radiographs are sometimes taken during fluoroscopy to provide a permanent record, or "still film." **Videofluoroscopy** refers to recording the fluoroscopic study on videotape. Increasingly, the use of digital recordings is common. *Videofluoroscopic swallow studies* (VFSS) are recorded fluoroscopies of barium swallows following some kind of prescribed protocol. The VFSS is a modification of the radiologist's "barium swallow," and may be called a *modified* barium swallow. VFSS, UGI, lower gastrointestinal (LGI), and air contrast studies (described earlier) are used to evaluate swallowing ability and esophageal, gastric, and intestinal structures and motility. **Cinefluoroscopy** (motion picture filmed recordings) can be used in a manner similar to videotaping and has some advantages because it provides a frame-by-frame analysis with images superior to videotape.

Manofluoroscopy is a technique that combines computerized manometry (see description of manometry in Chapter 5) and fluoroscopy to measure intrapharyngeal and esophageal pressure differences as they relate to bolus flow. Fluoroscopy studies are often used to evaluate cardiac motion and the structural and dynamic features of the GI tract and pulmonary abnormalities, and to identify optimal positioning for radiography (still films). Another method used for measuring the dynamic pressure changes in the esophagus is **intraluminal multiple electrical impedance**. It is a relatively new procedure that measures the electrical resistance in the esophagus to determine the volume of material passing through and clearing the esophagus.

D. Angiography

To obtain an x-ray image of blood vessels, a drug containing iodine is injected into the vessel either directly by needle or by a catheter passed percutaneously through the femoral or axillary arteries. Angiography is used for arterial, venous, and lymphatic circulation studies.

E. Pneumoencephalography

The **pneumoencephalograph (PEG)** is occasionally used to delineate the cisterns and the ventricular system. The PEG is especially useful for the evaluation of the posterior fossa tumors, suprasellar tumors, and third ventricular tumors.

F. Tomography

Tomography is a technique that permits imaging of a section or layer of the body. A computed, or computerized, **tomogram** (CT) is an image produced by a computer after processing x-ray data fed from detectors. To perform the scan, an x-ray tube is rotated in a complete circle, allowing x-rays to pass through the patient at overlapping, multiple intervals. The x-ray detectors provide data on these multiple measurements of a body section to the computer, which then calculates the radiodensities of the structures and creates a corresponding image from the data.

The radiodensities ascribed to a volume of tissue in the body are called **voxels**, for *volume elements.* A voxel is the smallest unit of tissue volume that can be imaged by a CT scan. A **pixel**, for *picture element*, is the smallest unit of surface that the computer can display. Because the thickness of the voxel is usually larger than the size of the pixel, the CT's reconstructed image lacks the precise detail found in MRIs.

CT images are made in *transverse* (axial) sections of about 1 to 10 mm (Figure 7-1 shows an illustration of brain CT scans). After the CT image data are stored in the computer, radiodensities can be selectively adjusted, or exaggerated, to provide a larger "viewing window." Adjusting the "viewing lever" and "viewing width" controls allows the desired tissues to be visualized more clearly. The introduction of rapid intravenous infusion of iodinated contrast media also assists in examination of intracranial structures. CTs are taken *without contrast* ("dry") followed by *with contrast* ("enhanced") scans. By disrupting the **blood-brain barrier**, a mechanism that normally prevents certain substances from passing from the blood into brain tissue, the contrast medium will be "taken up" in areas where pathologic processes exist. These areas will be shown to be "enhanced" (appear lighter) on the CT scan. "Enhancing" lesions are usually vascular and "nonenhancing" lesions are nonvascular.

G. Magnetic Resonance Imaging

Magnetic resonance images (MRIs) and the various magnetic imaging technologies such as **magnetic resonance angiography (MRA), magnetic resonance venography (MRV), magnetic resonance spectrography (MRS), diffusion-weighted magnetic resonance imaging (DWI), perfusion-weighted magnetic resonance imaging (PWI),** and **functional magnetic resonance imaging (fMRI)** provide highly detailed, dynamic, color images of the structures of the body. **Biochemical spectral analysis** is also possible from MRI data. Both **positron emission**

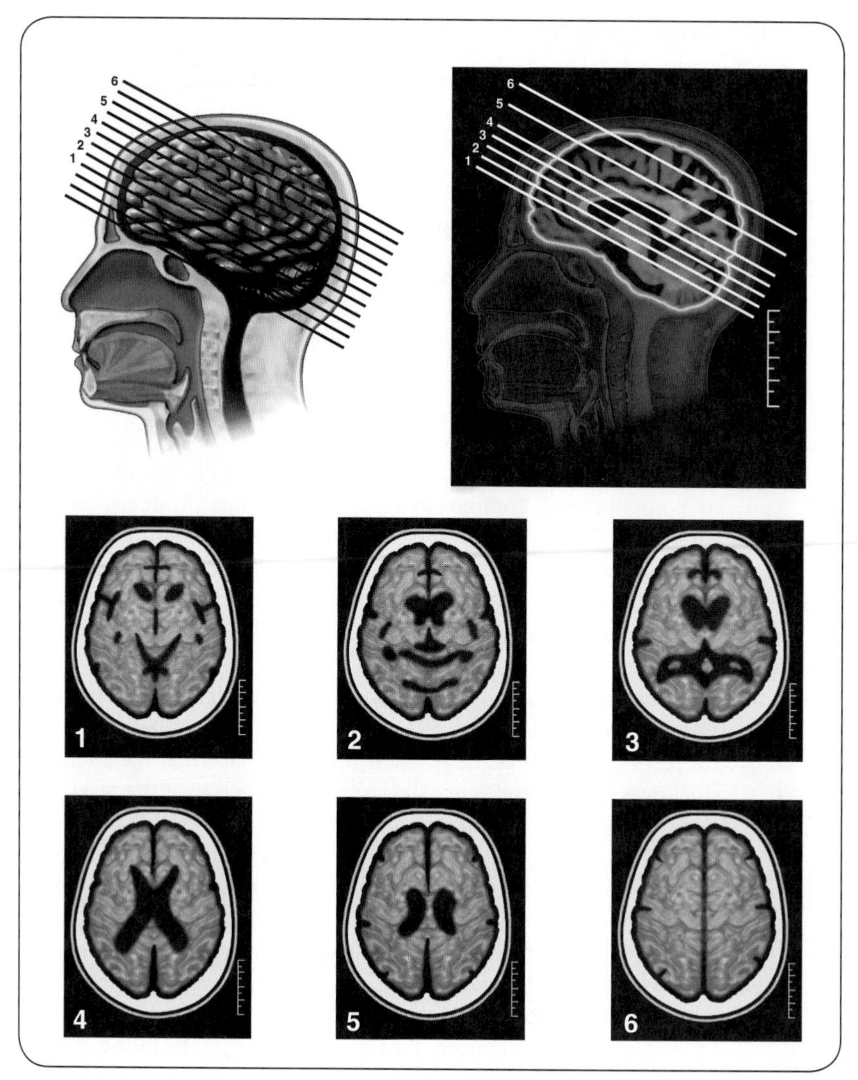

FIGURE 7–1 Illustration of brain CT scan sections. Based on Source: Naeser, M. A, & Hayward, R. W. (1978). *Lesion localization in aphasia with cranial computed tomography and the Boston Diagnostic Aphasia Exam.* Neurology, 28, 545–551.

tomography (PET) (see later) and fMRI are referred to as *functional* (brain) *activation studies*, in that they are used to examine brain physiology while the individual is engaged in a functional mental activity. Figure 7-2 provides a series of MRI images, demonstrating the emergence of the image of a sizable tumor in the deep structures of the left hemisphere (Seikel, King, & Drumright, 2005).

An MRI is a *relatively* lower risk procedure than a CT scan in that it does not use isotopes or x-rays, and it can provide higher resolution images than a CT scan. An MRI has some risks, however; for example, it often uses a contrast medium containing adolinium, which has been associated with a fibrosing condition of the skin and other tissues in patients with kidney disease. In addition, patients with claustrophobia may have difficulty tolerating

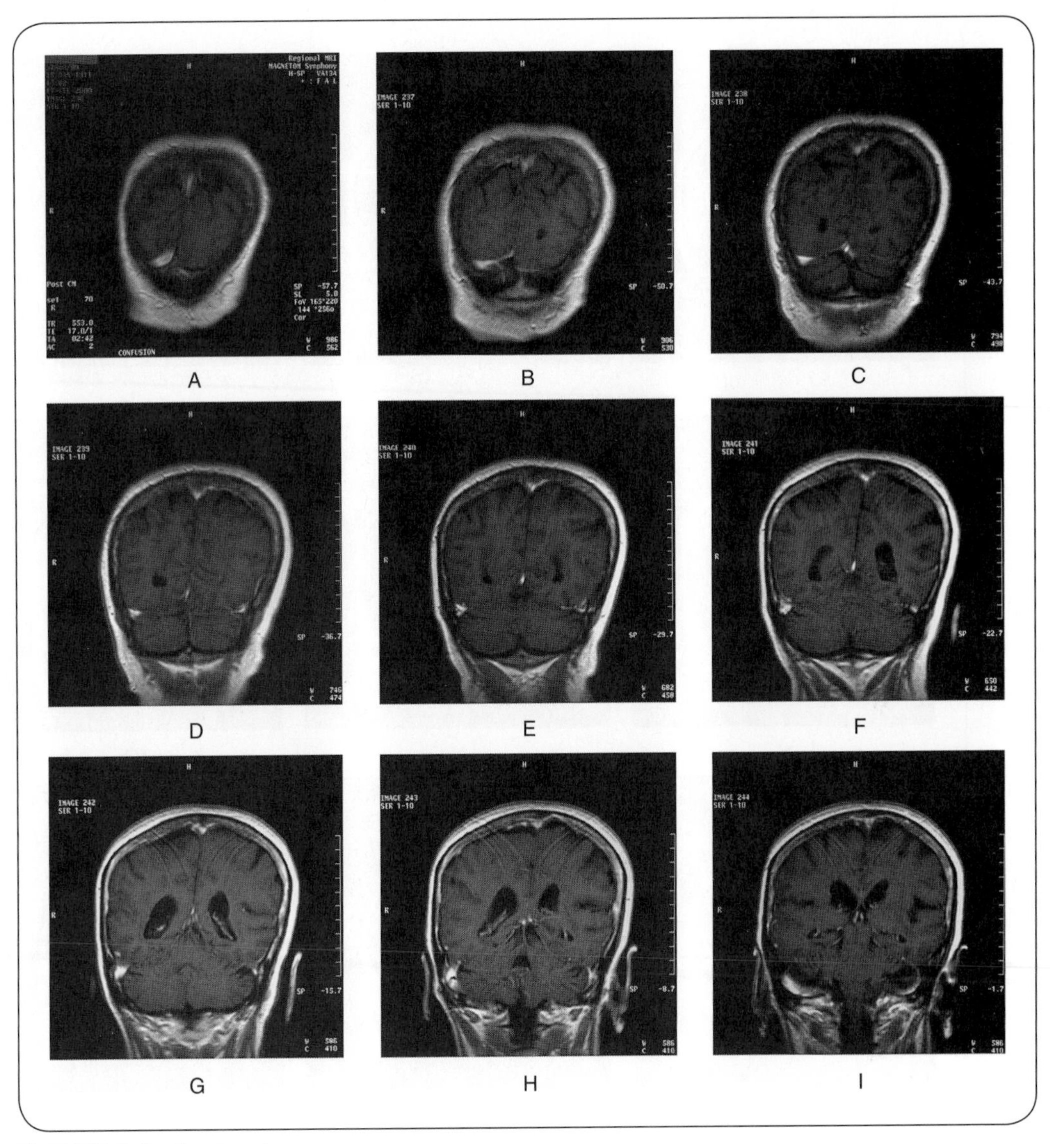

FIGURE 7–2 *(continues)*

the study because it requires lying in a small, enclosed space for an extended period. CT scans are considerably less expensive studies than MRIs and are usually sufficient for many diagnostic purposes. Additionally, MRIs cannot be used with certain people (such as individuals with artificial implants, heart valves, or stents, or who are highly claustrophobic). In brain imaging, magnetic imaging procedures are used most often with suspected strokes (typically within 6 hours of onset) or to examine for brain tumors, posterior fossa abnormalities, white matter diseases, or lacunar infarctions. fMRI is used to identify regional blood oxygenation activity (indicating heightened metabolic activation of a particular part of the brain, or lack

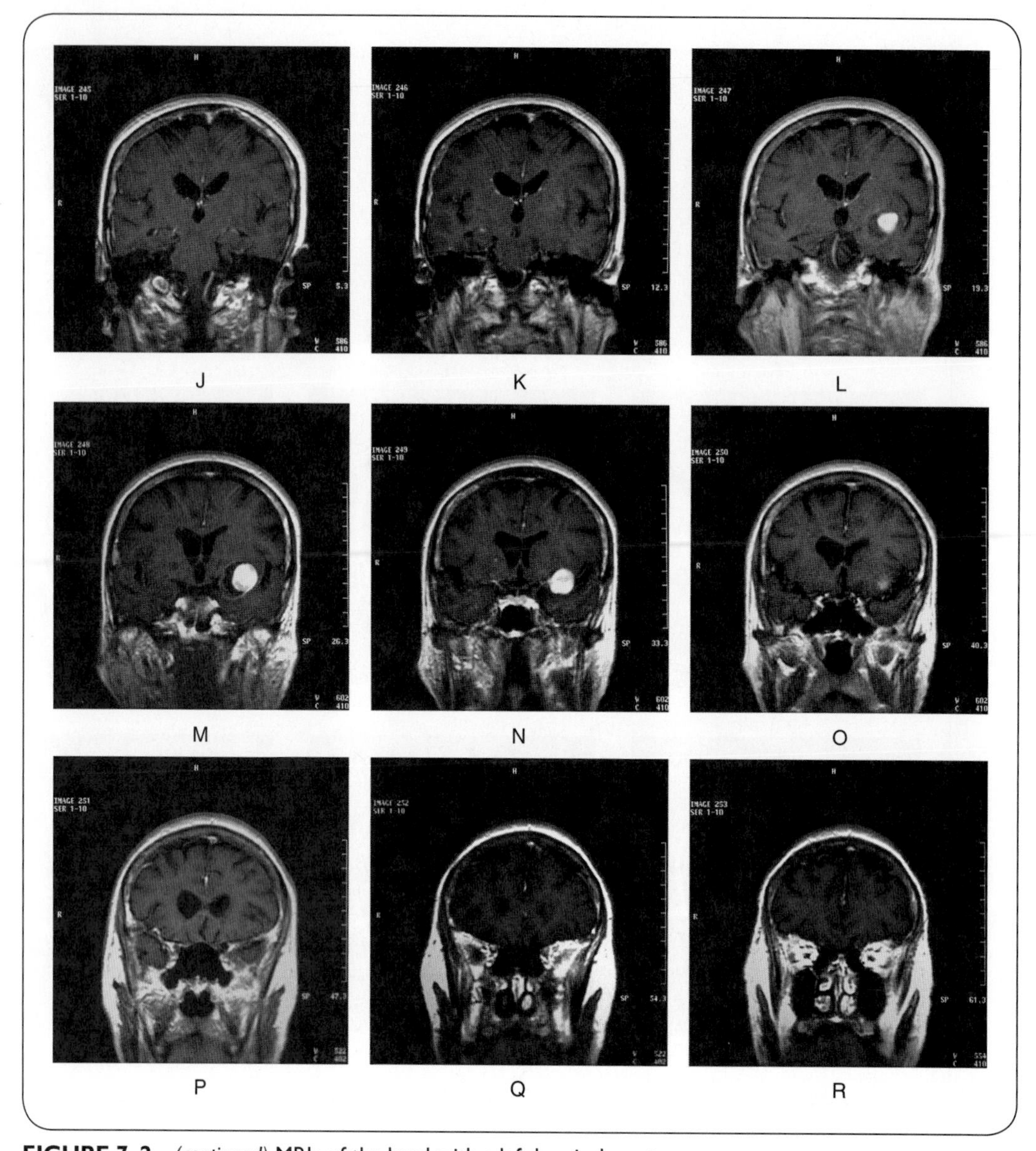

FIGURE 7–2 *(continued)* MRIs of the head with a left hemisphere tumor. Source: Delmar/Cengage Learning

of activation) during some sort of mental activity. fMRI has been applied in research related to language functions and other cognitive processes. Similarly, DWI and PWI have been used in the neuropsychological research, including the study of cortical and subcortical aphasia recovery relative to the physiologic (blood flow and metabolism) status of the brain (e.g., Hillis et al., 2004). An MRS study can detect the chemical composition of tissues and thus has been used in the study of the influence of drugs on the central nervous system, dementing diseases, brain tumors, and epilepsy.

The MRI is based on principles of magnetism and electromagnetic radiation. To produce a magnetic resonance image, hydrogen atoms in the water substrate of the body are exposed to a strong magnetic field that aligns the atoms. Radio frequency electromagnetic waves are then introduced and disrupt the alignment of the atoms. After the waves are turned off, the atoms release electromagnetic energy as they realign themselves with the magnetic field. This energy, or **magnetic resonance**, is then detected, localized, and measured by a computer to reconstruct a corresponding image. Depending on the methods used to sequence the electromagnetic radiation, different images and patterns will be elicited from the body's magnetic resonance. The changes in the magnetic vectors of the nuclei are measured as T-1 (the longitudinal relaxation time of changes in the z axis) and T-2 (the transverse relaxation time for changes in the x, y plane). The differences between T-l and T-2 measurements are the data used by the computer to construct the MRI image. The MRI image photograph and report will state the T weightings as "T-l weighted images" (the image is dependent on T-l differences for visual contrast) or "T-2 weighted images" (the image is dependent on T-2 differences for visual contrast). In T-l images the ventricles appear dark. T-l images are used to delineate *anatomy*. In T-2 images the ventricles appear white. T-2 images are used to demonstrate *pathology*. The MRI report will also specify the *pulse sequence*. The most common pulse sequence is termed "spin echo." "Inversion recovery," "saturation recovery," and "partial saturation" are additional, more recent, pulse sequences. Usually a description of the computation values is designated on the MRI "hardcopy" (photographic image) or in the radiologist's report (e.g., "T-1-weighted, repetition time 500–600 ms; echo time 20–30 ms").

The usual positions for MRI scans are transverse, sagittal, oblique, and coronal. The sagittal plane is frequently used to examine for posterior fossa and spinal cord abnormalities (refer to Figure 4–11). Although dental fillings and prostheses are not considered a problem during an MRI, as mentioned earlier, vascular clips, artificial valves and stents, pacemakers, and cochlear implants are contraindicated because the magnetism will cause them to displace.

H. Sonography

The **sonography** uses high-frequency sound waves promulgated through a body structure and reflected back to a crystal transducer. Sound waves are stopped by either air or bone (anechoic); thus, sonography is best suited for studies of soft tissue. Systems for **ultrasonography** include real-time scanners, phased-arrayed systems, or linear array systems. Different methods for recording images will be applied, including *A mode* (creates a linear graph), *B mode* (creates a two-dimensional image), and *M mode* (demonstrates the motion of a structure of the body, such as the motion of a heart valve). In **echocardiography**, the image is usually recorded in the M mode. Two-dimensional echocardiography, referred to as a **2-D echo**, is a study in the motion mode in which a wedge, or sector, of cardiac activity can be viewed. Picture images are created from sonographic data and will be saved as a digital or photographic record in the medical chart.

I. Tracer and Emission Imaging

Diagnostic imaging uses **radiotracers** (technetium-99m, iodine-131, xenon-133, thallium-201, and gallium-167) to image or treat diseases. These radioactive drugs can be used to mimic nonradioactive drug activity or to examine metabolic activity (as in thyroid studies). For example, xenon-133 gas distributes in the lungs in a manner similar to nitrogen and, thus, permits imaging of respiratory functions in pulmonary ventilation and perfusion scans. Tracer imaging provides metabolic, physiologic, and anatomic information.

Most of the radionuclides used in tracer imaging are **gamma ray emitters.** Images are detected by a rectilinear scanner, or a gamma camera, also called an Anger camera after the inventor, Hal Anger. Positron emitters are also used for imaging, as with *positron emission tomography* (PET) and **single proton emission computed tomography (SPECT).** After positrons interact with the electrons in their path, measurements can be made of the radioactive decomposition. These data are analyzed by a computer, which then generates an image. When images are formed by external detection of radiation emitted from an internally administered radioactive compound, the study will be called an *emission scan.* **Emission computer tomography (ECT)** is the study of a slice across a variety of planes (transaxial, coronal, or sagittal).

The radionuclides used in tracer scans and tomograms mimic metabolic activity. Thus, tracer scanning and emission tomography permit the neuroradiologist to look directly at cerebral glucose metabolism (i.e., how rapidly glucose is used by neural cells). This is the principle underlying PET scanning. This technique uses radioactive fluorine, F-18, attached to an altered glucose molecule (deoxyglucose), which is injected into a vein. The radioactive fluorine emits a positive electron, or positron, which combines with a negative electron to produce gamma rays. These rays are then read by radiation detectors to construct dynamic (changeable) tomograms of the brain. Similarly, regional **cerebral blood flow (rCBF)** and **local cerebral blood flow (LCBF)** studies use the radioactive gas xenon-133 injected into the carotid artery, and permit gamma radiation detection from the brain's surface. PET, SPECT, and rCBF studies are particularly useful in research that examines neuronal metabolic activity under various stimulus conditions and in the clinical evaluation of cerebral dysfunction. Abnormalities in blood flow and brain metabolism can be revealed in brains that appear structurally intact by CT scanning. (See Chapter 4 for additional discussion and a review of functional MRIs.)

IV. RADIATION ONCOLOGY

A. Methods of Administration

Radiologic oncology refers to medical treatment for cancerous tumors, or other undesirable tissues, with alpha, beta, gamma, or x-rays while attempting to preserve healthy tissues. Internal radiation methods can include either *sealed* (implantation of sealed containers near the tumor) or *unsealed* (intravenous administration of radionuclides) techniques. Sealed-type radiotherapy, called **brachytherapy**, uses radioactive rods, pellets, or beads or interstitial needles, sutures, or wires. Unsealed types of infusion therapies use **intravenous infusion** or **intracavitary infusion** of radioactive phosphorus-32. Intravenous injections are absorbed by bone marrow and are effective agents in the treatment of leukemia and **polycythemia**. Intracavitary methods are not absorbed by bone marrow. Oral ingestion of iodine-131 is used to treat **hyperthyroidism.**

External radiation, or teletherapy, administers doses calculated by the size, site, and depth of the lesion for maximal destruction of malignant cells. To accomplish external radiotherapy, a Cobalt 60 teletherapy unit, a 2 MeV Van de Graaf generator, or a low megavoltage linear accelerator is used.

The radiotherapy treatment regimen for cancer varies by site and cancer tissue type. Radio-therapy for glottic carcinoma, for example, generally ranges from 6000 to 7000 radiation absorbed doses, or "rads," with dosage calculated in fractions over 6½ weeks. Preferred dosages are determined depending on the size, location, and type (histopathology) of the tumor. The field of radiation can be altered with techniques such as wedge filters and rotations. The site of maximal radiation is precisely determined, and *isodose curves* are computed based on the dosage, size of the portal (width of the beam), and treatment technique used. For example, wedges are used to enhance radiation to a particular area and to eliminate "cold spots," which are areas receiving insufficient doses of radiation. Radiation therapy is often an adjuvant therapy used prior to or after surgery and/or chemotherapy (refer to Chapter 12).

B. Problems and Side Effects

To achieve a therapeutic, cumulative dose of radiation, unwanted side effects sometimes result. These can include **induration** (hardening) of the radiated soft tissues, **anorexia** (loss of appetite), **alopecia** (loss of hair), **necrosis** (death) of the bone, **diarrhea**, **vomiting**, **erythema** (reddening), **stomatitis** (irritation of the mouth), **xerostomia** (dry mouth), **mucositis** (irritation of the mucous membranes), and **malaise** (generally feeling weak and ill).

Radiation to the laryngeal area can, although rarely, cause **radiochondronecrosis** when the dosage has exceeded 7000 rads. Transient edema of the arytenoids occasionally occurs following laryngeal radiation, and subcutaneous fibrosis with **telangiectasis** (dilatation of a group of capillaries) may occur.

Radiation treatment for brain tumors will be affected by the "radio resistance" of neoplastic (tumor) cells. In vitro studies of hypoxic cells have shown them to be less sensitive to radiation than normally oxygenated cells. To overcome the hypoxic condition, biologically enhanced doses of radiation have been applied to treat brain tumors, such as malignant astrocytomas. Enhancement methods have included the use of a **hyperbaric oxygen chamber**, whole body **hyperthermia**, and **bromodeoxyuridine**.

V. CLINICAL COMPETENCIES

The learner outcomes, skills, and competencies gained from information contained in this chapter include the ability to:

- Read, interpret, and use terminology and abbreviations related to radiology studies and imaging procedures.
- Discuss the basic principles and potential problems involved in the use of contrast media for radiologic studies.
- Differentiate between still films and dynamic studies (e.g., fluoroscopies).
- Discuss the basic principles of computed tomography (CT) scans, magnetic resonance imaging, and sonography.
- Differentiate between tracer and emission imaging methods.
- Describe the methods of administration and side effects of radiation oncology.

VI. REFERENCES AND RESOURCES CONSULTED

Anderson, D. (Ed.). (2003). *Dorland's illustrated medical dictionary* (30th ed.). Philadelphia: W. B. Saunders.

Davies, J. J. (2008). *Essentials of medical terminology* (3rd ed.). Clifton Park, NY: Delmar Cengage Learning.

Freeman, M. (Ed.). (1988). *An introduction to clinical imaging.* New York: Churchill Livingstone.

Hillis, A. E., Barker, P. B., Wityk, R. J., Aldrich, E. M., Restrepo, L., Breese, E. L., et al. (2004). Variability in subcortical aphasia is due to variable sites of cortical hypoperfusion. *Brain and Language, 79*, 495–510.

Hunter, T. B., & Taljanovic, M. S. (2003). Glossary of medical devices and procedures: Abbreviations, acronyms, and definitions. *Radiographics, 23*, 195–213.

Jablonski, S. (2005). *Dictionary of medical acronyms and abbreviations* (5th ed.). Philadelphia: Elsevier Saunders.

Johnson, A. H., & Jacobson, B. H. (Eds.). (2007). *Medical speech-language pathology: A practitioner's guide* (2nd ed.). New York: Thieme.

Jones, B., & Downs, M. W. (1991). *Normal and abnormal swallowing: Imaging in diagnosis and therapy.* New York: Springer-Verlag.

Juhl, J. H., & Crummy, A. B. (1987). *Paul and Juhl's essentials of radiologic imaging* (5th ed.). Philadelphia: J. B. Lippincott.

Kirkwood, J. R. (1995). *Essentials of neuroimaging* (2nd ed.). New York: Churchill-Livingstone.

Naeser, M. A., & Hayward, R. W. (1978). Lesion localization in aphasia with cranial computed tomography and the Boston Diagnostic Aphasia Exam. *Neurology, 28*, 545–551.

Plausic, B. M., Robinson, A. E., & Jeffrey, R. B., Jr. (1992). *Gastrointestinal radiology: A concise text.* New York: McGraw Hill.

Rice, D. H., & Spiro, R. H. (1989). *Current concepts in head and neck cancer.* New York: The American Cancer Society.

Seikel, J. A., King, D. W., & Drumright, D. G. (2005). *Anatomy and physiology for speech, language, and hearing* (3rd ed.). Clifton Park, NY: Delmar Cengage Learning.

Shapshay, S. M., & Ossoff, R. H. (Eds.). (1985). Squamous cell cancer of the head and neck. *The Otolaryngologic Clinics of North America, 18.*

Squire, L. F., & Novelline, R. A. (1988). *The fundamentals of radiology* (4th ed.). Cambridge, MA: Harvard University Press.

CHAPTER 8

Infectious Diseases and Infection Control

All health care personnel must follow infection precautions when they have contact with patients. The facility's **Environment of Care (EOC)** policies and procedures are intended to ensure that all employees actively avoid and prevent exposure of others and themselves to contagious and potentially infectious diseases. Certain patient populations, such as neonates, burn patients, critically ill patients, elderly patients, and patients preparing for or undergoing transplants, are especially susceptible to infection; however, standard precautions apply regardless of whether or not a risk for infection is known. Everyone in a health care facility can present a risk for the spread of infection; consequently, all employees are expected to understand and apply **universal precautions**.

It is advisable for anyone with a contagious disease or an **exudative** (open, oozing) lesion on the skin to avoid physical contact with patients. Additionally, clinicians must be especially careful to ensure that nondisposable equipment used in or near the mouth (such as special feeding nipples and bottles, penlights and oral examination mirrors, tracheoesophageal puncture prosthesis fitting devices, endoscopic scopes and tubes, etc.) has been properly cleaned of fluids and tissues and sterilized according to infection control guidelines between uses. Any equipment that has been loaned to patients needs to be **decontaminated** and in some cases sterilized before it is reused by others. Augmentative communication devices loaned to a patient, for example, should be decontaminated after use.

In inpatient settings, speech-language pathologists (SLPs) move from ward to ward and patient to patient. They see patients in intensive care units and burn units and patients who have infection control precautions in place due to immune suppression. They have frequent contact with patients who have tracheostomies, intravenous (IV) lines, or are receiving enteric feeding via feeding tubes. SLPs are in close contact with patients who have had head and neck surgeries and patients who require oral feeding assistance. SLPs are especially vulnerable to exposure to potentially infectious body fluids and can also potentially contribute to the spread of infectious diseases; thus, medical SLPs need to be vigilant about infection control practices.

I. CHAPTER FOCUS

This chapter reviews terminology and abbreviations encountered when discussing infectious diseases and infection control. Infection prevention and the characteristics of common infectious diseases are described. This review is intended to inform clinicians about how infectious diseases are prevented and managed to emphasize the SLP's role and heighten the clinicians' awareness regarding a responsibility to themselves and their patients in reducing, preventing, and avoiding exposure to hospital-related infections.

II. TERMINOLOGY AND ABBREVIATIONS

A. Terminology

Additional terminology related to hematologic factors is found in Chapter 9, and further discussion of laboratory tests to detect infectious diseases is found in Chapter 3.

Acid fast bacilli (AFB) isolation. Infection control practice to prevent the spread of the organism that causes tuberculosis.

Acquired immunodeficiency syndrome (AIDS). Refer to the discussion of human immunodeficiency virus and HIV (see later).

Aerobic. With oxygen.

AIDS-related complex (ARC). A term previously used to refer to symptoms of night sweats, diarrhea, and wasting in association with HIV infection.

Airborne transmission. Air route for the spread of pathogens.

Anaerobic. Without oxygen.

Antibiotic. Drug used to treat infection.

Antimicrobial agent. Chemical used to kill or inhibit the growth of microorganisms.

Antiseptic. Chemical used to kill or inhibit the growth of microorganisms that is usually safe to apply on living tissue.

Asepsis. Lack of infection.

Autoclave. An apparatus for pressurized steam sterilization.

Autoclave film. A continuous roll of transparent plastic tubing or bags for packaging items exposed to autoclave sterilization.

Autoclave tape. A tape with ink that is sensitive to heat or chemical agents and visible only after exposure to sterilization. The ink changes to a dark color during the sterilization process.

Bacteremia. When bacteria are present in the blood.

Bacteria. Single-celled organisms that reproduce asexually and multiply rapidly. Bacteria are classified by their shape: *cocci* are spherical, *bacilli* are rodlike, and *flagella* have whiplike extensions. Bacteria that require oxygen to multiply are called **aerobic**, and those that do not require oxygen to function and reproduce are called **anaerobic**. Some types of bacteria are essential to normal body functions, such as the normal flora (bacteria) in the intestinal tract.

Bacteriostatic. Chemicals used to prevent or inhibit the growth of microorganisms and are safe to use on living tissues.

Barrier. Technique, instrument, or garment used to block the transfer of pathogens.

Blood and body fluid precautions. Method of infection control that prevents contact with blood or body fluids; for example, this method is used with patients who have HIV infection or the hepatitis B virus.

Candidiasis. A white, patchy appearing fungal infection, commonly referred to as thrush, or a yeast infection; frequently seen in individuals with immature or compromised immune systems or in those who have used antibiotics or steroids.

Cat-scratch disease. A subacute regional lymphadenitis caused by exposure to *Bartonella henselae* that appears after a cutaneous inoculation following an animal bite or scratch.

Centers for Disease Control and Prevention (CDC). The government agency located in Atlanta, Georgia, that conducts and collates research data related to infectious diseases.

***Clostridium difficile* (C-diff).** An "overgrowth" organism that causes colitis or enteritis, characterized by watery diarrhea usually brought on by repeated enemas, prolonged nasogastric tube insertion, or gastrointestinal (GI) surgery. The overuse of antibiotics, especially penicillin (ampicillin), clindamycin, and cephalosporins, may also alter the normal intestinal flora and increase the risk of developing this condition. C-diff is common and difficult to manage in children who have a long history of enteral feeding and repeated infections.

Colonization. Growth of microbial agents; a stage of infection.

Communicable. Contagious, transferable from one person to another.

Contact isolation. Procedures applied to eliminate physical contact with infected individuals and any articles they have touched.

Contact route. Contact with infection that can come directly through touching an infected person, indirectly through contaminated surfaces or objects, and by droplets when in close proximity to a patient's breath or expectorate.

Contaminate. To expose to pathogens or desterilize.

Cultures. Examinations of bacteria in body fluids, cells, and samples, including throat sputum, cerebrospinal fluid, urine, pus, wounds, drains, genital secretions, and stool.

Deinfestation, disinfestation. Elimination of parasitic insects.

Direct fluorescent antibody (DFA) test. Test for syphilis.

Disease-specific isolation. Special treatment and isolation procedures for designated infectious diseases.

Disinfectant. Chemical that kills microorganisms but not necessarily their spores.

Double-bagging technique. Procedure used with patients who have infectious diseases. It involves placing a bag that holds contaminated items into a clean bag that has not been in contact with the isolation (contaminated) room or the patient.

Drainage and secretion precautions. Procedures applied to eliminate contact with infected wounds and body secretions; used primarily with burn patients and patients with conjunctivitis.

Empyema. Collection of pus within a body cavity.

Encephalitis. Acute viral or other infectious causes that produce inflammation of the central nervous system; characterized by fever, headache, and stiff neck.

Endocarditis. Infection involving the lining of the membrane of the cardiac chambers or a cardiac valve.

Enteric precautions. Procedures applied to eliminate contact with infected feces; used primarily with patients who have the hepatitis A virus.

Envenomations. Poison exposures resulting from spider and snake bites or hymenoptera (bees, hornets, yellow jacket) stings.

Eosinophilic esophagitis. A condition in which the cellular structure of the walls of the esophagus have a much higher than normal number of eosinophils. These cells are thought to be increased in response to allergens and bacteria (see Chapter 5).

Epiglottitis. Usually refers to an aggressive disease that occurs in young children in which a sore throat, copious oral secretions, severe pain of the pharyngeal area without reddening, and respiratory difficulty develop.

Fever. Condition in which the body temperature is above a normal range, usually in excess of 37.8°C or 100.2°F. Causes of fever can include infections (viral, bacterial, or fungal), tissue injury, drugs, malignancy, immune-mediated disorders, endocrine disorders, and other inflammatory disorders.

Flora. Bacteria that are normally present in a given location.

Hepatitis. Inflammation of the liver.

Hepatomegaly. Enlargement of the liver and spleen; indicative of infection.

Host. Person (or animal) carrying an organism.

Human immunodeficiency viruses (HIV-1, HIV-2). Referring to the viral agents of acquired immune deficiency syndrome (AIDS), formerly called *human T-lymphotropic virus type III (HTLV-III)* or *lymphadenopathy-associated virus (LAV)*. HIV is transmitted through the exchange of body fluids, such as between a mother and fetus, within breast milk, sharing contaminated needles, receiving contaminated blood products, and sexual intercourse. HIV causes the individual to be susceptible to opportunistic infections due to several immunological changes that occur. **Lymphopenia** with a decreased helper T-lymphocyte to suppressor lymphocyte (T 4 to T 8) ratio is characteristic of HIV infections. Patients may acquire **cytomegalovirus (CMV)**, **Epstein-Barr virus (EBV)**, and **herpes simplex virus (HSV)**. For further discussion see Section IX, HIV-Positive Patients.

Humidifier. A method for saturating gas with vapor.

Iatrogenic infection. Infection that inadvertently results from a medical or surgical procedure. Health care acquired infections, or **hospital-acquired infections (HAI)** are usually the result of iatrogenic risk factors, such as pathogens transferred in the hands of medical personnel or with invasive procedures (e.g., indwelling vascular lines, urine catheterization, intubation) (also see Section VIII, Nosocomial Infections).

Infectious mononucleosis. Cervical lymphadenopathy presenting with fever, malaise, tonsillar pharyngitis, and hepatosplenomegaly; the *Epstein-Barr virus* is the causative agent.

Infectious period. Time when pathogens can be transmitted from a host.

Interferons. A family of proteins produced by lymphocytes, fibroblasts, epithelial cells, and macrophages that provide a major host defense against viruses.

Ludwig's angina. A condition characterized by *cellulitis* of the floor of the mouth usually due to an odontogenic infection. The tongue may be pushed upward with induration (firm hardening) of the submandibular space; patients have difficulty swallowing and may complain of chest pain.

Mantoux test; purified protein derivative (PPD). A screening skin test for tuberculosis that is required annually in health care settings.

Meningitis. An inflammation of the *leptomeninges* (pia and arachnoid) caused by infectious or noninfectious processes (e.g., cancer, hemorrhage). The types of infectious meningitis include bacterial meningitis, aseptic meningitis, herpes simplex, viral meningitis, and tubercular meningitis. Additional discussion is found in Chapter 10, Neurologic and Psychiatric Disorders.

Microorganisms. Minute forms of life capable of causing diseases.

Mononuclear phagocyte. Macrophages that degrade and kill bacteria directly and in antibody-dependent reactions.

Myelitis. Inflammation of the spinal cord; several viruses, such as varicella zoster, are associated with myelitis.

Natural killer (NK) cells. Lymphocytes that are defined by their ability to lyse (break down) certain tumors.

Nebulizer. Device producing an aerosol.

Neutropenic. Having a low neutrophil (white) cell count and at risk for infection.

Neutrophils. Cells that ingest bacteria and kill them.

Nonpathogenic organism. Harmless microorganism.

Otitis externa, otitis media. Referring to infections of the external auditory canal and the middle ear, respectively.

Pathogenic organism. Microorganism that is contagious or can cause an infection.

Pediculosis. Lice infection.

Pharyngitis. Referring to inflammation of the pharyngeal mucosa. The causes of pharyngitis include viruses (respiratory viruses, herpes simplex, Epstein-Barr virus, coxsackievirus A), bacteria (Group A streptococcus, Vincent's fusospirochetes, *Corynebacterium diphtheriae*, *Corynebacterium hemolyticum*), and gonorrhea.

Pneumonia. Referring generally to an inflammation of the lungs caused by bacteria, viruses, or chemical and physical agents. Pneumonia may also result from other causes, such as acute and chronic lung disease and congestive heart failure (CHF). Acute pneumonia is synonymous with *lobar pneumonia*, or *pneumococcal pneumonia*, usually brought on by pneumococcus bacteria. **Aspiration pneumonia** results from bacteria growth on inhaled secretions. Aspiration of normal oropharyngeal flora may lead to **necrotizing pneumonia**. Some degree of aspiration is normal and common, especially during sleep.

The adverse effects of minimal amounts of aspiration depend on the individual's immune and mechanical defenses, including cough and mucociliary clearance. A condition called **hypostatic pneumonia** can result in poorly ventilated areas of the lungs in people who lie in the same positions for long periods. A condition called **mycoplasmal pneumonia** is caused by the *Mycoplasma pneumoniae* organism, which causes a chronic, severe cough. Milder forms are sometimes called "walking pneumonia." ***Pneumocystis carinii*** pneumonia is an often fatal lung disease occurring most frequently in premature infants, neonates, individuals receiving immunosuppressant drugs, and individuals with HIV disease. (Also see Section VIII, Nosocomial Infections, later in this chapter.)

Portal of entry. Site of infection entry.

Prophylaxis. Any measures taken to prevent injury or acquiring a disease; immunizations for childhood diseases, or for hepatitis B and **tetanus**, are forms of prophylaxis.

Quinsy. A unilateral peritonsillar abscess. This condition may require surgical drainage to prevent glottal edema and respiratory distress.

Reservoir. Site where microorganisms reproduce or sequester.

Resistant organisms. Infectious organisms that do not respond to antibiotics.

Respiratory isolation. Procedures applied to prevent the spread of contagious diseases through airborne means; used with patients who have *rubeola (*measles), *rubella* (German measles), *pertussis* (whooping cough), *mumps*, and *tuberculosis.*

Retropharyngeal space abscess, lateral pharyngeal space abscess. Soft tissue infections in the back and sides of the pharyngeal walls, respectively. A lateral pharyngeal space abscess can be life threatening if erosion of the carotid artery occurs, resulting in *carotid exsanguination.*

Reverse isolation. Procedure applied to prevent the spread of infection to a noncontagious but highly susceptible patient; used with certain cases of leukemia, burn patients, transplant patients, premature infants, and other immunosuppressed patients.

Rhinitis. Watery nasal discharge.

Rickettsiae. A group of organisms that are larger than viruses but smaller than bacteria. Some rickettsiae cause human disease (e.g., typhus and Rocky Mountain spotted fever).

Secondary infection. Infection resulting from another condition.

Sepsis, septicemia. A systemic response to infection in which there is intravascular inflammation in response to toxins and microorganisms. Patients will be said to be "septic." Sepsis with severe hypotension and other catastrophic systemic dysfunctions, including impaired perfusion of vital organs, is called **septic shock**.

Seroconversion. A conversion from a negative status in blood analysis for a given antibody to positive status, indicating that infection is present.

Seropositive. An indicator in blood analysis of exposure to a virus.

Spore. A microbial state that allows survival until a growth environment is provided.

Sterile field. An area where all surfaces are sterile and kept free of microorganisms and their spores.

Sterile technique. Application of procedures to keep instruments and surfaces free of microorganisms and their spores.

Sterilization. A process for destroying microorganisms and their spores; sterilization is the highest level of decontamination.

Stomatitis. Inflammation of the mouth. **Aphthous stomatitis** refers to shallow, painful ulcers on the labial or buccal mucosa. **Vincent's stomatitis** is an ulcerative infection of the gingival mucosa due to an anaerobic *fusobacteria* and *spirochetes.* This condition is characterized by foul breath and purulent gray ulcerations. Other conditions associated with oral ulcers and vesicles include **herpangina** (a childhood disease that causes tiny ulcerations of the soft palate due to infection with the *coxsackievirus A*), fungal diseases, and systemic illnesses.

Strict isolation. Procedure used to limit contact with patients who have highly contagious diseases; used with patients who have smallpox, chickenpox, or diphtheria, and with patients who are extreme risks for infections, such as burn patients.

T-cells. T-lymphocytes are cells that originate from bone marrow and mature as a product of processes in the thymus gland and are present in the immune system to combat infections; HIV attacks T-lymphocytes, specifically the OK T4 ("helper") lymphocytes.

Thrush. Infection of the oral mucosa by *Candida*; see *Candidiasis.*

TORCH. Acronym for an infectious disease panel examining for ***t***oxoplasma, ***o***ther infections, ***r***ubella, ***c***ytomegalovirus, and ***h***erpes virus type 2. Sometimes the acronym includes ***s***yphilis; therefore, STORCH.

Vaccine. Derivative given to promote the body's immune defenses against a contagious disease.

Vector. The entity (person, animal, insect) that spreads pathogenic microorganisms.

Vehicle of transmission. The transmission method or media of pathogens can occur through *airborne means* (by exposure to air particles containing pathogens), *vector borne* means (by exposure to animals or insects carrying pathogenic microorganisms), and *contaminated substances* (e.g., blood, food, water, or drugs).

Viruses. Viruses are not living organisms. They are large nucleoprotein particles that are capable of entering specific types of cells. Viruses are nearly as small as a single molecule of protein. Many of the infections caused by viruses can create a lasting immunity; thus, inoculation (vaccination) with weakened forms of a virus can help to prevent infection (see Section VI, Viral Infections).

B. Abbreviations

Ab. Antibody

AFB. Acid-fast bacilli

AIDS. Acquired immune deficiency syndrome

AIHA. Autoimmune hemolytic anemia

ARC. AIDS-related complex (now usually referred to simply as HIV)

AZT. Azidothymidine

CDC. Centers for Disease Control and Prevention

CNS. Coagulase negative staphylococcus

EBV. Epstein-Barr virus *E. coli. Escherichia coli*

ELISA. Enzyme-linked immunosorbent assay

FUO. Fever of unknown/undetermined origin

GC. Gonococcus (gonorrhea)

GNR. Gram-negative rod

GN, G–. Gram negative

GNB. Gram-negative bacillus

GNID. Gram-negative intracellular diplococci

GP, G+. Gram positive

GVHD. Graft versus host disease

HAA. Hepatitis-associated antigen

HAV. Hepatitis A virus

HBc. Hepatitis B core antigen

HBeAg. Hepatitis B e antigen

HBsAg. Hepatitis B surface antigen

HBIG. Hepatitis B immune globulin

HBV. Hepatitis B virus

HCV. Hepatitis C virus

HIV, HIV-1, HIV-2. Human immunodeficiency virus, type 1, type 2

HIVD. Human immunodeficiency virus disease

HSV. Herpes simplex virus

ID. Infectious disease

Inf. Infected, infectious

MBC. Minimum bactericidal concentration

MIC. Minimum inhibitory concentration

MMR. Measles, mumps, rubella

MO. Multiple organisms

MRSA. Methicillin-resistant *Staphylococcus aureus*

MSSA. Methicillin-sensitive *Staphylococcus aureus*

O & P. Ova and parasites

OPV. Oral polio vaccine

PAIDS. Pediatric AIDS

PCP. *Pneumocystis carinii* pneumonia

PML. Progressive (cranial nerve) multifocal lymphencephalopathy

PPD. Purified protein derivative

RT. Rubella titer

STD. Sexually transmitted disease

Syph. Syphilis

TB. Tuberculosis

TBC. Tuberculin calibrated (syringe)

Tdap. Tetanus toxoid-diphtheria-acellular pertussis (vaccines)

TDT. Tetanus-diphtheria toxoid

TOPV. Trivalent oral polio vaccine

TORCH. Toxoplasma, other (syphilis), rubella, cytomegalovirus, and herpes virus

URI. Upper respiratory infection

UTI. Urinary tract infection

VD. Venereal disease

VDRL. Venereal Disease Research Laboratory (test)

III. UNIVERSAL PRECAUTIONS

Health care facilities in the United States apply what are called *universal precautions (UP)*, meaning *everyone* (patients, family, visitors, volunteers, and staff) in the facility is considered an infectious risk. This approach to infection control is based on the following presumptions:

- Infectious agents are present before symptoms are present.
- Multiple resistant organisms may be present before they are detected.
- Airborne and bloodborne infections are always potential hazards to staff and patients.

Special precautions for infection controls are required for highly contagious conditions, such as tuberculosis, multiresistant bacterial infection or colonization, herpes simplex, varicella zoster, scabies (pediculosis), measles, and mumps. When UP are part of the infection control policies, all patient contact requires the following:

- Thorough **handwashing** with soap and water, or use of an antimicrobial handwashing agent, *before and after* patient contact.
- Disposable **gloves worn** if there is any contact with body fluids, mucous membranes, or broken skin.
- Disposable **gowns worn** if clothing is likely to become soiled or if required by posted precautions.
- Eye and face **personal protective equipment**, such as masks, worn if any expectorant, blood, or body fluid splashes are likely.
- All disposable intact needle/syringes and sharp instruments are placed in the "**sharps disposal**" container, and any other disposable items that have been exposed to infectious fluids are placed in a biohazard (red) bag.

In addition, EOC standards restrict all clinical staff from eating or drinking in patient care areas. Fingernails are to be kept clean and neatly trimmed. Clinical staff who work in patient care settings are usually required to have only natural nails (e.g., no acrylic nails). Shoes must be closed toed (to reduce exposure risk to stray "sharps" or other items on the floor).

IV. PROTECTION METHODS

A. Handwashing and Gloves

Handwashing has been demonstrated to be the *single most important procedure for preventing nosocomial* (facility acquired) *infections.* To emphasize the importance of handwashing, a feature of "Tracer Methodology" (see Chapter 2) in The Joint Commission's site visit might include questions to patients such as, "Did you observe your therapist/nurse/doctor wash his/her hands before and after working with you today?" When UP are applied, hands must be cleaned with an antimicrobial agent or washed with soap and water before and after contact with *every patient* and immediately after contact with blood or body fluids. Handwashing is mandatory after eating, drinking, grooming, or trips to the toilet. A suggested handwashing technique for routine protection is described next, followed by instructions for donning and removing sterile gloves.

1. Routine Handwashing

- Remove or push up the wristwatch and sleeves from the wrist and remove jewelry.
- Turn the water on and off using a clean paper towel on the faucet.
- Wet hands and apply a liquid disinfecting soap.
- Rub hands and forearms vigorously in a circular motion for at least 30 seconds (sing the "Happy Birthday" song twice) or for a full minute or longer if directly exposed to contamination.

- Rinse and dry with clean paper towels.
- Use a clean paper towel to push open the door, or turn the doorknob, when entering or leaving the room.

2. *Gloves*

Gloves should be worn any time there is a risk of contact with a person who has a known infectious disease, especially when contact with blood or body secretions is likely. Gloves need to be put on in such a way as to *avoid touching the outside of the glove* with your bare skin. Although a *sterile technique* is not routinely required for SLP procedures, the techniques for donning and removing sterile gloves are described next.

Putting on Sterile Gloves.

- Open the glove package without touching the gloves.
- Touching only the folded cuff of the glove, lift the right hand glove and place it on your hand, avoiding touching the outside surface of the glove.
- With the gloved right hand, insert your fingers under the outside edge of the cuff of the left glove to lift it.
- Place it on the left hand, avoiding any contact between the outside surface of the clean glove and the bare skin of the left hand.
- Carefully fold back the glove cuffs without touching bare skin or the inside of the gloves.

Removing Contaminated Gloves.

- With your gloved right hand, grasp the wrist fold of your left glove and remove the glove, rolling it inside out; dispose of the glove in the appropriate container.
- With your now-bare left hand, reach into the inside of the right glove and remove the glove without touching the outside of the glove, peeling off or rolling the glove inside out; dispose of the contaminated glove in the appropriate container, according to the facility policy.

B. Personal Protective Equipment

Masks and eye protectors, or *personal protective equipment*, must be provided for all personnel. They are to be worn with any patient likely to transmit fluids or pathogens through airborne means or splashing (e.g., a laryngectomy with an uncovered stoma). The use of plastic eye protectors, or face masks with clear plastic eye protectors attached, is encouraged, because the eye can provide a portal of entry for infection.

C. Sterile Gowns and Hair and Shoe Coverings

Sterile gowns are worn in surgery or when required by *isolation precautions*, which are usually posted at the patient's closed door. Sterile gowns may be made of cloth or disposable paper and usually are provided outside or just inside the patient's room for donning upon entry. Sterile masks, gloves, and hair and shoe coverings are used to protect an infection-susceptible patient (such as a burn patient) from exposure to pathogens or in cases where the patient has a highly contagious disease. Sterile coverings must be disposed of in the appropriate container immediately upon leaving the contaminated room.

Donning a Sterile Gown

- After applying a mask and hair and shoe coverings, pick up the sterile gown by the neck area.
- Shake it or allow it to unfold and insert your arms *without touching the outside* surfaces with your bare hands, and do not extend your hands out from the sleeves.
- Ask an assistant who is wearing sterile gloves to secure the neck and to pull up on the sleeves to allow you to extend your hands.
- Apply sterile gloves in the manner described earlier.

D. Obtaining Signatures

Patients who are susceptible to or have an infectious disease can sign documents by placing a clean paper towel beneath the document paper and another clean paper towel on top of the paper, exposing the surface as necessary to be read. The patient can then rest his or her hand on the paper towel and sign without touching the document. See Figure 8–1 for an illustration.

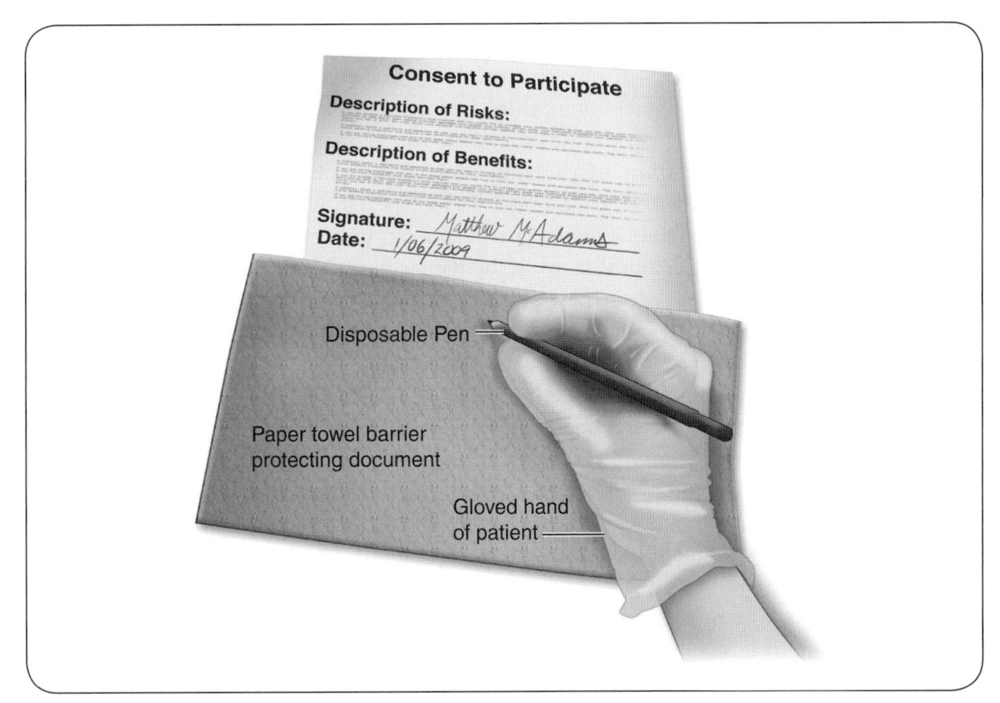

FIGURE 8–1 Illustration of a barrier technique used to obtain an informed consent signature from a patient with contact precautions. Source: Delmar/Cengage Learning

E. Contaminated Devices and Equipment

1. Decontamination

Medical treatment areas are kept clean, or decontaminated, with various cleaning agents. Some areas require at least *low- to medium-level decontamination*; other areas, such as surgical suites, require a sterile environment, or *high-level decontamination.* Pediatric clinics have a "toy cleaning" policy, which requires that toys have solid surfaces (no plush toys), allowing them to be cleaned in hot, soapy water or a dishwasher. Table tops in play area surfaces are cleaned and wiped with disinfecting agents between uses.

2. Disinfecting

Disinfecting refers to a process that destroys most microorganisms but may not destroy their spores; thus, cleaning with disinfecting agents does not necessarily eliminate a risk for infection. **Quaternary ammonium compounds**, or "Quats," are commonly used as low-level disinfectants. Chlorine (household bleach) and iodine are **halogens** and are considered medium-level disinfectants. Soaking in isopropyl alcohol solution or wiping surfaces with alcohol wipes or hydrogen peroxide offers little more than low-level disinfection. The facility's infection control policies state the appropriate agents and cleaning procedures to use for various surfaces.

3. Sterilization

High-level decontamination, or *sterilization,* is directed toward destroying both the pathogenic microbes and their spores. Sterilization requires special methods that usually include heat, ethylene oxide gas, or chemical immersion agents. Dry heat is used to sterilize sharp instruments and reusable syringes. Pressurized steam, or an autoclave, is considered a dependable method for destroying microorganisms and their spores but it cannot be used with sharp instruments or devices that are affected by moisture.

Hospital infection control practices include washer-sterilizers, which provide medium- to high-level disinfection. Ultrasound washers are used to agitate and loosen tiny particles from instruments, which is a process called "cavitation."

Chemical gas sterilization is useful when instruments or equipment would be damaged by other methods. Ethylene oxide gas can penetrate outer coverings well and is advantageous when equipment would be damaged by heat or liquid. Instruments that have been contaminated require heat or gas sterilization or a prolonged chemical cleaning before they can be reused. Chemical agents, such as *hexachlorophene* ("Cidex"), *phenolic compounds,* and *glutaraldehyde solutions,* are not considered as effective as gas or heat sterilization; thus, prolonged immersion (several hours) is advised. Some instruments, such as the end piece of a stroboscope, may be damaged by prolonged immersion in compounds like Cidex. The facility's infection control officer, or the infectious disease (I.D.) nurse practitioner, should be consulted for guidelines on an adequate immersion cleaning time. Contaminated disposable items and cleaning fluids need to be placed in the designated receptacles for disposal. Any material contaminated by a significant amount of blood or other body fluids must be disposed of in proper "infectious waste" (biohazard) bags, which are usually red, heavy gauge plastic bags. Items such as Band-Aids, 4 × 4 swabs, or tissues with only a trace or small amounts of body fluids are not typically required to be placed in red bags. Disposing of hospital waste in red bags requires handling and disposal and is costly to the facility, so these special infectious waste receptacles should be used judiciously and according to the facility policy.

V. INFECTION CONTROL PRACTITIONERS

Every medical facility has an **Infection Control Committee**, which usually is chaired by an **infection control officer** or **infection control practitioner (I.C.P.)**. The I.C.P. may be an I.D. physician or an I.D. nurse practitioner. The Infection Control Committee is responsible for ensuring that the hospital's EOC standards are upheld by all staff to minimize the exposure of both the patient and staff to infectious complications. This group monitors and reports the occurrence data for hospital-related infections and identifies sources of contamination or risks. The Infection Control Committee develops policies and procedures for infection prevention and systematic reporting of hospital infections and infectious complications. The Infection Control Committee's policies and procedures typically cover *admission screening*; *visiting policies;* staff *immunization policies; isolation policies*; *cleaning procedures*; *insertion and disposal instructions* for at-risk procedures, such as the use of intravascular devices and their dressing changes; *serologic testing*; *maintenance of dialysis equipment*; *timing of equipment changes*; *preparation and delivery of enteral feeding solutions*; *new staff orientation* and annual *EOC education*; *infection communications*; *incident reporting*; and *oversight of the management of nosocomial infections* (see Section VIII).

VI. COMMON INFECTIONS AND DISEASES

A. Bacterial Infections

Bacterial infections are classified clinically based on the result of the **Gram stain**. This test consists of exposing specimens to a series of staining chemicals and examining for color changes or decolorization. **Gram-positive organisms** include **staphylococcus** (*S. aureus* and S. epidermidis), **streptococcus** (*S. pneumoniae, S. viridans,* and *enterococci*), and some **bacilli** (*bacillus, listeria, corynebacterium*). **Gram-negative organisms** include **Pseudomonadaceae** (*P. aeruginosa* and *P. mallei*), **hemophilus**, **legionella**, and various bacilli (including *shigella, salmonella, proteus*, and others).

B. Viral Infections

Viral infections that are frequently found among critically ill patients include HSV; varicella-zoster; CMV; EBV; hepatitis A, hepatitis B, and hepatitis C virus; and retroviruses (HIV). Hospital workers who routinely come in contact with body fluids are strongly recommended to undergo **hepatitis B** vaccination. Patients with hepatitis are typically jaundiced and fatigue easily. Patients may have hepatitis from noninfectious causes, such as **autoimmune hepatitis** or **alcohol-related hepatitis**.

C. Fungal Infections

Fungal conditions often found among critically ill and immune-compromised patients include **candidiasis**, **aspergillus**, ***Cryptococcus neoformans***, and **histoplasmosis**.

VII. NEUROLOGIC INFECTIONS

Meningitis can result from **bacterial causes** (*Neisseria meningitidis*, *Haemophilus influenzae*; gram-negative bacilli; gram-positive bacilli, including tetanus; *S. aureus*, *S. epidermidis;* nocardia;

syphilis; and meningitides); **viral causes** (HIV; CMV; enterovirus, such as coxsackievirus; measles; mumps; HSV; and varicella-zoster virus); **fungal causes** (histoplasma, candida, aspergillus, Mucoraceae, coccidioides, cryptococcus); **tuberculosis**; or **parasitic causes** (toxoplasmosis). The clinical manifestations vary depending on the type of organism responsible for causing the infection and the neurologic structures affected. Cerebrospinal fluid (CSF) findings, blood cultures, and computerized tomography (CT) scans are usually ordered for the diagnosis (see Chapters 3 and 4). The CSF findings are examined for their *appearance*, the amount of *protein and glucose present*, the number of *lymphocytes* and other cells per cubic millimeter, and any *increase in CSF pressure.*

Another neurologic manifestation of infection is **septic shock**. Septic shock is the systemic response to an infectious process and results in hypotension, fever or hypothermia, impaired mental status, metabolic abnormalities, impaired organ perfusion, and **multiple organ systems failure (MOSF).**

Tuberculosis and poliomyelitis (polio) are infectious diseases known to attack cranial (and spinal) nerves. Recurrent symptoms have been found in some patients who were treated for and presumably recovered from poliomyelitis decades earlier.

VIII. NOSOCOMIAL INFECTIONS

Health care acquired, or hospital-acquired infections (HAI) are called *nosocomial* infections. They are *iatrogenic* in that they occur in the hands of, or as a result of, medical care. These infections can include wound infections following surgeries or infections secondary to decubitus ulcers. Other common types of hospital-associated infections include urinary tract infections (UTIs), upper respiratory infections (URIs), pneumonia, contamination of enteral formula, or intravascular (IV) infections. *Aspiration pneumonia* is a complication common to patients who receive tube feedings or have tracheostomies and translaryngeal intubation. The risk for aspiration pneumonia increases with depressed levels of consciousness. **Enteric gram-negative aerobic bacteria (EGNAB)**, the flora from the GI tract, are the organisms of nosocomial pneumonia that tend to colonize in the elderly and chronically ill patient. The patient's immobility, when coupled with any preexisting respiratory disease, is a primary contributor.

Patients vary widely in their susceptibility to pneumonia following aspiration of the bacteria-laden secretions in the oropharynx. The clinical manifestations of aspiration pneumonia include increased production of purulent sputum, fever, and progressing pulmonary infiltrates. Some patients have "silent," or small volume, aspiration tendencies that can be identified through a **modified barium swallow (MBS)**, videofluoroscopic swallow study (VFSS), or similar study if the patient is alert enough to participate. Other methods for determining aspiration risks include **methylene blue** ("blue dye") tests, which can be performed on patients with tracheostomies, and **fiberoptic endoscopic examination of swallowing safety (FEESS or FEES)** (see Chapter 5). Frequently, silent aspiration is surmised after the development of fever and a chest x-ray revealing new infiltrates. Aspiration consequences depend on the volume and size of the particles in the aspirate, the pathogenic organisms, the pH of the material aspirated, and the patient's immune status and ability to mechanically clear the material.

IX. HIV-POSITIVE PATIENTS

The risk of HIV infection to health care providers is not as widely discussed in the popular press as in past decades. Health care providers are expected to approach **all patients** as if they present a risk for infection, and universal precautions are just that—universal. Infection control precautions are applied with every patient contact without prejudice. This approach to patient care minimizes both the risk for HIV exposure to health care providers and exposure of HIV-positive patients to opportunistic infections from health care providers and other patients. As the term *immunodeficient* implies, patients found to have antibodies to HIV are at risk for opportunistic infections. The etiology for this disease is a *retrovirus*, which selectively enters OK T4 ("helper") lymphocytes and becomes integrated into the genome of the host. A severe deficit in cellular immunity is ultimately manifested. Serologic testing for HIV is done with an **enzyme-linked immunosorbent assay**, or ELISA, followed by a confirming **Western blot test** (see Chapter 3). The natural history for infections associated with HIV is still not entirely understood; however, medical management with a combination of drugs known as "antivirals" has been highly effective in keeping HIV in check and allowing infected individuals to live with this disease. These drugs generally work at the nucleic acid level to stop viral replication.

Patients who are *seropositive* for HIV ultimately develop what was previously called "AIDS-related complex" (ARC) (now referred to simply as *HIV positive*). HIV is manifested by unexplained fevers, weight loss, fatigue, diarrhea, viral leukoplakia and/or oral candidiasis, and lymphadenopathy. Patients who are diagnosed to have HIV-AIDs are those who have *Pneumocystis carinii* pneumonia and Kaposi's sarcoma, as well as other opportunistic infections and lymphomas. The neurologic complications associated with HIV-AIDS include progressive dementia with disorientation, cognitive problems, and, sometimes, focal neurologic signs; encephalitis; meningitis; space-occupying lesions, including metastatic Kaposi's sarcoma and primary and systemic lymphoma; and peripheral neuropathies, including inflammatory polyneuropathy, transverse myelitis, and cranial nerve involvement. The acquisition and progression of opportunistic infections in association with HIV differ between children and adults.

X. INFECTIONS IN NEWBORNS

Infections in newborns are classified as **transplacental** (transferred to the fetus during gestation), **transvaginal** (occurring during birth), or **acquired** (occurring after birth). HIV can be transferred to the fetus during gestation. Transplacental infections tend to be viral and usually include toxoplasmosis, CMV, rubella, and syphilis. Although the source of infection is the mother, she may be asymptomatic. CMV is a member of the herpes virus family. It is a common virus worldwide and is usually harmless and rarely causes illness. However, CMV infection does present risks for newborns of women who have had a first-time CMV infection during pregnancy. CMV-infected newborns may develop severe vision, hearing, and developmental disorders over time. CMV antibody testing is recommended for pregnant women, including pregnant women who work with infants and children, and for persons with weakened immune systems (cancer patients on chemotherapy, transplant patients, and individuals with HIV). The herpes virus also can be transmitted during passage through the birth canal, through a transvaginal mode.

Most *acquired* postdelivery infections are bacterial. The most common mode of infection in the neonatal intensive care unit is the same as that in adult intensive care units, which is transmission via the hands of the staff and caregivers; thus, the UP emphasized throughout this chapter apply across the age span.

XI. CLINICAL COMPETENCIES

The learner outcomes, skills, and competencies gained from information contained in this chapter include the ability to:

- Read, interpret, and use terminology, abbreviations, and descriptions of procedures related to infectious diseases and infection control.
- Describe reasons why SLPs are particularly vulnerable for exposure to infections and for the spread of infections among hospitalized patients.
- Discuss the role of the infection control officer.
- Demonstrate proper handwashing techniques.
- Demonstrate the proper method for donning and doffing sterile gloves and gowns.
- Define and describe the importance of universal precautions.
- Describe how handwashing might be audited by The Joint Commission site visitor as a part of "Tracer Methodology."
- Describe the difference between bacteria and viruses.
- List the types of pneumonia.
- Define "nosocomial" pneumonia.
- Demonstrate how signatures for informed consent might be obtained from a patient with a contagious disease or contact precautions.
- Describe the differences among decontamination, disinfection, and sterilization.
- List some of the common types of nervous system infections.
- Describe the methods in which newborns might become infected.

XII. REFERENCES AND RESOURCES CONSULTED

Anderson, D. (Ed.). (2003). *Dorland's illustrated medical dictionary* (30th ed.). Philadelphia: W. B. Saunders.

Avery, M., & Imdieke, B. (1984). *Medical records in ambulatory care.* Rockville, MD: Aspen.

Ayres, S. M., Schlichtig, R., & Sterling, M. J. (1988). *Care of the critically ill* (3rd ed.). Chicago: Yearbook Medical.

Davis, M. A., Gruskin, K. D., Chiang, V. W., & Manzi, S. (Eds.). (2005). *Signs and symptoms in pediatrics: Urgent and emergent care.* Philadelphia: Elsevier Mosby.

Fein, I. A., & Strasberg, M. A. (1987). *Managing the critical care unit.* Rockville, MD: Aspen.

Gray, B. H., & Field, M. J. (Eds.). (1989). *Controlling costs and changing patient care?* Washington, DC: National Academy Press.

Haller, R. M., & Sheldon, N. (1976). *Speech pathology and audiology in medical settings.* New York: Stratten International Medical Book.

Hendricks, K. M., & Duggan, C. (Eds.). (2005). *Manual of pediatric nutrition* (4th ed.). Hamilton, Ontario: BC Decker.

Jablonski, S. (2005). *Dictionary of medical acronyms and abbreviations* (5th ed.). Philadelphia: Elsevier Saunders.

Lewis, L. W., & Timby, B. K. (1988). *Fundamental skills and concepts in patient care* (4th ed.). Philadelphia: J. B. Lippincott.

Miller, R. M., & Groher, M. E. (1990). *Medical speech pathology.* Rockville, MD: Aspen.

Nicolosi, L., Harryman, E., & Kresheck, J. (1983). *Terminology in communication disorders* (2nd ed.). Baltimore: Williams & Wilkins.

Persons, C. G. (1987). *Critical care procedures and protocols.* Philadelphia: J. B. Lippincott.

Wolper, L. F., & Pena, J. J. (Eds.). (1987). *Health care administration.* Rockville, MD: Aspen.

CHAPTER 9

Cardiac, Pulmonary, and Hematologic Functions

Patients, both children and adults, with a history of cardiac, pulmonary, and hematologic diseases or disorders often have associated communication and swallowing disorders. A substantial proportion of the speech-language pathologist's (SLP's) caseload in a medical setting includes patients who have been admitted to the cardiology, pulmonary, or hematology (Heme-Onc) bed services. To appreciate the nature of the medical conditions that brought these patients to the hospital and how communication and swallowing management might be complicated by those conditions, SLPs should have a fundamental knowledge of the systems, principles, procedures, studies, terminology, and abbreviations encountered with patients who have cardiovascular, pulmonary, and hematologic diseases and disorders.

I. CHAPTER FOCUS

This chapter expands on topics introduced in Chapter 3, Vital Signs and Physical Examination, with additional terminology, abbreviations, and procedures. Much of the information contained in this chapter can be cross-linked to discussions found in other chapters, including Chapter 5, Nutrition, Hydration, and Swallowing, where the relationship between cardiopulmonary conditions and dysphagia, particularly in children, is discussed. In Chapter 7, Imaging Studies and Radiologic Oncology, specific radiologic and imaging techniques used to examine cardiovascular and pulmonary functions are described in greater detail. Chapter 10, Neurologic and Psychiatric Disorders, provides descriptions of cerebrovascular diseases; Chapter 11, Acute and Critical Illnesses, provides descriptions of acute and critical illnesses, including cardiac, pulmonary, and hematologic conditions; and Chapter 13, Surgeries and Other Procedures, includes a discussion of some of the airway, gastrointestinal (GI), thoracic, and vascular surgeries that patients with cardiopulmonary diseases may have had.

II. TERMINOLOGY, ABBREVIATIONS, FUNDAMENTAL PRINCIPLES, AND PROCEDURES IN CARDIOLOGY

A. Terminology

Aneurysm. A widening or ballooning-out of a weakened blood vessel wall.

Angina. Organ pain during ischemia (reduced blood flow to an organ). Some people will have a sensation of choking during *cardiac angina* attacks due to ventricular dysfunction. Angina is usually clinically described by levels of pain, using the following scale: 1+ = light or barely noticeable; 2+ = moderate, bothersome; 3+ = severe and very uncomfortable; and 4+ = most severe pain ever experienced.

Angiocarditis. Inflammation of the heart and its vessels.

Aorta. Largest artery of the body; receives blood pumped from the left ventricle as the initial point of circulation to the rest of the body.

Artery. Blood vessels that carry blood away from the heart to various parts of the body.

Arrhythmia. A lack of rhythmic heartbeats resulting from ischemia, metabolic dysfunction, drug toxicity, or atrial distention. Various forms of arrhythmia include *atrial fibrillation, atrial flutter, paroxysmal atrial tachycardia* (PAT), *atrioventricular nodal arrhythmias, ventricular arrhythmias*, and conduction disturbances.

Arteriosclerosis. Induration or hardening of the arteries; **athrosclerosis** is a form of arteriosclerosis in which fatty plaques are formed along the walls of the arteries, restricting blood through the affected region.

Atria. Smaller, upper heart chambers.

Atrial septal defect. Congenital abnormality in which there is a communicating opening between the atria.

Atrioventricular bundle (bundle of His). Part of the conducting system of the heart with fibers extending from the *atrioventricular* (AV) node into the intraventricular septum, causing ventricular heart contractions (see Figure 9–2).

Atrioventricular node (AV node). Point between the upper and lower chambers of the heart where electrical excitatory impulses from the *sinoatrial* (SA) node are promulgated onto the ventricular heart muscle (see Figure 9–2).

Bicuspid valve. Heart valve located between the left atrium and ventricle; mitral valve.

Bovine graft. Biologic prosthetic body part, such as a heart valve, derived from a cow.

Bradycardia. Slow heartbeat.

Capillary. Tiny networks of blood vessels that connect the venules and arterioles.

Cardiac arrest. Cessation of heart muscle action (contraction).

Cardiac arrhythmias. Irregularities of heart rate and rhythm action due to disturbances in conduction. Arrhythmias include **atrial arrhythmias** (atrial fibriliation; atrial flutter; and PAT); **atrioventricular nodal arrhythmias**; and **ventricular arrhythmias** (*ventricular fibrillation*; *premature ventricular contractions*, PVCs; and *ventricular tachycardia*, or "V tach").

Cardiac tamponade. Compression on the heart, usually by hemorrhage or effusion in the pericardium.

Cardiomegaly. Enlarged heart.

Cardioplegia. Paralysis of the heart muscle.

Cardiopulmonary arrest. Sudden cessation of respiration and circulation.

Carditis. Inflammation of heart tissues.

Claudication. An impaired ability to walk due to pain from inadequate blood supply to the muscles of the legs.

Coarctation of the aorta. Narrowing of the aorta.

Conduction disturbances. Heart abnormalities resulting from disturbances in myocardial neural impulses, including *atrioventricular block* (first-, second-, or third-degree heart block); *bundle branch block* (BBB); *hemiblock*; *Stokes-Adams syndrome* (cardiac stasis); and *Wolff-Parkinson-White syndrome*, or WPW (a congenital conduction disorder).

Congestive heart failure (CHF). Condition in which the heart is unable to pump adequately to supply the body's tissues. Left-sided failure with left ventricular dilatation leads to pulmonary congestion, edema, cerebral hypoxia, and coma. Right-sided failure involving the right ventricle leads to portal system involvement, causing ascites and enlargement of the liver and spleen. Patients with CHF often have an associated fluid accumulation in the lungs, resulting in pneumonia.

Coronary arteries. Arteries supplying the heart muscle; includes the **left main coronary artery (LMCA)**, **left anterior descending artery (LADA)**, **circumflex artery**, and **right coronary artery (RCA)**. It should be noted that *coronary artery bypass grafts* (CABGs) are grafting anastomoses surgeries that are most often performed on these four heart arteries.

Coronary atherosclerotic disease. Condition in which fibrous fatty plaques have accumulated on the walls of the arteries that supply the heart muscle, potentially causing ischemic heart disease.

Cor triatriatum. Congenital condition in which the heart has three atrial chambers.

Cor triloculare. Congenital condition in which the heart has three chambers due to a lack of interatrial or interventricular septa.

Cyanosis. Having a blue appearance to the skin due to a lack of oxygenation.

Dextrocardia. Having the heart on the right side of the body.

Diastole. Relaxation of the ventricular heart muscle.

Embolus. A particle, air bubble, or clot carried in the bloodstream.

Endocardium. The inner lining of the heart.

Extracorporeal therapy. Circulation of blood outside the body, as in hemodialysis or plasmapheresis.

Extrasystole. Heart contraction that is not initiated by the sinoatrial node.

Hypertension. High blood pressure; *essential* hypertension is idiopathic (of unknown cause), whereas *secondary* hypertension is a condition resulting from an associated disease such as glomerulonephritis, pyelonephritis, or adenoma of the adrenal cortex.

Hypotension. Low blood pressure.

Infarction. Tissue death caused by lack of adequate oxygenation due to impaired blood supply.

Ischemia. Inadequate blood supply to tissues.

Isolated pulmonary stenosis. A congenital defect characterized by stenosing (narrowing) of the pulmonary valve.

Murmur. A rasping heart sound heard during auscultation (listening with a stethoscope) of cardiac blood flow.

Myocardial infarction (MI). A condition usually caused by atherosclerotic disease of the vessels that supply the heart muscle characterized by intense, constrictive chest pain with *diaphoresis* (profuse sweating), pallor, hypotension, *dyspnea* (shortness of breath), nausea, vomiting, and fainting.

Myocardium. The heart muscle (middle layer of the heart).

Occlusion. Blockage.

Patent. Open.

Patent ductus arteriosus (PDA). A congenital condition in which the communicating duct between the pulmonary artery and aorta fails to close following birth. In newborns, PDA is sometimes associated with **infant respiratory distress syndrome (IRDS).**

Pericardium. Pertaining to the sac covering the heart.

Petechiae. Small, pinpoint hemorrhages on the skin.

Phlebitis. Inflammation of a vein.

Pulmonary artery. The artery that carries (deoxygenated) blood from the heart to the lungs to be oxygenated.

Pulmonary vein. The vein that carries oxygenated blood from the lungs to the heart.

Pulse sites, peripheral pulse sites. Body locations that provide good access to arterial pulses for checking heart rate and rhythms; includes *radial pulse* (thumb side of the wrist), *brachial pulse* (in the antecubital space of the elbow), *high brachial pulse* (inside the upper arm), *carotid pulse* (on the sides of the neck), *temporal pulse* (at the temple), *femoral pulse* (located on either side of the groin), *popliteal pulse* (behind the knee), *posterior pedis pulse* (ankle), and *dorsalis pedis pulse* (in the instep of the foot) (see Figure 3–3).

Pulsus paradoxus. The disappearance of a Korotkoff's sound during blood pressure measurement (see Chapter 3).

Reynaud's phenomenon. Episodes of pallor and numbness of the extremities associated with emotional stress, cold, or smoking.

Rheumatic heart disease. Valvular heart disease or damage to the endocardium after rheumatic fever.

Septum (cardiovascular). The partition between the right and left sides of the heart.

Sinoatrial node (SA node). Site in the right atrium where a heartbeat is initiated; the pacemaker of the heart (see Figure 9–2).

Stengtaken-Blakemore tube. A triple lumen device used to control esophageal hemorrhage from *varices* (bleeding from ulcerated varicose veins, usually in the lower esophagus).

Systole. Contraction phase of the ventricular heart muscle.

Swan-Ganz catheter. A multilumen central venous catheter used to measure cardiac output and hemodynamic pressures.

Tachycardia. A fast heartbeat.

Tetralogy of Fallot (TOF). A syndrome of congenital heart defects that includes *ventricular septal defect, pulmonary stenosis, transposition of the aorta toward the right,* and *hypertrophy of the right ventricle.*

Tricuspid valve. Heart valve located between the right atrium and ventricle that has cusps, or flaps.

Valves. Structures in the heart or veins that close to prevent backflow of blood. Valvular abnormalities or dysfunctions in heart valves can include **atresia** (congenital absence or closure); **prolapse** (typically of the mitral valve, where the valve cusp falls back into the atrium during systole); **regurgitation** (an incompetent, or insufficient, valve allowing backflow); and **stenosis** (stiff and fibrotic valve obstructing passage of blood flow).

Varicose veins. Condition in which the valves in the veins fail to prevent the backflow of blood, resulting in abnormally swollen veins, occurring particularly in the legs.

Vasoconstriction. Narrowing of a blood vessel.

Vasodilatation. Widening of a blood vessel.

Vasospasm. Contraction of a blood vessel.

Vegetations. Growths within or on a structure. For example, damaged heart valves are vulnerable to bacterial vegetation growth.

Veins. Blood vessels that carry blood toward the heart.

Venae cavae. The superior vena cava and inferior vena cava that carry blood from the upper and lower body, respectively, to the right atrium of the heart (see Figure 9–1).

Ventricles. Larger, lower chambers of the heart.

Ventricular septal defect (VSD). Congenital heart defect in which there is a partial or complete absence of the ventricular septum.

B. Abbreviations

AAA. Abdominal aortic aneurysm

ABF; AGF. Aortobifemoral bypass graft; aortofemoral bypass graft

ACD; AICD. Automatic cardioverter defibrillator (implanted); automatic implanted cardioverter defibrillator.

ACG. Angiocardiography

ACLS. Advanced Cardiovascular Life Support

AD. Aortic dissection (also see Chapter 11)

AHA-ASA. American Heart Association-American Stroke Association

AI. Aortic insufficiency

AIF. Aorto-ileo-femoral (graft)

AMI. Acute myocardial infarction

AS. Aortic stenosis

ASD. Atrial septal defect

ASH. Asymmetrical septal hypertrophy

ASHD. Atherosclerotic heart disease

AST. Aspartate aminotransferase

AV. Atrioventricular

AVR. Aortic valve replacement

BBB. Bundle branch block

BLS. Basic Life Support

BP. Blood pressure

BPM. Beats per minute

CABG. Coronary artery bypass graft

CAD. Coronary artery disease

CC. Coronary catheterization

CCA. Circumflex coronary artery

CCU. Coronary care unit

CHF. Congestive heart failure

CK. Creatinine kinase

CO. Cardiac output

CPB. Cardiopulmonary bypass

CPR. Cardiopulmonary resuscitation

CVAC. Central venous access catheter

CVC; VAD. Central venous catheter; vascular access device

CVP. Central venous pressure

DVT. Deep vein thrombosis

ECC; ECTx. Extracorporeal circulation; extracorporeal therapy

EKG/ECG. Electrocardiogram

ESR. Erythrocyte sedimentation rate

FHS. Fetal heart sounds

G1, G2, G3, G4, G5, G6. Grade one, grade two, and so on (referring to extra heart sounds)

HDL. High-density lipoproteins

HL Tx. Heart and lung transplant

IHSS. Idiopathic hypertrophic subaortic stenosis

JVD. Jugular venous distention

KVO. Keep vein open

LA. Left atrium

LAC. Left atrial catheter

LADA. Left anterior descending artery

LAP. Left atrial pressure

LBBB. Left bundle branch block

LD, LDH. Lactic dehydrogenase

LDL. Low-density lipoproteins

LHF. Left heart failure

LMCA. Left main coronary artery

LV. Left ventricle

LVAD. Left ventricular assist device

MI. Myocardial infarction

MS. Mitral stenosis

MUGA. Multiple Gated Acquisition (scan)

MVP. Mitral valve prolapse

NSR. Normal sinus rhythm

OHS. Open heart surgery

PAC. Premature atrial contractions, or *pulmonary artery catheter* (Swan-Ganz catheter)

PAT. Paroxysmal atrial tachycardia

PDA. Patent ductus arteriosus

PM. Pacemaker

PMI. Point of maximal impulse

POOH. Postoperative open heart (surgery)

PPS. Postperfusion syndrome

PTCA. Percutaneous transluminal coronary angioplasty

PVC. Premature ventricular contraction

RA. Right atrium

RAE. Right atrial enlargement

RCA. Right coronary artery

RHF. Right heart failure

RV. Right ventricle

S1, S2, S3, S4. Sound one, sound two, and so on (basic heart sounds)

SA. Sinoatrial

SBE. Subacute bacterial endocarditis

SCD. Sudden cardiac death

SGOT. Serum glutamic-oxaloacetic transaminase

tPA. Tissue plasminogen activator

TEE. Transesophageal echocardiogram

2-D echo. Two-dimensional echocardiogram

VCG. Vectorcardiogram

VLDL. Very low-density lipoproteins

VSD. Ventricular septal defect

C. Fundamental Principles

1. *Circulation*

The heart is a fist-sized organ with four chambers that pumps deoxygenated blood to the lungs and oxygenated blood to the tissues of the body. The two upper chambers of the heart are the atria; the two lower chambers are the ventricles. Deoxygenated blood enters the right atrium from the inferior and superior venae cavae, where it is pumped through the tricuspid valve into the right ventricle. From the right ventricle, the blood is pumped into the pulmonary arteries to the lungs for oxygenation and removal of carbon dioxide. Blood returning from the lungs enters through the pulmonary veins into the left atrium. It then passes through the mitral (or bicuspid) valve into the left ventricle and is then pumped through the aortic valve into the aorta and on to the body. Figure 9–1 illustrates the circulation of the heart.

2. *Conduction*

The excitation of a heartbeat and maintenance of rhythmic contractions (systoles) and relaxations (diastoles) are regulated by neuroelectrical nodes within the myocardium.

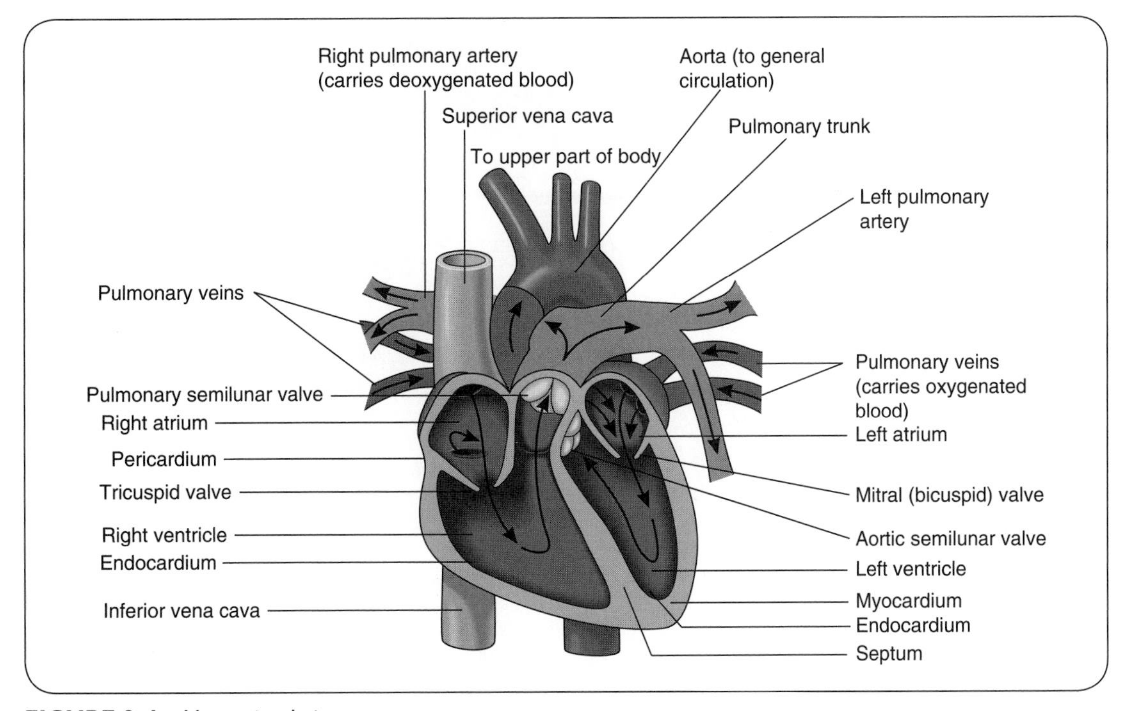

FIGURE 9–1 Heart circulation. Source: Delmar/Cengage Learning

These impulses originate from the parasympathetic and sympathetic nerves of the autonomic nervous system, primarily from the vagus nerve (CN X).

The **sinoatrial (SA)** node, or pacemaker of the heart, is located in the right atrium near the superior vena cava. The SA node stimulates simultaneous contractions of the atria. Electrical impulses from the SA node are projected to the **atrioventricular (AV)** node located in the **interatrial septum**. Impulses from the AV node are then directed to a region deep in the ventricular wall, the **bundle of His**, or **atrioventricular bundle**, which elicits contractions of the ventricles. Ventricular contraction is called the **systole**, and ventricular relaxation is called the **diastole**. Figure 9–2 illustrates the locations of these nodal impulses. Damage to the heart that causes an interruption in the conductive impulses arising from the AV node and extending to the right ventricle is called a **right bundle branch block (RBBB)**; damage in the conduction of impulses from the AV node extending to the left ventricle is called a **left bundle branch block (LBBB)**.

3. *Electrocardiograms*

The electrocardiograph (EKG, ECG) is a recording of the neuroelectrical conduction activity across the heart muscle. The EKG has five characteristics in its wave pattern, which are designated by the letters **P, Q, R, S,** and **T**, representing phases in conductive activity.

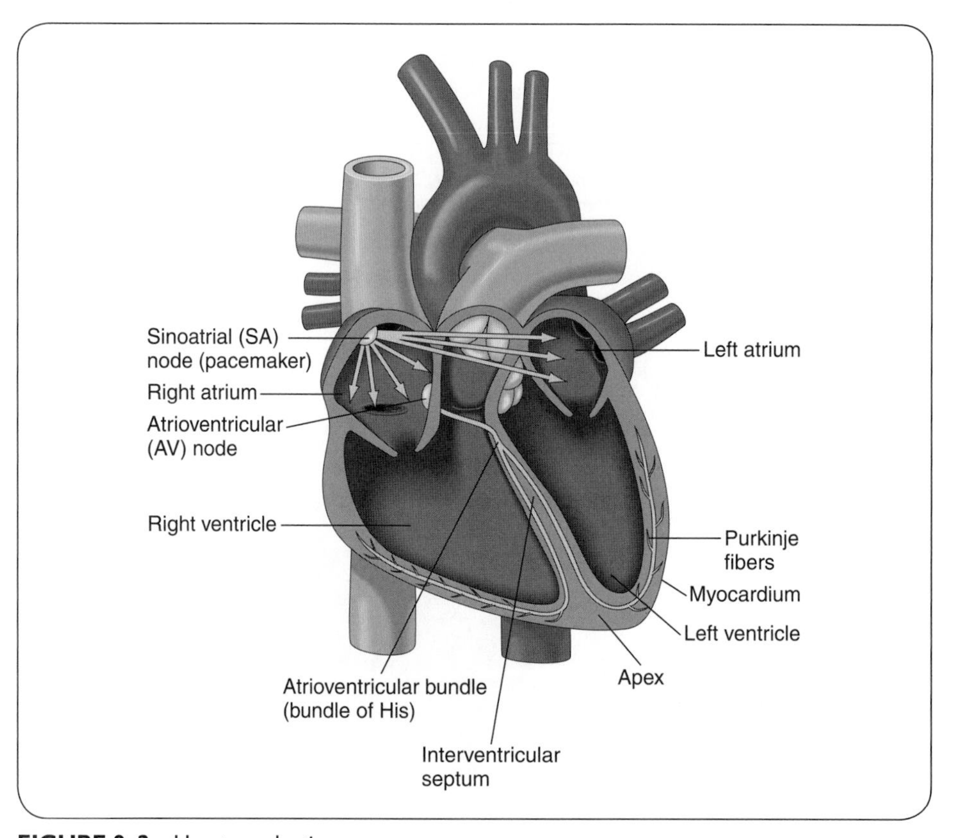

FIGURE 9–2 Heart conduction. Source: Delmar/Cengage Learning

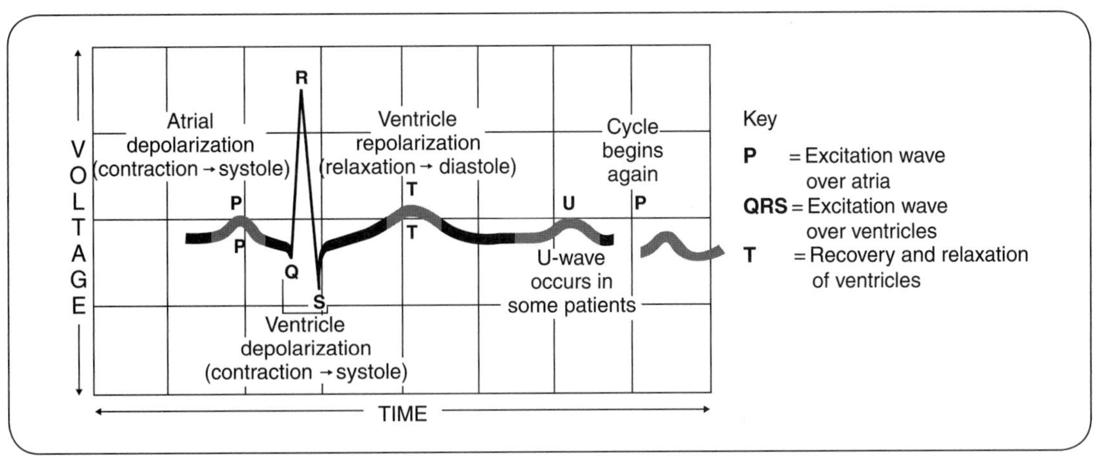

FIGURE 9–3 EKG tracing. Source: Delmar/Cengage Learning

The "P" wave occurs with depolarization of the atria as the impulse passes from the SA to the AV nodes. The "Q," "R," and "S" waves, or **QRS complex**, represent the spread of excitation elicited by the bundle of His, causing contraction of the ventricles. The "T" wave represents repolarization, or the relaxation, of the ventricles. Figure 9–3 illustrates a normal EKG tracing.

D. Procedures and Studies

Anastomosis. Two vessels attached together, usually referring to a surgical procedure.

Aneurysm repair. Aneurysms can occur in any vessel, large and small. With smaller vessels, the surgeon may remove the aneurysm and replace it with a vein grafted from another vessel, usually from the leg. Larger arteries, such as the aorta, require a man-made grafted patch. Aneurysms such as those in the head, may be corrected with clips or small clamps, or the neurosurgeon may thread a tiny plastic or metal coil through the blood vessels and fill the ballooned space.

Angiogram. Radiographic study using a contrast medium to reveal dimensions of the heart and its vessels.

Angioplasty. Surgical correction of a blood vessel defect.

Arterial puncture. A procedure used for blood gas sampling or when arterial blood is needed for chemistry studies. Arterial puncture involves using a *heparinized* needle to aspirate blood from the radial, femoral, or brachial arteries.

Artificial pacemaker. An electronic device implanted to provide rhythmic electrical stimulation of the heart.

Auscultation. Listening to sounds of the heart, blood vessels, lungs, or gastrointestinal tract, usually with a stethoscope.

Cardiac monitor. An electronic device that monitors and reveals heart functions and permits detection of arrhythmias. *Hardwire monitoring* involves the use of a three- or five-lead EKG cable attached to a bedside, hardwire monitor connected to a computerized central monitor. *Telemetry monitoring* involves continuous monitoring of cardiac rhythm through the use of a portable transmitter in the ambulatory patient, who stays within the vicinity of the monitor to document cardiac dysrhythmias. **Holter monitoring** refers to the trade name of an ambulatory cardiac monitoring device with which a cardiac rhythm recording is made while the patient is involved in his or her normal activities, usually away from the hospital, for an extended period. The information recorded in the monitoring device is later transferred to a computer for analysis.

Cardiocentesis. A surgical puncture into the heart.

Cardiopulmonary bypass. A technique for diverting blood temporarily from the heart so the surgeon can operate directly on the heart or its vessels.

Cardiopulmonary resuscitation (CPR). Revival of cardiac and respiratory functions through rescue techniques, mechanical means, drugs, or electrical stimulation, as with an **automatic external defibrillator** (AED).

Cardioversion (defibrillation). Application of direct electrical current to the chest to correct abnormal rhythms back to normal sinus rhythms.

Coronary artery bypass grafts (CABGs). Surgery to improve the blood supply to the heart by anastomoses (joining together) of other arteries to the coronary arteries. The notations "CABG × 2," "CABG × 3," "CABG × 4," "CABG × 5," and so on, refer to the number of bypass grafts done, not to the number of vessels operated on. In other words, a single coronary vessel may have more than one graft. The way to describe the number of vessels that received bypass grafts is: "2 vessel CABG," "3 vessel CABG," and so on.

Doppler echocardiogram. Ultrasound study of cross valvular pressure gradients and blood flow patterns; part of the workup for valvular disease.

Doppler flow and pressure assessments. An evaluation of peripheral vascular disease and routine blood pressure measurements. This assessment uses a Doppler flow monitor and blood pressure cuff.

Echocardiography, transesophageal echocardiography (TEE), two-dimensional echocardiography (2-D echo). Diagnostic imaging techniques for studies of the heart's structure and activity using ultrasound.

Electrocardiography (ECG, EKG). A measurement of the electrical and conductive activity of the heart muscle (see Section III, C and Figure 9–3).

Endarterectomy. Surgical removal of fatty deposits (atheromas) along the walls of arteries.

Multiple Gated Acquisition (MUGA) scan. A dynamic cardiac imaging procedure performed by attaching technetium-99, a radioactive substance, to red blood cells then injecting the red blood cells into the patient's bloodstream and imaging the heart's movement by a special camera (a gamma camera).

Percutaneous transluminal coronary angioplasty (PTCA). A procedure that uses a balloon catheter to expand the lumen of a blood vessel to the heart to improve blood flow.

Scalp monitoring (internal). A method for assessing fetal heart rate patterns during labor to determine if there is fetal distress.

Stent (cardiac). A metal wire coil used in angioplasty to open a blocked coronary artery and improve blood flow. Some stents are coated with medication (drug-eluting stents).

Stress test. A study of the heart's activity (along with blood pressure and respiratory rate) during physical exertion, such as jogging on an inclined treadmill.

Thrombolytic therapy. The use of **tissue plasminogen activator (t-PA)**, **recombinant tissue plasminogen activator (r-tPA)**, and drugs, such as *streptokinase*, to prevent clotting and improve survival after a myocardial infarction and stroke.

Valve replacements, valve bioprosthetics. Surgical removal of a stenotic or incompetent valve and replacement with either a valve from a normal cadaver or a prosthetic valve, or the creation of a **biological prosthetic** valve. A biological prosthetic valve is generally made of porcine or bovine material that is supported by a metal or plastic frame. Although bioprosthetics are less *thrombogenic* (likely to produce a clot) than mechanical prostheses, they often degenerate over time and must be replaced.

Venipuncture (phlebotomy). Needle puncture into a vein.

Venoclysis. Intravenous drip; injecting medication or other fluids into a vein.

Ventricular assist devices (VAD). A mechanical pump surgically implanted and used to assist a heart that is too weak to pump blood sufficiently and often serves as a "bridge to transplant" device while the patient awaits a heart transplant. There are essentially three types of devices. A **left ventricular assist device (LVAD)** helps the left side of the heart push blood to the aorta. This is the most common type of heart pump and may also be called a *left ventricular assist system* (LVAS). A **right ventricular assist device (RVAD)** pulls blood from the right side of the heart and sends it to the lungs. A **biventricular assist device (BVAD)** helps both sides of the heart pump blood.

III. TERMINOLOGY, ABBREVIATIONS, FUNDAMENTAL PRINCIPLES, AND PROCEDURES IN PULMONOLOGY

A. Terminology

Abscess (pulmonary). A localized area of necrosis and suppuration of the lung tissue.

Actinomycosis of the sinus. Fungal infection of the nasal sinus.

Acute respiratory failure (ARF). A sudden, life-threatening condition characterized by difficulty breathing and excessively low levels of oxygen and excessively high levels of carbon dioxide in the blood.

Adult respiratory distress syndrome (ARDS). A form of pulmonary edema resulting from marked, widespread damage to the alveolar-capillary membrane, sometimes a feature of septic *shock* (see Chapter 8).

Aerophore. A device for inflating the lungs of stillborn infants.

Aerosolization. Suspending droplets of water into a gas.

Airway. The passages through which air passes in and out of the lungs.

Alveoli. Air sacs at the end of bronchioles in the lungs (see Figure 9–4).

Anoxia. Lack of oxygen.

Apex (pulmonary). Top of the lung.

Aplasia (pulmonary). Lack of lung development.

Apnea. Temporary cessation of breathing.

Asphyxia. A depletion of oxygen from the blood.

Aspiration. The movement of material from one cavity to another, or in or out of a cavity, by means of suction. Secretions or other substances in the hypopharynx can be aspirated, or drawn, into the lungs. Aspiration can also refer to the *removal* of substances out of the body, for example, by means of a vacuum suction machine or syringe (e.g., a needle biopsy).

Asthma. Bronchial airway obstruction.

Atelectasis. Collapsed, airless portion of the lung; lack of pulmonary dilation.

Atomization. Suspending and spraying large droplets into the air.

Bag-mask. Face mask for resuscitation equipment.

Base (pulmonary). Lower portion of the lung.

Bennett respirator. Trade name for a popular model of mechanical ventilation device.

Bird respirator. Trade name for a popular model of mechanical ventilation device.

Bronchi. Branches of the trachea that pass into the lungs. The mainstem bronchi are the initial (left and right) branches into the lungs.

Bronchial hyperactivity. Reactive airway disease.

Bronchiectasis. Bronchial dilatation.

Bronchioles. Smallest branches of the bronchi.

Bronchitis. Inflammation of the bronchi.

Bronchogenic carcinoma. Lung cancer originating in the mainstem bronchus.

Bronchopulmonary dysplasia (BPD). A progressive lung disease seen in infants who have received high concentrations of oxygen during mechanical ventilation.

Bronchopulmonary segment. One of the divisions of the lungs. The right lung has 10 divisions; the left lung has 9.

Carina. Point at which the trachea branches into the right and left bronchi.

Cheyne-Stokes respiration (CSR). Rhythmic breath cycles followed by periods of apnea lasting from 10 seconds to 1 minute before breathing resumes.

Choana. Opening of the nasal cavity into the pharynx.

Choanal atresia. A rare congenital condition identified in infants in which there is a partial or complete obstruction of the posterior nasal cavity, causing respiratory distress.

Cilia. Hairlike structures lining the mucous membranes of the respiratory tract.

Complemental air. The amount of air that can be forcibly inspired beyond normal inspiration; also referred to as *inspiratory reserve.*

Coryza. Common cold.

Cracking. A technique used by respiration therapists and nurses that involves releasing a burst of oxygen into a tank to clear particles from the outlet.

Crepitus. Crackling sounds (in the lungs or joints).

Croup. Acute respiratory obstruction resulting from infection, allergy, or a foreign body in the glottis; characterized by respiratory distress, hoarseness, and a "barking" cough.

Cuff pneumometer. Gauge for measuring the pressure within an inflated tracheostomy cuff (balloon).

Cystic fibrosis (CF). An inherited condition that affects the respiratory system as well as the pancreas and sweat glands.

Dyspnea. Difficulty with breathing.

Edema. Swelling; fluid retention in the tissues.

Effusion. Dispersement of fluid into a tissue.

Emphysema. A chronic progressive pulmonary disease marked by a loss in elasticity of lung tissues, eventually causing the bronchioles to become obstructed with mucus. Emphysema is often related to smoking or exposure to industrial hazards.

Endolaryngeal carcinoma. Malignant epithelial cancer of the laryngeal structures.

Epiglottis. Cartilaginous covering of the trachea located at the base of the tongue, providing aspiration protection during swallowing.

Epistaxis. Nosebleed.

Eupnea. Normal or good respiration.

External respiration. Gas exchanges within the lungs.

Fremitus. A vibration, or "thrill sound"; heard during auscultation of lung sounds or felt with touch (tactile fremitus).

Functional residual capacity. The air left in the lung after normal expiration.

Glottis. Opening into the trachea. The rima glottis refers to the space between the true vocal folds.

Hemothorax. Blood in the chest cavity.

Histoplasmosis. A fungal disease sometimes associated with the formation of calcifications in the pulmonary tissues, evident on CXR.

Humidification. Adding moisture to the air.

Hypercapnia, hypercarbia. An excess of carbon dioxide in the blood. The abnormally high carbon dioxide tension causes overstimulation of the respiratory center in the medulla.

Hyperpnea. Rapid respirations.

Hypoplasia of the epiglottis. Incomplete development of the epiglottis.

Infiltrates. Radiodensities in the lungs indicating permeation of substances into the lung spaces.

Internal respiration. Gas exchanges within the tissue cells.

Kussmaul's breathing. A respiratory pattern associated with metabolic acidosis in which there is a deep gasping breathing pattern with slow, very deep breathing; also called "air hunger."

Lobes (pulmonary). Referring to lung divisions. The right lung has three divisions (right upper lobe, right middle lobe, and right lower lobe). The left lung is smaller to accommodate the heart and has two divisions (the left upper lobe and the left lower lobe).

Mediastinum. Chest cavity between the lungs.

Mesothelioma. A malignant tumor of the serous membrane of the pleural sac.

Minimal air. Air remaining in the alveoli.

Narcosis. A reversible state of sleepiness or incomplete unconsciousness due to reduced oxygenation or anesthesia, or too much carbon dioxide (CO_2), that is, *CO_2 narcosis.*

Nares. Nostrils. One nostril is called a "naris."

Nebulization. Transforming liquid into a fog or mist.

Orthopnea. Inability to breathe comfortably unless sitting up.

Oxyhood. A head box used to deliver oxygen to infants requiring oxygen therapy.

Paranasal sinuses. Cranial sinuses located above the nasal cavity; includes the *ethmoidal sinus,* the frontal sinus, the *maxillary sinus*, and the *sphenoid sinus.*

Parietal pleura. Outermost fold of the pleura lying close to the ribs.

Paroxysmal nocturnal dyspnea (PND). Respiratory difficulties occurring at night usually associated with heart disease.

Perichondritis. Inflammation of the perichondrium, the fibrous connective tissue surrounding the trachea.

Persistent fetal circulation (PFC), persistent pulmonary vascular obstruction of the newborn (PPVON), progressive pulmonary hypertension in the newborn. A group of related cardiopulmonary disorders in newborn infants.

Pertussis. Whooping cough.

Phthisis. (Pronounced /tIs-Is/,) Wasting of tissue, usually referring to pulmonary phthisis related to tuberculosis. Phthisis is often preceded by an adjective, such as *renal phthisis* or *diabetic phthisis.* Lung sounds are described as *phthisic* (tIz-Ik) when there is an asthmatic condition related to lung tissue wasting.

Pleura. Double-folded lubricating sac surrounding the lungs.

Pleural adhesions. Fibrosities binding the visceral pleura to the parietal pleura.

Pleural effusion. Fluid in the pleural spaces.

Pleural exudate. Serum or pus in the pleural spaces.

Pleurisy. Inflammation of the pleura.

Pleuritic pain. Intercostal pain provoked by moving the pleura, such as with deep inspiration or coughing.

Pneumonia. Inflammation with exudation of the lung tissues. *Nosocomial* (hospital-acquired) pneumonias are usually caused by gram-negative organisms, discussed in Chapter 8.

Pneumothorax. Air in the pleural space.

Pollinosis. Hay fever.

Pulmonary edema. Fluid in the lungs.

Pulmonary interstitial emphysema (PIE). A condition that sometimes occurs in infants who have received mechanical ventilation.

Pulmonary parenchyma. Cells of the lungs.

Pyothorax. Infection with pus in the chest cavity.

Rales. Crackling or bubbling sounds heard during auscultation of the lungs.

Rescue breathing. Breathing for an unconscious person who has a pulse but is not breathing by providing respiratory support via direct, mouth-to-mouth or with a personal resuscitation mask, a **bag valve mask**, **BVM** (or **Ambu bag**), or with a mechanical resuscitator/ventilator. When a patient has had support with a BVM or Ambu bag, the patient will be said to have been "*bagged.*"

Respiratory acidosis. A condition in which the blood pH is abnormally low (below 7.35) due to a deficiency in respiratory ventilation and CO_2 retention, most often caused by emphysema, pulmonary obstructions, or pneumonia.

Respiratory alkalosis. A condition in which the blood pH is abnormally high (above 7.45) due to an increase in respiratory ventilation and loss of CO_2 most often related to anxiety hyperventilation, elevated temperature, liver failure, or drug intoxication.

Retinopathy of prematurity (ROP). A complication of long-term oxygen therapy with newborns in which there is obliteration of the retinal vessels after hyperoxia.

Rhinorrhea. Drainage from the nose.

Rhinovirus. One of the viruses that causes the common cold.

Septum (nasal). Partition between the right and left sides of the nasal cavity.

Siderosis. Inflammation of the lungs due to inhalation of iron oxide, causing chronic bronchitis and emphysema.

Silicosis. Industrial disease due to inhalation of silica dust.

Speaking trach valves. Devices that can be attached to tracheostomy tubes to permit phonation by allowing air to be directed through the glottis (e.g., see Figure 9–9).

Status asthmaticus. Prolonged state of severe asthma.

Stridor. Harsh sound heard when there is obstruction of the upper (laryngeal) airway, for example, due to vocal fold paralysis or a foreign body obstruction.

Supplemental air. The amount of air that can be forcibly expired following normal expiration; *expiratory reserve.*

Tachypnea. Rapid breathing.

Total lung capacity (TLC). The maximal volume of air in the lungs after maximal inspiration.

Tracheoesophageal fistula (TEF). An opening between the esophagus and the trachea.

Tracheopleural fistula (TPF). An opening between the trachea and the pleura (sometimes the result of pressure necrosis from an inflated tracheostomy cuff).

Ventilator. Respirator; a mechanical device that provides assistance with breathing. Ventilator machines used in most hospitals are equipped with a *breathing circuitry,* a *heated humidification* and *sterile water distribution system*, *oxygen* and *air sources*, an *oxygen analyzer* (oximeter), a *manual resuscitator*, a *stethoscope*, **a sphygmomanometer** (for blood pressure measurement), and a *suction machine.* Ventilator controls regulate and measure **tidal volume**, **respiratory rate**, and the **percent of concentration of oxygen**. Audible and visible alarms are activated when respiratory parameters are outside of the control settings, due to a change in the patient's respiratory status, a problem with the machine, or during any disconnection process (see Figure 11–1 for an illustration of an intensive care unit (ICU) patient on a ventilator).

Ventilator dependent. Requiring mechanical support to breathe.

Ventriculogram. Contrast study usually of the left ventricle.

Visceral pleura. Innermost fold of pleura lying close to lung tissues.

B. Abbreviations

A. Alveolar (gas)

a. Arterial (gas)

ABGs. Arterial blood gases

AFB. Acid-fast bacilli

ARD. Acute respiratory disease

ARDS. Adult respiratory distress syndrome

BH. Bronchial hyperactivity

BiPAP. Bilevel positive airway pressure

BPD. Bronchopulmonary dysplasia

BS. Breath sounds

c. Capillary

CDAP. Continuous distending airway pressure

CF. Cystic fibrosis

CNH. Central neurogenic hyperventilation

COAD. Chronic obstructive airway disease

COLD. Chronic obstructive lung disease

COPD. Chronic obstructive pulmonary disease

CPAP. Continuous positive airway pressure

CPTPD. Chest physiotherapy and postural drainage

CXR. Chest x-ray

D. Dead (space gas)

E. Expired (gas)

ECMO. Extracorporeal membrane oxygenation.

ERV. Expiratory reserve volume

ET. Endotracheal

ETT. Endotracheal tube

F. Fractional (concentration of)

FEF. Forced expiratory flow

HBOT. Hyperbaric oxygen therapy

H & L. Heart and lungs

HMD. Hyaline membrane disease

I. Inspired (gas)

IMV. Intermittent mandatory ventilation

IPPB. Intermittent positive-pressure breathing

IRDS. Infant respiratory distress syndrome

IRV. Inspiratory reserve volume

MBC. Maximal breathing capacity

MVV. Minimal voluntary ventilation

OTB. Old tuberculosis

P. Pressure (in blood gases)

PAP. Pulmonary artery pressure

PEEP. Positive end-expiratory pressure

PFT. Pulmonary function test

PIE. Pulmonary interstitial emphysema, pulmonary infiltration with eosinophilia

PND. Postnasal drip

PPD. Purified protein derivative

ppd. Packs (of cigarettes) per day

R. Respiration

RD. Respiratory disease

RDS. Respiratory distress syndrome

RLF. Retrolental fibroplasia

SIDS. Sudden infant death syndrome

SIMV. Synchronous intermittent mandatory ventilation

SOB. Short of breath

T. Tidal (gas)

T & A. Tonsillectomy and adenoidectomy

TB. Tuberculosis

TLC. Total lung capacity

URI. Upper respiratory infection

V. Volume (of gas)

VC. Vital capacity

V/Q. Ventilation-perfusion

C. Fundamental Principles

1. Respiratory Tract

The respiratory tract begins with the nasal and oral cavities where air passes into the *nasopharynx*, *pharynx*, and *hypopharynx* (Figure 9–4). The nares (pronounced "nareez"), or nostrils, of the nose open into two chambers divided by the nasal septum. Within these cavities are three passages—the superior, inferior, and middle meati—which are connected to the middle ears through the **eustachian tube**, to the paranasal sinuses, and to the pharynx. The respiratory tract is sometimes called the **aerodigestive tract** because oral, pharyngeal, and upper laryngeal structures are shared by these systems. The **epiglottis** is a laryngeal cartilage located at the base of the tongue. It is part of the protective mechanism for venting oral secretions, food, and liquid away from the airway toward the esophagus and preventing aspiration during swallowing. The recesses on either side of the epiglottis are the **valleculae**; the recesses on the lateral sides of the glottis, or true vocal folds (Figure 9–5) are the **pyriform sinuses**. Pooling and stasis of material in these recesses is recognized as indicators for risk of aspiration.

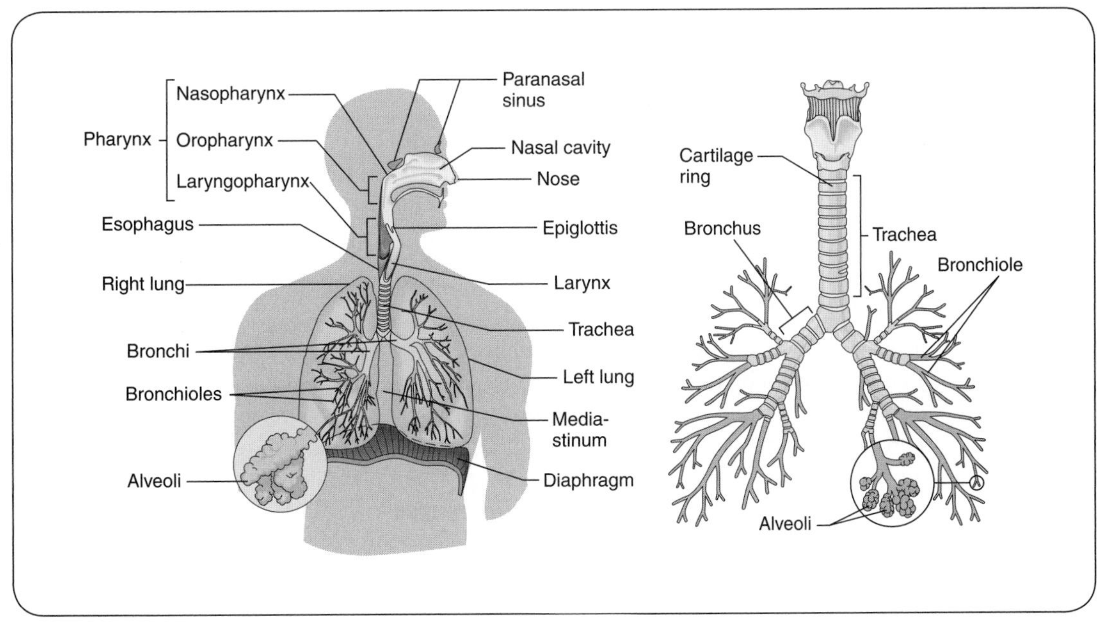

FIGURE 9–4 Respiratory tract. Source: Delmar/Cengage Learning

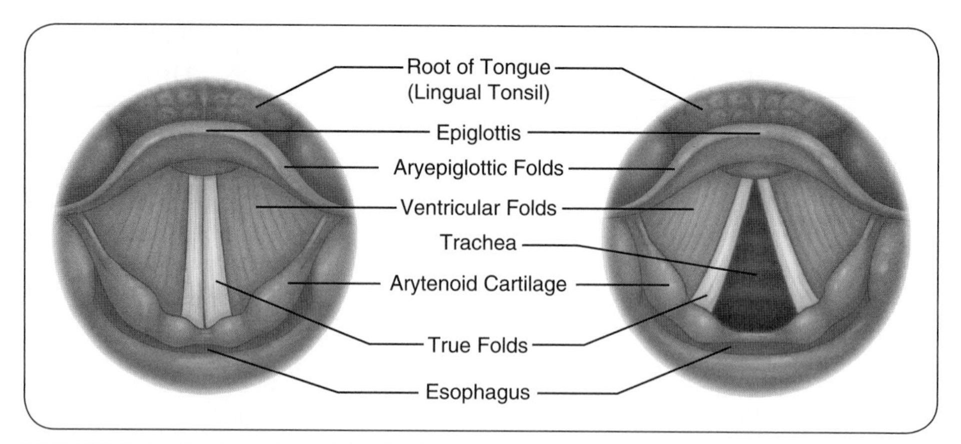

FIGURE 9–5 Superior view of the glottis. Source: Delmar/Cengage Learning

Entry into the lungs begins at the **larynx**. The elevation and rotation of the larynx and constrictive closure of the endolaryngeal musculature during swallows serve to prevent unwanted material from passing into the airway. Coughing helps clear material from the larynx, trachea, and endolaryngeal mucosa. The **endolarynx** has three divisions: *supraglottic* (above the vocal folds), *subglottic* (below the vocal folds), and *glottic* (at the level of the vocal folds). The **rima glottis** refers to the space between the vocal folds

The trachea, which is attached to the larynx at the **cricoid cartilage**, is a flexible tube of 18 to 20 C-shaped cartilages. In adults, it is about 1 inch in diameter and 4 to 5 inches long. The trachea terminates in a bifurcation, called the **carina**, where it opens into the two **mainstem bronchi** of the lungs. The bronchi branch into progressively smaller **bronchioles**, terminating in the **alveolar sacs** (see Figure 9–4). The alveoli are the tiny air sacs that contain pulmonary capillaries that bring air into contact with blood, allowing for the exchange of oxygen and CO_2. This exchange of gases within the lungs is referred to as **external respiration. Internal respiration** refers to the process of oxygen and CO_2 exchange from tissue cells through the capillaries.

The alveoli are supported by the lung's network of elastic tissues. The lungs are enclosed in the **visceral**, or pulmonary, **pleurae** (each lung having its own pleural sac). The right lung is larger than the left, which has a medial indentation to accommodate the heart, the *cardiac depression.*

2. *Respiration*

The air inhaled during respiration contains about 21% oxygen, and about one-fourth of that is taken up by the lungs. Expired air contains about 16% oxygen as well as a small amount of CO_2 (about 5%) and moisture. Because expired air retains a fairly substantial percentage of oxygen, **rescue breathing** (in which a rescuer expires his or her own lung air into a stricken person to inflate the lungs when breathing has stopped) can provide ventilatory support during **cardiopulmonary resuscitation (CPR)**, which is discussed later in this chapter.

Respiration is both a neuromuscular and a neurometabolic phenomenon. Respiratory centers in the medulla and pons are sensitive to changes in oxygen and carbon dioxide levels in the blood and correct any imbalances by activating respiratory musculature.

3. *Respiratory Centers*

Respiration is controlled by neural centers in the brain stem. The **medullary center** is responsible for initiation and maintenance of spontaneous respiration; the **pneumotaxic center** in the pons coordinates respiration cycles. Chemoreceptors in the brain's respiratory centers work together to monitor and correct metabolic abnormalities. Respiratory failure can be the result of a variety of *extrapulmonary* causes, including respiratory muscle weakness, upper airway obstruction, efferent disruption of impulses to respiratory musculature chest wall disorders, and dysfunction of the respiratory centers. *Neurogenic* causes of efferent disruption of impulses to the diaphragm via the *phrenic nerve* include high spinal cord lesions (C2, C3), which can diminish or abolish innervation to the diaphragm and intercostal muscles. Other neurogenic causes of disruptions in respiration include **anterior horn cell disease** (such as amyotrophic lateral sclerosis), **peripheral neuropathies** (e.g., Guillain-Barré syndrome), and **neuromuscular junction disease** (e.g., myasthenia gravis) (see Chapter 10). Obstructive causes include **obesity-hypoventilation syndrome** (Pickwickian syndrome); pleural disease; skeletal deformities; and **upper airway obstructions** (paralysis, foreign body obstructions, tracheal stenosis or tracheal malacia, laryngomalacia, and obstructive apnea). Common pulmonary and airway disorders in neonates and children are discussed further in Chapter 5.

4. *Respiratory Patterns*

Examination of respiratory patterns is helpful in determining the extent and location of lesions and disorders involving the brain stem. Large (usually deep and bilateral) *supratentorial* lesions or metabolic disturbances give rise to a breathing pattern termed **Cheyne-Stokes respiration (CSR)**, in which there is a pattern of rapid respirations followed by **apnea** (cessation of breathing) lasting 10 seconds or longer. The CSR phenomenon is attributed to disruption of controls from the cerebrum to the brain stem's respiratory centers, causing hyperventilation. Hyperventilation causes the CO_2 levels in the blood to drop, and this drop is sensed by the respiratory centers, which then are stimulated to stop breathing to correct the imbalance. CSR may also be related to the effects of low levels of oxygen in arterial blood in conditions such as congestive heart failure. Lesions in the upper *pontine tegmentum* and lower midbrain may cause **central neurogenic hyperventilation (CNH)**, in which there is an increase in both rate and depth of respiration, potentially leading to respiratory alkalosis (also see the discussion of ICU monitoring in Chapter 3).

Basilar artery occlusion causing low *pontine lesions* sometimes produces **apneustic breathing**, which may be called **"short cycle" respirations (SCRs)** characterized by short pauses after deep inspirations. In some cases, the patterns include intermittent quick shallow breaths; in other cases, there is an occasional omission of inspiration, referred to as **respiration alternans**. Lesions in the dorsimedial region of the medulla may cause each breath to vary in rate and depth. This pattern is variously described as **Biot breathing**, chaotic breathing, and sometimes—inappropriately—ataxic breathing.

5. *Neurolaryngologic Factors*

The inspiratory contractions of the glottal opening, particularly the **posterior cricoarytenoid (PCA)** muscle activity, are controlled by laryngeal innervation through the branches of the vagus nerve and are also influenced by physiologic pulmonary mechanisms. Damage to the nerves that innervate the larynx will affect glottal closure (see Cranial Nerve discussions in Chapter 4). Procedures, such as the presence of a tracheostomy tube, can also cause glottal dysfunction. Tracheostomy tubes can cause tube-induced abrasions and infections and their presence reduces stimulation of the PCA receptors. Patients with prolonged tracheotomies who have experienced reduced respiratory resistance to the glottis sometimes have an inadequate glottal closure initially following decannulation (removal) of the tracheostomy tube (see Kirchner, 1987 for discussion). For that reason, it may be necessary to introduce air resistance through the glottis gradually to reestablish phonation following tracheotomies (Kirchner, 1987)

D. Procedures and Studies

Ambu bag. One of the self-inflating breathing bags and masks used for emergency artificial ventilation of the lungs.

Antrotomy. Removal of the antral wall of the nasal cavity.

Assisted ventilation. A mechanical ventilation technique in which the initiation of each inspiration comes from the patient's own effort.

Bilevel positive airway pressure (BiPAP). BiPap, or **variable positive airway pressure (VPAP)** provides two levels of pressure (inspiratory and expiratory) for respiratory support and is used in hospitals with patients who are in congestive cardiac failure, have respiratory failure, or have an acute exacerbation of obstructive airways disease (notably COPD and asthma).

Bronchial brushing, brush biopsy. Method for establishing a diagnosis in a lung mass in which a radiopaque catheter is passed under fluoroscopic guidance into the bronchial passage where the mass is located. Minute nylon brushes then take scrapings of cells for analysis.

Bronchogram. Radiologic study of the bronchial branches using a radiopaque contrast material.

Cervicomediastinotomy. An excision in the mediastinum of the neck region to obtain a biopsy of the lymph node.

Continuous positive airway pressure (CPAP). A respiratory therapy maneuver producing positive airway pressure throughout the respiration cycle. A CPAP device may be used for treating patients with sleep apnea at home by delivering a stream of compressed air via various types of masks or a nasal pillow.

Cordectomy, laryngofissure. Incision made to separate the vocal folds or remove part of the vocal folds.

Decannulation. Removal of the tracheostomy tube.

Downsize. Progressively adjusting tracheostomy tubes to smaller sizes.

Extubation. Removal of an endotracheal or tracheostomy tube apparatus.

Fiberoptic bronchoscopy. An endoscopic examination of the right and left mainstem bronchi and the carina.

Fowler's positioning. Placement of the patient in a sitting position to facilitate breathing.

Heimlich maneuver. A technique using a brisk, posterior and upward compression of the abdomen subdiaphragmatically (above the navel) of a choking individual to expel an airway obstruction (see Figures 9–11A, 9–11B, 9–12A, and 9–12B). Techniques to expel foreign body obstructions vary depending on the age, pregnancy status, and level of consciousness of the stricken individual.

Hemilaryngectomy. Surgical removal of one-half of the laryngeal structures.

Incentive breathing spirometers. Devices used in respiratory therapy to prevent *atelectasis* and improve lung volumes.

Intermittent mandatory ventilation (IMV). Respiration therapy maneuver in which the patient breathes on his or her own with intermittent intervals of ventilator support as part of the weaning process in respiration therapy.

Intermittent positive-pressure breathing (IPPB). Administration of gases or drugs by mechanical means using pressures above atmospheric pressure to force deeper inspirations. This therapy uses commercially available machines that are portable for home use.

Intubation. Insertion of an endotracheal tube (from the oropharyngeal cavity into the trachea) or tracheostomy tube (directly into the trachea) (see Figure 13–2).

Laminography. Tomograms, or planigrams, taken of the lung, providing a sectional study of lung tissues and the underlying and surrounding structures.

Laryngectomy. Removal of the larynx (see Figure 13–1).

Lobectomy. Complete removal of a pulmonary lobe.

Lung biopsy. Removal of a small specimen of lung tissue to examine for carcinogenic, bacteriologic, or other pathologic conditions.

Lung resection. Partial removal of a portion of the lung.

Needle biopsy, percutaneous needle biopsy. Insertion of a biopsy needle into a lesion, usually through the skin, to aspirate cells to examine for cytologic, bacteriologic, and other pathologic conditions.

Oxygen delivery. Oxygen may be delivered by a *mask*, *oxygen tent*, *nasal catheter*, *nasal cannula*, or directly into a *tracheostomy tube*, or *intubation* apparatus (through a **T-piece**, see Figure 9–10). Oxygen may be piped from a pressurized tank or directly from a wall vent (see Figure 11–1 for an illustration). An **oxygen flowmeter** is used to control the amount of oxygen delivered at a liter-per-minute rate. These rates are required (by The Joint Commission) to be converted into *equivalent percentages* according to the delivery method. For example, a mask delivering 6 liters of oxygen per minute has a percent equivalent of 60% oxygen flow, whereas a **nasal cannula** delivering 6 liters of oxygen per minute has a percent equivalent of 44% oxygen flow. Some masks, such as a **Venturi mask**, deliver precise mixes of oxygen and room air. Because oxygen dries mucous membranes, delivery devices direct the oxygen gas through a bottle of sterile water, which humidifies the oxygen before delivering it to the patient.

Percussion. A technique for loosening lung secretions by rhythmic gentle blows across the chest with a cupped hand.

Positive end-expiratory pressure (PEEP) therapy. A respiratory therapy maneuver used to increase the functional residual capacity of the lungs.

Postural drainage. Technique that uses positioning to promote gravitational drainage of secretions from areas of the lungs.

Pulmonary function studies. Laboratory studies of the respiratory functions, including lung volumes, ventilation, and oxygen consumption.

Rescue breathing. Mouth-to-mouth (or mouth-to-tracheostoma) artificial ventilation.

Respirometry. Use of a respirometer to measure exhaled tidal volume. This device may be attached to the endotracheal tube of an unconscious patient.

Rhinoplasty. Plastic surgical reconstruction of the nose.

Silverman-Anderson score. System for scoring the degree of respiratory distress.

Sinus lavage. Method for removing purulent material from the sinuses using flushing and suctioning.

Spirometry. Measurement with graphic recording of lung capacities. *Bronchospirometry* measures the relative differences between the two lungs' capacities.

Stroboscopy, videostroboscopy. Method for endoscopic (usually with videotaped or digitized imaging recording) visualization of laryngeal activity using flashes of light in synchrony with the phases of vibratory cycles of the vocal folds.

Suctioning. Using a vacuum (wall unit or freestanding device), suction tip, and catheter to clear secretions, primarily from the airway. Suctioning is done to remove secretions that have accumulated when the patient is unable to clear his or her own air passages. Table 9–1 describes suctioning methods.

TABLE 9–1 Tracheostomy and oropharyngeal suctioning

STEP	PROCEDURE
1.	Determine the need for suctioning.
2.	Explain to the patient why and how suctioning will be done.
3.	Assemble the necessary equipment.
4.	Turn on the suction machine and set the pressure gauges. **Suction vacuum settings** usually are around: **80–120 mmHg** for *adults*, **80–100 mmHg** for *children*, and **60–100 mmHg** for *infants*.
5.	Place the patient in a Fowler's (sitting) or semi-Fowler's position (leaning back between 45–60°), or lying on the side if unconscious.
6.	Remove the sterile catheter without contamination.
7.	Don sterile or clean gloves.
8.	Turn on the suction machine with the nondominant hand.
9.	Test the suction in normal saline solution.

continues

STEP	PROCEDURE
10.	Lubricate the tip with a water soluble lubricant.
11.	Introduce the suction catheter into the tracheostomy or toward the base of the pharynx; patient may want to and should be encouraged to cough.
12.	Occlude the catheter vent or one end of a Y-tubing connector with the gloved thumb to create a vacuum in the catheter lasting about 10–15 seconds.
13.	Rotate and twist the catheter as it is being withdrawn to collect additional secretions.
14.	Remove the thumb from the catheter vent when ready to release the suctioned material into a collection basin.
15.	Continue until the suctioning process is completed; remove the glove while holding the catheter, pulling the glove off inside out, and dispose of the catheter and the glove in the appropriate receptacles.
16.	Reassess status of the patient and record procedure in the medical chart.

Source: Adapted from Lewis, L. W., & Trimby, B. K. (1988). *Fundamental skills and concepts in patient care* (4th ed.). Philadelphia: J. B. Lippincott; and Persons, C. G. (1987). *Critical care procedures and protocols.* Philadelphia: J. B. Lippincott.

Thoracentesis. Surgical procedure that involves introducing a tube into the thoracic cavity to remove fluid.

Thoracostomy. Excision of a rib segment to allow for drainage of an *empyema* (pus-filled space).

Thoracotomy. An incision into the chest.

Tracheostomy. An opening into the trachea, usually for placement of a **tracheostomy tube.**

Tracheostomy care. Techniques for cleaning tracheostomy tubes. Usually this is done every 6 or 8 hours (see Table 9–2).

Tracheostomy tubes. Tracheostomy tubes, or "trachs," vary in dimensions and characteristics and are selected based on the ventilatory needs of the patient. Figure 9–6 illustrates the parts and features of a metal (**Jackson-type**) tracheostomy tube. Figure 9–7 illustrates the parts of a cuffed tracheostomy tube. Figure 9–8A illustrates the inflated and deflated **cuffed, trach tube**, and Figure 9–8B illustrates airflow through a fenestrated tracheostomy tube. Figure 9–9 illustrates a **Passy-Muir™** speaking valve, one of the devices available to permit phonation when attached to tracheostomy tube. Lung air must be allowed to flow around the trach, or through a fenestration, and up through the glottis to achieve phonation; thus, patients must be able to tolerate having the cuff of their tracheostomy tube deflated during use (see Figure 9–9), These devices are sometimes called "speaking trachs" or "speaking valves." Table 9–3 provides general guidelines for SLPs training ventilator-dependent patients to use speaking trachs and valves, such as the Passy-Muir™ speaking valves.

TABLE 9–2 Tracheostomy care

STEP	PROCEDURE
1.	Assemble equipment, including a basin of hydrogen peroxide, a basin of sterile water, and a receptacle for soiled items.
2.	Wash hands thoroughly and don sterile gloves.
3.	Remove the stoma dressing.
4.	Swab the stoma area with sterile hydrogen peroxide followed by sterile water.
5.	Unlock and remove the inner cannula and clean it thoroughly with a brush and hydrogen peroxide before placing it in sterile water.
6.	Dry the inner cannula with sterile gauze and resecure.
7.	Reapply a sterile dressing and tie the tracheostomy tube in place avoiding knots that might press on the neck.
8.	Dispose of all contaminated items.

Source: Adapted from Lewis, L.W., & Trimby, B. K. (1988). *Fundamental skills and concepts in patient care* (4th ed.). Philadelphia: J. B. Lippincott; and Persons, C. G. (1987). *Critical care procedures and protocols.* Philadelphia: J. B. Lippincott.

Tracheostomy collar, or T-piece. Flexible tubing for humidification or oxygen delivery that may be attached to the trach tube of a tracheostomized patient; sometimes called a Brigg's adapter. Figure 9–10 provides an illustration.

Tracheotomy. An incision into the trachea (see Figure 13–2).

Transantral ligation of the maxillary artery. The application of vascular clips to the maxillary artery to control severe, recurrent nosebleeds (epistaxis).

Tuberculin (TB) skin tests. Tests of exposure or sensitization to tuberculosis. TB screening is usually done by the **Mantoux test**, or PPD (an interdermal tuberculin test using purified protein derivative). Other screening tests, such as the **Tine test** (interdermal test using a four pronged device, dipped in attenuated TB, for puncturing the skin), **Heaf test** (uses multiple punctures for interdermal TB testing), and **Mono-Vacc** (screening test using multiple punctures), currently are not as commonly used.

Ventilatory management. Use of a machine to provide adequate ventilatory support.

Vibration. Loosening lung secretions using firm, circular motions applied to the chest with open hands to produce wavelike vibrations within the chest.

Water-seal drainage management. In cases where drainage of accumulated fluids in the lungs is necessary, a water-seal drainage system is used to ensure that air is not permitted to contact the fluids being drained and to prevent back movement of air. Hospitals normally use a commercially available system, such as a "Pleur-evac" (Deknatel Corporation). (See Chapter 3 for further discussion and Figure 11–1 for an illustration.)

Weaning (respiratory). Gradual elimination of mechanical support for respiration.

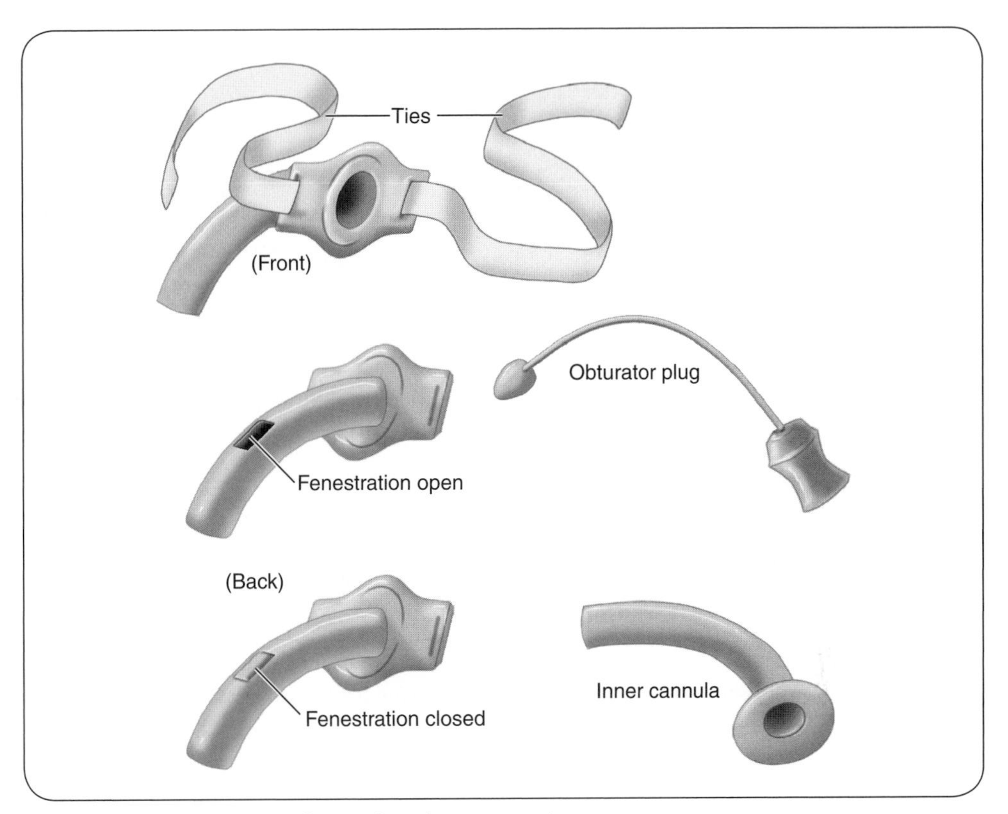

FIGURE 9–6 Illustration of a metal tracheostomy tube. Source: Delmar/Cengage Learning

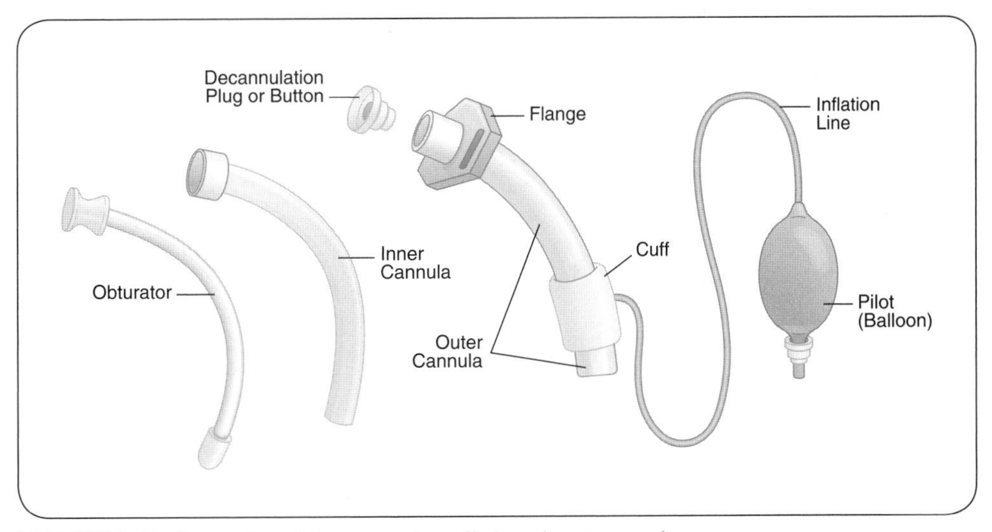

FIGURE 9–7 Illustration of the parts of a cuffed tracheostomy tube. Source: Delmar/Cengage Learning

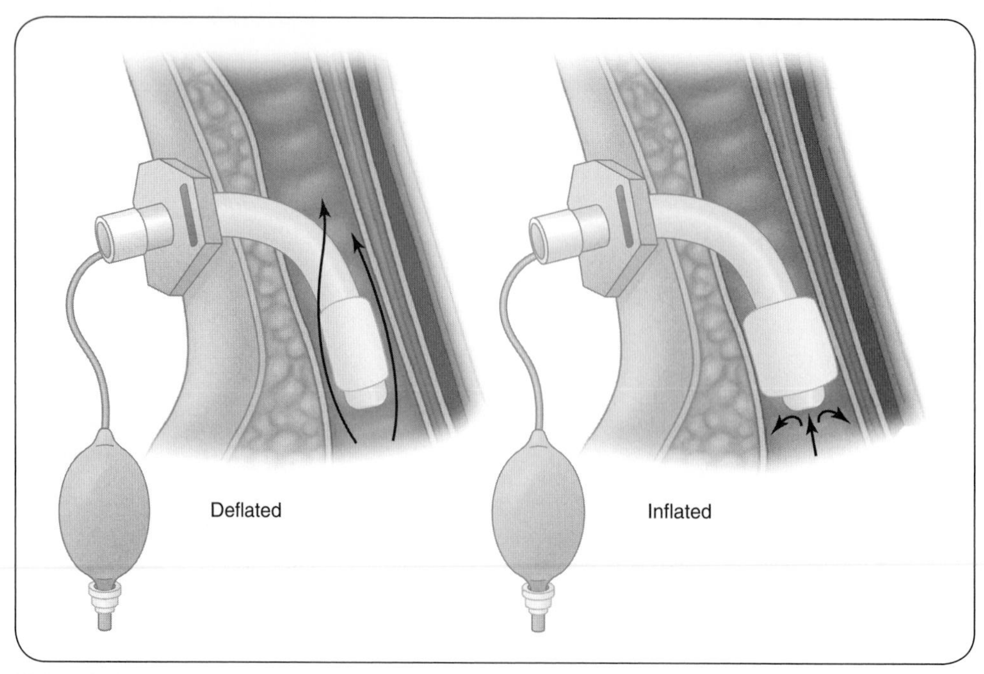

FIGURE 9–8A Inflation and deflation of a cuffed tracheostomy tube. Source: Delmar/Cengage Learning

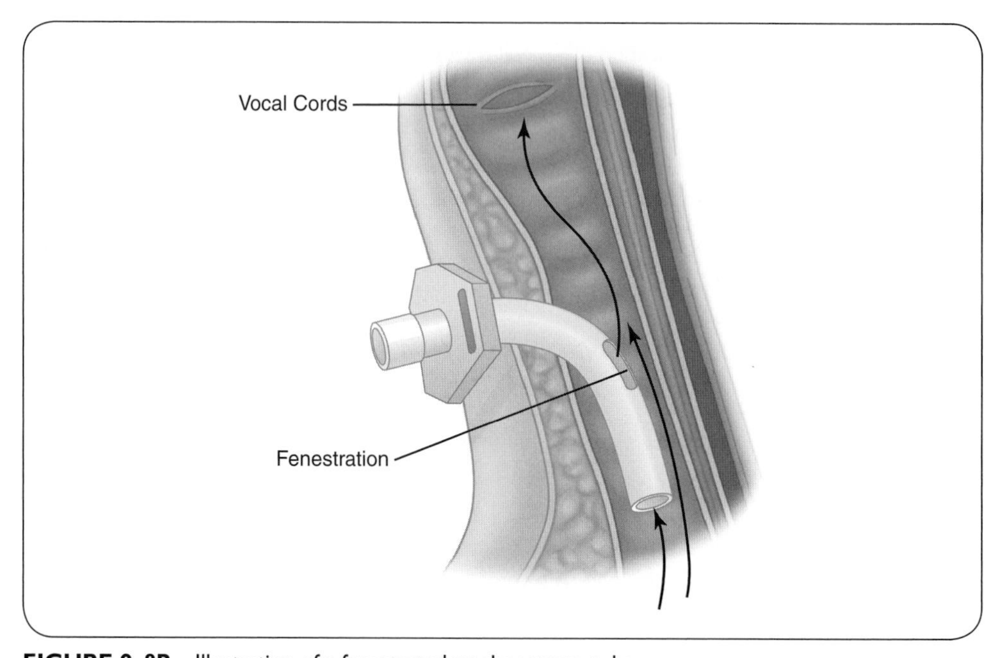

FIGURE 9–8B Illustration of a fenestrated tracheostomy tube. Source: Delmar/Cengage Learning

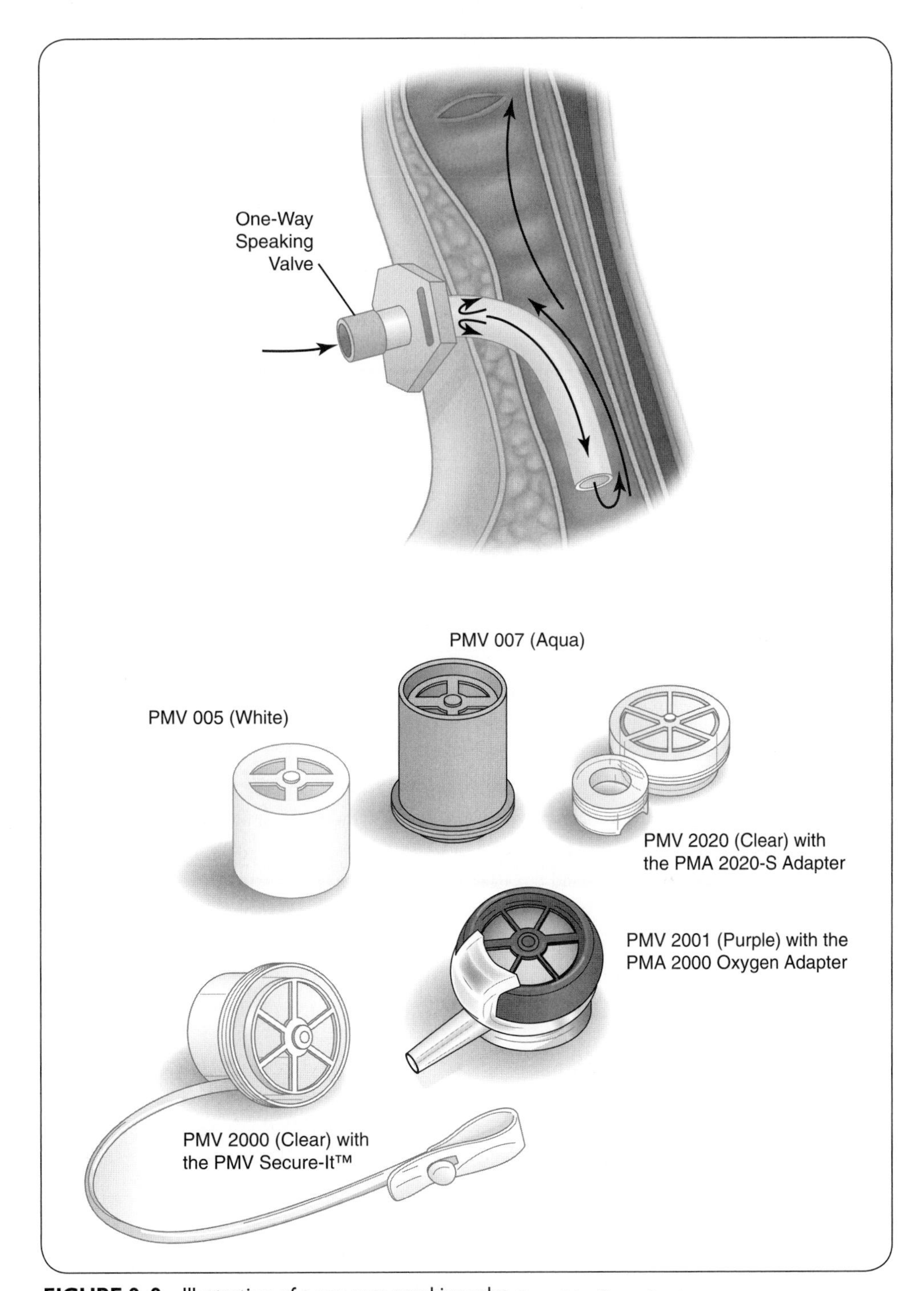

FIGURE 9–9 Illustration of a one-way speaking valve. Source: Delmar/Cengage Learning

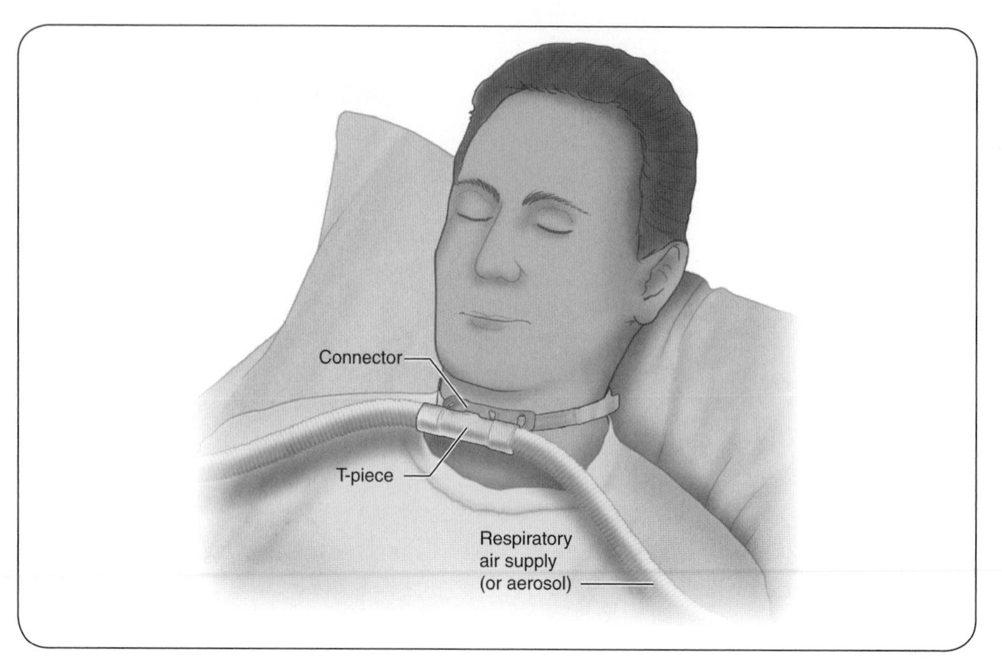

FIGURE 9–10 Illustration of a T-piece. Source: Delmar/Cengage Learning

TABLE 9–3 Guidelines for working with ventilator dependent patients using speaking valves

- Inform the primary nurse and/or respiratory therapist (R.T.) of your session and plans.
- Encourage the primary nurse to observe how the speaking valve functions.
- Check oximeter level and take precautions to ensure that adequate oxygen saturation in the blood is maintained throughout the session (recommended level is 88% or above), it is prudent to use an oxygen saturation monitor throughout the sessions.
- Take a resting heart rate. If pulse increases to 20 beats above the resting rate, the patient may be in distress.
- *High pressure alarms* may be triggered when tubing is occluded, coughing is present, or suctioning is needed.
- *Low pressure alarms* may be triggered if the tubing is disconnected or if the circuitry is disconnected from the patient or from the ventilator.
- If the speaking valve requires deflating the cuff, as with a Passy-Muir valve, the low pressure alarm will be triggered. The respiratory therapist or nurse will need to assist with any changes in the pressure settings.
- Check with the nurse and/or R.T. before deflating the trach cuff.
- Cuff inflation pressures are usually recommended to be 24 cm water pressure.
- Document your observations and the results of the session in the medical chart. Be sure to note any concerns that may affect prognosis for using the device successfully or adjustments that may improve the patient's potential for using the device without compromising ventilatory status.

IV. TERMINOLOGY, ABBREVIATIONS, FUNDAMENTAL PRINCIPLES, AND PROCEDURES IN HEMATOLOGY

A. Terminology

ABO typing. An international system for typing the main blood groups.

Acquired immune deficiency syndrome (AIDS). A condition resulting from acquiring a human immunodeficiency virus (HIV), causing a patient's immune defenses to become compromised and allowing opportunistic infections (see Chapter 8.)

Albumin. A blood protein. The measurement of albumin levels in the blood, or serum albumin, aids in determining nutrition status.

Anemia. Low red blood cells.

Antibodies. Proteins synthesized by lymphoid tissue in the presence of antigens (foreign or invading substances) that destroy or inactivate the antigens that have stimulated its formation.

Anticoagulant. A substance that inhibits the formation of blood clots.

Antigens. Substances that cause the formation of antibodies.

Autohemotherapy. The use of a patient's own blood for his or her treatment.

B-cells. Lymphocytes that are capable of forming antibodies.

Bilirubin. Orange-yellowish pigment derived from the hemoglobin in blood; released by the liver after red cell destruction.

Bleeding time. Time taken for a wound to form platelets and clot. Bleeding time is clinically determined by measuring the time required to stop the flow of blood following a puncture (usually done on the earlobe or forearm).

Chyle. Fats in lymph fluids that are absorbed from the small intestine.

Coagulation time. Time taken for the formation of a clot in the bloodstream.

Corpuscle. Blood cell.

Creatinemia. Excessive creatine in the blood.

Disseminated intravascular coagulation (DIC). A group of disorders with accelerated coagulation and activation of the fibrinolytic mechanisms, resulting in both hemorrhages and thromboses (see Chapter 11).

Electrophoresis. Use of an electric force to separate out proteins in plasma.

Embolus. Thrombus or clot, air bubble, or particle that has migrated within the circulatory system; a potential cause of blockage.

Erythrocyte. Red blood cell.

Erythrocytosis. Condition in which there is an abnormally high number of red blood cells.

Erythropoiesis. Formation of red blood cells.

Exchange transfusion. Removing and replacing blood with fresh, whole blood from a donor.

Extravasation. A condition in which fluids have escaped into surrounding tissues.

Fibrin. Threads of protein that cause blood to clot.

Globulin. Plasma proteins that include alpha, beta, and gamma types.

Hematocrit (Ht, HCT, crit), packed cell volume (PCV). The fraction of blood volume that is composed of red blood cells when solids are separated from the plasma by a centrifuge.

Hematoma. A mass of blood that has hemorrhaged from a vessel into soft tissues.

Heme. Iron-containing portion of the hemoglobulin molecule.

Hemochromatosis. A blood disease in which there is a buildup of iron in the skin tissues and damage to the liver, pancreas, and heart due to a lack of iron metabolism.

Hemoglobin. The iron-containing portion of red blood cells.

Hemolysis. Red blood cell destruction.

Hemophilia. A sex-linked, inherited blood disease in which there is a tendency to bleed due to a prolonged coagulation time. Individuals with *hemophilia A* have a deficiency in blood factor VIII; individuals with *hemophilia B* have a deficiency in factor IX.

Hemorrhage. Gushing, excessive flow of blood.

Hemostasis. Stopping the flow of blood. In surgery, hemostats, or clamps, are instruments used to stop blood flow (see Figure 13–6).

Hypercapnia. Elevated levels in the pressure of arterial carbon dioxide ($PaCO_2$). A respiratory acid-base imbalance can develop, referred to as acidosis.

Hyperglycemia. Excessive amounts of glucose in the blood.

Hyperlipidemia. Excessive amounts of lipids (fats) in the blood.

Immunoglobulin (Ig). Blood proteins that act as antibodies (IgA, IgD, IgE, IgG, and IgM). Increases or decreases in Ig indicate disease.

Leukemia. A malignant blood condition that may be acute or chronic, characterized by an **overproduction of leukocytes** (white blood cells) but a lack of mature neutrophils (see Chapter 12 for additional discussion).

Leukocytopenia. A lack or diminished number of white blood cells.

Lymph. Clear liquid made up of water, salts, sugar, metabolic waste (such as urea and creatinine), lymphocytes, monocytes, platelets, and erythrocytes circulating in lymphatic vessels.

Lymphadenopathy. Enlarged or inflamed lymph glands.

Lymphedema. Accumulation of lymph due to poor tissue drainage, most often the result of surgery or radiation.

Lymph node. Collection of lymph tissue.

Mononucleosis. A higher than normal number of mononuclear white blood cells in the blood.

Multiple myeloma. Plasma cell malignancies of the bone marrow (discussed in greater detail in Chapter 12).

Neutropenia. A decreased number of neutrophilic (white) blood cells.

Packed cells. Blood component therapy in which most of the plasma has been removed; used after marked blood loss.

Pernicious anemia. A blood disease characterized by a reduction in red blood cells, reflecting a deficient absorption of vitamin B_{12}.

Phagocytes, histocytes. Cells that engulf and remove bacteria.

Plasma. The noncellular, fluid part of the blood. **Serum** is the fluid that separates from the fibrinogen (blood-clotting agents).

Plasmapheresis. A technique performed by circulating the blood extracorporeally through a centrifuge to separate the plasma from cells and then returning the cells to the patient. Plasmapheresis can be used to treat autoimmune and other conditions (e.g., Guillain-Barré syndrome) by removing excess antibodies from the blood.

Pneumocystis pneumonia, *Pneumocystis carinii* pneumonia (PCP). A form of pneumonia prevalent among individuals with severe immunodeficiencies, especially patients with HIV, caused by a *protozoan* infection.

Polycythemia, polycythemia rubra vera. A condition in which there is a greater than normal number of red blood cells.

Septicemia. Bacteria in the blood.

Seroculture. Bacterial blood culture.

Sickle cell anemia. An inherited blood disease found predominantly in individuals with African heritage, characterized by hemolysis and sickle-shaped erythrocytes.

Sideropenia. Lack of iron in the blood.

Spleen. Organ involved in blood cell production, storage, and elimination.

Splenomegaly. Enlarged spleen.

T-cells. Lymphocytes produced by the processes in the thymus gland; infection-fighting cells important to the body's immune defense system.

Thalassemia. An inherited, anemic condition occurring primarily in individuals with Mediterranean or Southeast Asian heritage.

Thrombocyte. Blood platelet, or clotting cell.

Thrombotic thrombocytopenic purpura (TTP). A group of clinical syndromes characterized by thrombocytopenia, hemolytic anemia, fever, renal dysfunction, and fluctuating neurologic abnormalities.

Thrombus. A blood clot formed around plaque deposits along blood vessel walls; a thromboembolic clot refers to a thrombus particle that has dislodged (become an embolus) and moved into the bloodstream. (Also see Chapter 10.)

Thymoma. Tumor of the thymus gland.

Thymus. One of a pair of endocrine glands, located in the mediastinum, important to fetal and early childhood growth, and a part of the lymphoid system; manufactures T-cells.

Tonsils. Lymphoid tissues located in the pharynx that aid in the formation of white blood cells. The tonsils include the palatine tonsils, nasopharyngeal (adenoidal) tonsils, and lingual tonsils.

Universal donor. Person with type O Rh negative blood, the blood type that has no agglutinogens to other blood types.

Universal recipient. Person with AB Rh positive blood.

B. Abbreviations

AABB. American Association of Blood Banks

Ab. Antibody

ABO. Blood groups

ACD. Acid-citrate-dextrose

Ag. Antigen

AHF. Antihemophilic factor VIII

AHG. Antihemophilic globulin (factor) VIII

AIDS. Acquired immune deficiency syndrome

AIHA. Autoimmune hemolytic anemia

ALL. Acute lymphoblastic leukemia

BAC. Blood alcohol concentration

Basos. Basophils

CBC. Complete blood count

CLL. Chronic lymphocytic leukemia

CML. Chronic myelocytic leukemia

diff. Differential (count)

EBV. Epstein-Barr virus

ELISA. Enzyme-linked immunosorbent assay

ESR. Erythrocyte sedimentation rate

FDP. Fibrin-fibrinogen degradation products

FR. Fibrin-fibrinogen related

FSP. Fibrin-fibrinogen split products

HAI. Hemagglutination-inhibition immunoassay

HCT, Hct, crit. Hematocrit

Hgb. Hemoglobin

HIV-1, HIV-2. Human immunodeficiency viruses

Ig. Immunoglobulin

ITP. Idiopathic thrombocytopenia

Lymphs. Lymphocytes

PA. Pernicious anemia

MCH. Mean corpuscular hemoglobin

MCHC. Mean corpuscular hemoglobin count

MCV. Mean corpuscular volume

monos. Monocytes

PCP. *Pneumocystis carinii* pneumonia

Polys, PMN. Polymorphonuclear (leukocytes)

PT. Prothrombin time

PTT. Partial thromboplastin time

RBC. Red blood cell (count)

Rh. Rhesus (factor)

RIA. Radioimmunoassay

SCA. Sickle cell anemia

Segs. Segmented(s) (mature red blood cells)

WBC. White blood cell (count)

C. Fundamental Principles

1. Blood and Lymph Circulation

Circulation of blood and lymph occurs through separate but interconnected vascular systems. The average person's blood volume is approximately 6 liters. Blood is made up of 40% "formed elements" and 60% plasma. The formed elements are the blood's cells, including **erythocytes** (red blood cells formed in the red bone marrow); **thrombocytes** (also called platelets); and **leukocyte**s, which include **granulocytes** (neutrophils, basophils, and eosinophils), **monocytes**, and **lymphocytes**. Lymph is rich in fats and contains two types of leukocytes, *lymphocytes*, and *monocytes*. Blood cells carry oxygen, hormones, and nutrients to body tissues.

2. *Protein Transport and Immune Protection*

Lymph transports proteins that have seeped out of the blood circulation (capillaries) back into the veins. Lymph absorbs fat from the small intestine and carries it to the bloodstream. The lymph system also provides the body's immune responses and responses to pathogens. The following section describes some of the studies of immune mechanisms as well as blood counts and blood cell morphology. Such studies are key indicators of infectious processes, cardiopulmonary status, and oncologic and hematologic diseases.

D. Procedures and Studies

Also see the list of commonly ordered laboratory studies in Section IV, Laboratory Tests and Assays to Identify Specific Conditions or Factors, in Chapter 3.

Antinuclear antibodies (ANA) test. Blood test for antibodies present in autoimmune diseases.

Aspirin therapy, ASA therapy. A prophylactic anticoagulation therapy to diminish risk factors for stroke and heart attack.

Blood gases. Measurements of blood to examine for indicators of deficiencies in tissue perfusion and lung function. Blood gas measurements include the pressure, or tension, of **carbon dioxide** ($PaCO_2$ for *arterial measurements* and $PvCO_2$ for *venous measures*), **blood acidity** (pH), and pressures of **oxygen** (PaO_2 and PvO_2).

Blood typing. Blood test to determine the **Rh factor** (Rh– or Rh+) and **blood type** (A, B, AB, and O).

Bone marrow aspiration, bone marrow biopsy. Removal of cells from the bone marrow to diagnose blood-related diseases or for donor purposes.

Complete blood count (CBC). A blood analysis that includes a *white blood cell (WBC) count; red blood cell (RBC) count; hemoglobin (Hg, Hbg); hematocrit (HCT, Hct, crit., Hemocrit); mean corpuscular hemoglobin (MCH); mean corpuscular hemoglobin count (MCHC); mean corpuscular volume (MCV)*; and the *red cell distribution.*

Coumarin derivative therapy. The use of an anticoagulant drug (Coumadin) to act as an antagonist to the coagulating properties of vitamin K.

Erythrocyte sedimentation rate (ESR), "sed rate." A blood test that measures the depth to which RBCs settle in a vertical tube following a specified time delay. Increased "sed rates" indicate pathologic conditions, such as infectious processes, inflammation, myocardial infarction, endocarditis, and neoplasm.

Heparin therapy. The use of an anticoagulant drug to inhibit platelet aggregation as a prophylactic treatment to prevent clotting.

Immunoglobulin (Ig) analysis. Serologic test to examine for the presence of immunoglobulin.

Partial thromboplastin time (PTT). A test of the time required for clotting in plasma; helps to determine heparin levels and to diagnose clotting disorders.

Red blood cell (RBC) count and morphology. Measurement of the number of erythrocytes present in the blood and identification of any abnormalities in cell characteristics (shape and maturity); useful in diagnosing liver diseases, anemias, and other hematologic conditions.

White blood cell (WBC) count and morphology. Measurement of the number of leukocytes in the blood and their cell characteristics (shape and maturity); useful in diagnosing blood diseases, such as leukemias and anemias, and other conditions, such as infections.

V. CARDIOPULMONARY RESUSCITATION (CPR)

A. Basic and Advanced Life Support

Nearly everyone who works in health service delivery is required to have biennial training in *cardiopulmonary resuscitation, or CPR.* **Basic Life Support (BLS)** training from the American Heart Association involves knowledge and skills acquisition in the techniques of CPR for *emergency cardiac care (ECC).* The purpose of this training is to prevent or diminish the adverse effects of cardiocirculatory or respiratory arrest, principally to prevent damage to the central nervous system. BLS and **Advanced Cardiac Life Support (ACLS)** training in hospitals are conducted by the American Heart Association (AHA) or professionals who received training in the AHA's programs, or through the Red Cross. These classes typically include readings, lectures, demonstrations, videotapes, and hands-on practice in foreign body airway management, resuscitation techniques, and the use of *automatic external defibrillators (AEDs)* with infants, children, and adults (using manikins). Minimum performance criteria and knowledge are required for "successful completion" of an AHA-approved course. Completing an AHA-approved BLS training program does not indicate that an individual is "licensed" or "certified" in CPR. Upon completion of the biennial training, health care providers receive a verification card, indicating that he or she has completed an approved course and demonstrated the cognitive abilities and technical skills required to pass the national AHA Healthcare Providers (CPR and AED) curriculum. The more advanced training, ACLS, is usually mandated only for individuals whose job descriptions require providing emergency cardiopulmonary care, for example, inpatient nursing staff, emergency medical technicians (EMTs), or individuals who work in settings where cardiopulmonary emergencies are likely (e.g., a cardiac rehabilitation unit). Further discussion of cardiopulmonary emergencies is found in Chapter 2.

B. ABCs of CPR

The sequence of emergency procedures applied during CPR is based on three basic concerns for management: **airway**, **breathing**, and **circulation**, referred to as the ABCs of CPR. Sometimes CPR is described as an ABC **D** procedure, in which "D" refers to **definitive** therapy, or access to cardiac care management (an admission to the cardiac care unit [CCU]). Optimal resuscitation emphasizes *early access* to CPR, defibrillation, and advanced care.

During CPR training, the health care providers are taught to follow a fairly scripted response sequence, starting with determining if the stricken individual is *conscious or responsive* by attempting to arouse the individual by gentle shaking and asking him or her, "Are you all right?" If the stricken individual is not responsive, the rescuer is instructed to call for assistance immediately (instructing someone in the vicinity to "Call 911!"), if possible, to obtain Emergency Medical Service. In a hospital setting, a "code" would be initiated to obtain emergency assistance from the facility's first responder, or **Code Blue Team** (see discussion later). If no phone is available, and there is no one in the vicinity to provide assistance to the rescuer, and it has been determined that the stricken person is neither responsive nor breathing, the rescuer is taught to position the head in a manner that would best prevent the tongue and epiglottis from obstructing the airway. The technique involves tilting the head back slightly and lifting the jaw up and forward with a **"jaw thrust" maneuver** and *visually* checking for airway obstructions. Rescuers are cautioned, however, to *not* attempt a blind finger sweep down the stricken individual's throat. If the stricken individual has not resumed breathing after positioning the head and ensuring as well as possible that the airway is cleared, the rescuer will begin **rescue breathing** (see definition). Rescue breathing can require mouth-to-mouth, mouth-to-nose (with the mouth closed), mouth over the mouth and nose (of a small child or infant), or mouth-to-stoma (with laryngectomees) ventilation. Ideally, rescue breathing is delivered through a protective mask with a one-way valve to reduce infection risks. The proper skills for rescue breathing techniques should be taught by a *trained, certified instructor* within an AHA or Red Cross resuscitation training program. Both inadequate and excessive rescue ventilation can be problematic.

Following airway clearance and after providing two of rescue breaths, the rescuer will attempt to determine the need for assistance with cardiac circulation. The resuscitator will palpate (feel) for a carotid (neck) pulse in adults or a high brachial (inside, upper arm) pulse in small children and infants. If no pulse is palpable, chest compressions are then initiated. The optimal pace, intensity, compression pressure, hand placement (adults), finger placement (infants), and procedures for administering chest compressions and rescue breathing sequences will vary depending on the age of the stricken individual and if another rescuer is available to assist. These skills are a part of the CPR training.

If an AED device is available, that device should be activated according to the device directions. Experience with AEDs for both children and adults is a part of the CPR training curriculum. All health care providers should note the location of AEDs in their work settings and elsewhere. AEDs are portable, computerized devices designed for use by individuals who are not medically trained. When activated, AEDs have step-by-step written or recorded spoken instructions for the rescuer to follow, describing where to place the two adhesive-backed pads on the stricken individual's chest and which buttons to push. Placement and pad sizes vary for adults and children. Once the pads are properly placed, the AED should be activated, and the device will automatically diagnose a life-threatening arrhythmia and inform the rescuer if electrical stimulation is required or not. If the need for electrical stimulation is indicated, the AED will verbally instruct the rescuer(s) to "clear" any contact with the stricken individual and then it will provide an electrical stimulation to the chest to elicit an effective heart rhythm. If there is no AED in the immediate environment, the rescuer is instructed to continue CPR (chest compression and rescue ventilation cycles) until the stricken individual has revived or recovered or emergency medical personnel have arrived.

The techniques used in CPR need to be *implemented correctly* and without delay. Recommended rescue procedures have evolved slightly in recent years as a function of new medical information related to outcomes. Basic cognitive and skills training and practice are essential for efficient actions during a resuscitation emergency. Rescuer knowledge, skill, and confidence can help to ensure efficient implementation of the optimal resuscitation procedures, which should enhance survivability; however, most CPR trainers advise us that even if we are uncertain if we are doing each step perfectly correctly, it is better to *do something* than to do nothing.

C. Codes

Most health care facilities have disaster plans, emergency alert processes, emergency paging procedures, and **codes**. These procedures, taught during the safety orientation and annually, are well-known to the staff and are intended to elicit a swift and efficient response in an emergency. For example, a "Code Red" alert may refer to a fire emergency; "Code Orange" may refer to a weather emergency; "Code Walker" may refer to a wandering patient; and "Code Blue" may be the alert for a cardiopulmonary emergency.

Patients will be said to have been "coded" if they have had a cardiopulmonary event that required calling the first responders team, or Code Blue Team, or others to perform resuscitation emergently. When calling a cardiopulmonary code in a hospital or hospital-based clinic, the typical actions are:

- **Activate the cardiopulmonary code** according to the facility's procedures (usually the procedure involves calling a dedicated telephone response line number and providing specific verbal information, including the exact location of the stricken individual).
- If the stricken individual is not responsive, not breathing, and has no pulse (see earlier) **provide CPR** until the first responder team arrives.
- If there is a **Crash Cart** in your area, make sure it is readily available for the team and placed next to the stricken individual.
- If needed, make sure that a staff member is available to **help the code team** locate the stricken individual (e.g., post someone outside the clinic door to direct the team).
- When the team arrives, **get out of the way** and keep the area clear of bystanders to eliminate distractions and to allow the team sufficient room to care for the patient.
- **Provide any needed assistance** (e.g., hold an elevator on the floor to be ready for transportation).

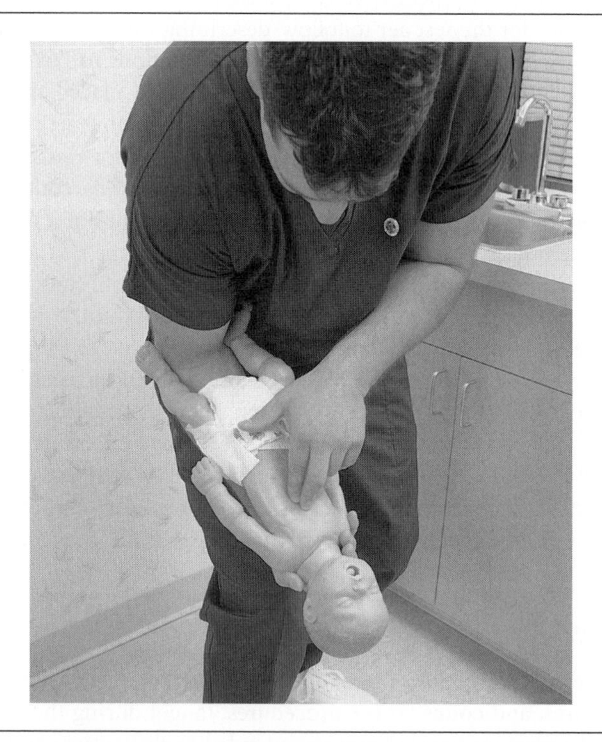

FIGURES 9–11A Foreign body airway management with an infant lying on the forearm (give five chest thrusts). Source: Delmar/Cengage Learning

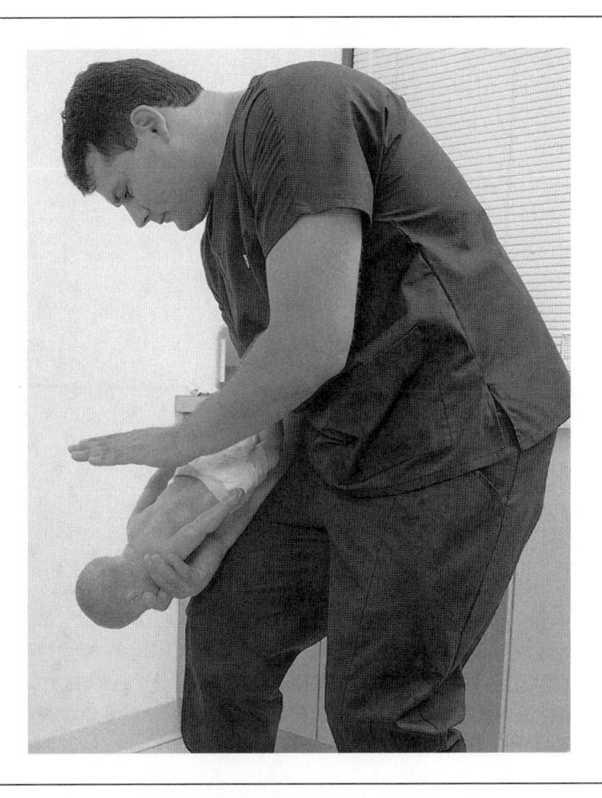

FIGURE 9–11B Foreign body airway management with an infant face down on the forearm (give five back blows). Source: Delmar/Cengage Learning

When sudden "cardiac death," or cardiac arrest, has occurred, respiration will cease. After four minutes of hypoxia, irreversible damage to the brain begins. The rare, reported exceptions to this can be found in cases of near-drownings or other conditions in which hypoxia occurs within conditions of extreme cold (when metabolic rate is slowed). In most cases, without CPR, biological death will occur so oxygen perfusion must be initiated immediately. When the heart has ceased to beat and no ventilation is apparent, clinical death has occurred; however, this state is potentially reversible. Consequently, even though the probability of needing to use CPR rescue techniques in a hospital is low, clinicians should always be prepared.

D. Foreign Body Obstruction

Familiarity with the *subdiaphragmatic abdominal thrust*, or the so-called Heimlich maneuver, is important for health care personnel and laypersons alike. It is an especially important safety technique when working with children and adults with dysphagia and individuals who have oral, pharyngeal, or laryngeal weakness. Figures 9–11A, 9–11B, 9–12A, and 9-12B provide illustrations of emergency management of an airway obstruction with children and adults. Emergency management of a foreign body obstruction in adults, children, infants, pregnant women, and unconscious individuals is a part of the AHA's Basic Life Support for Healthcare Providers training.

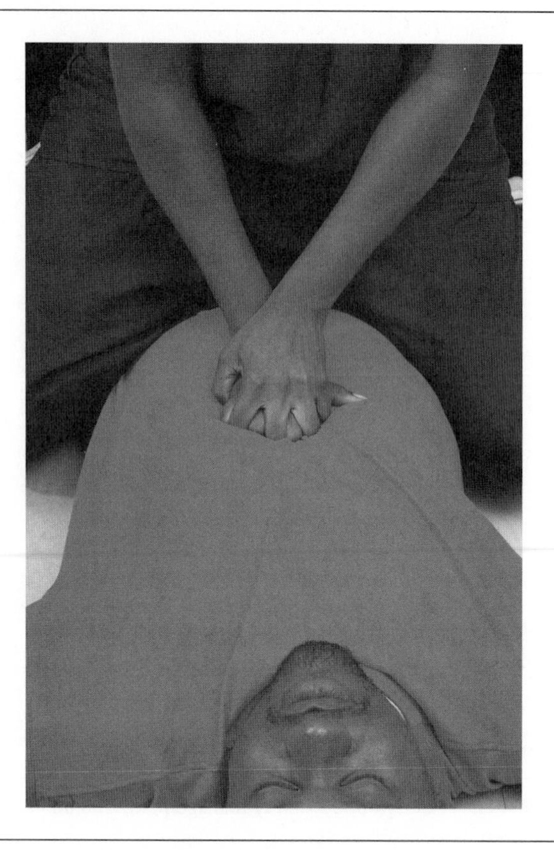

FIGURE 9–12A Foreign body airway management for an unconscious adult with abdominal thrusts. Source: Delmar/Cengage Learning

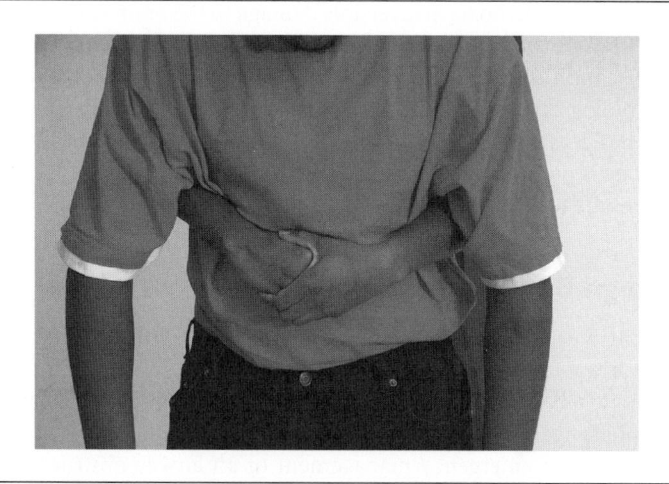

FIGURE 9–12B Foreign body airway management with an adult: hand placement for an abdominal thrust (Heimlich maneuver). Source: Delmar/Cengage Learning

VI. CLINICAL COMPETENCIES

The learner outcomes, skills, and competencies gained from information contained in this chapter include the ability to:

- Read, interpret, and use terminology and abbreviations related to cardiology, pulmonology, and hematology.
- Discuss the basic principles of blood circulation and heart conduction.
- Describe the wave features of an electrocardiogram (EKG/ECG) and to what heart activity each feature corresponds.
- List some of the common diagnostic heart studies and therapeutic procedures.
- Illustrate and label the structures of the respiratory tract.
- Identify the anatomy of the larynx and structures and functions involved in airway protection.
- Describe the basic principles of respiration.
- List the neural control centers for respiration.
- Describe aberrant respiration patterns and the disorders or diseases they indicate.
- List the steps and precautions applied in tracheostomy and oropharyngeal suctioning.
- Demonstrate the techniques used in tracheostomy care.
- Define what is meant by "cuffed" and "fenestrated" trachs.
- List some of the potential complications of prolonged use of tracheostomy tubes.
- Describe basic precautions when using a Passy-Muir ™ valve with a patient who has a cuffed trach.
- Explain the principles of lymphatic circulation and drainage.
- Define what is meant by the "ABCs of CPR."
- Describe the two purposes of an AED.
- Describe the cardiopulmonary code procedures in your work setting or an affiliated training facility.
- Demonstrate the appropriate steps for the SLP to take after calling in a cardiopulmonary "code."
- Demonstrate the emergency procedures for foreign body airway obstruction (choking) management in an unconscious adult and a 6-month-old infant.

VII. REFERENCES AND RESOURCES CONSULTED

Albarran-Sotelo, R., Flint, L. S., & Kelly, K. J. (1988). *Healthcare provider's manual for basic life support.* Dallas, TX: American Heart Association.

Anderson, D. (Ed.). (2003). *Dorland's illustrated medical dictionary* (30th ed.). Philadelphia: W. B. Saunders.

Andreoli, T. A., Carpenter, C., & Grigg, R. C. (Eds.). (2007). *Cecil essentials of medicine* (7th ed.). Philadelphia: W. B. Saunders.

Ayres, S. M., Schlichtig, R., & Sterling, M. J. (1988). *Care of the critically ill* (3rd ed.). Chicago: Yearbook Medical.

Bleile, K. M. (1993). *The care of children with long-term tracheostomies.* San Diego, CA: Singular.

Budassi, S. A., & Barber, J. M. (1981). *Emergency nursing: Principles and practice.* St. Louis, MO: C. V. Mosby.

Davis, M. A., Gruskin, K. D., Chiang, V. W., & Manzi, S. (Eds.). (2005). *Signs and symptoms in pediatrics: Urgent and emergent care.* Philadelphia: Elsevier Mosby.

Davis, J. J. (2008). *Essentials of medical terminology* (3rd ed.). Clifton Park, NY: Delmar Cengage Learning.

Fein, I. A., & Strasberg, M. A. (1987). *Managing the critical care unit.* Rockville, MD: Aspen.

Fogle, P. (2008). *Foundations of communication sciences and disorders.* Clifton Park, NY: Delmar Cengage Learning.

Freeman, M. (Ed.). (1988). *An introduction to clinical imaging.* New York: Churchill Livingstone.

Hirano, M., Kirchner, J. A., & Bless, D. M. (Eds.). (1987). *Neurology: Recent advances.* San Diego, CA: Singular.

Hunter, T. B., & Taljanovic, M. S. (2003). Glossary of medical devices and procedures: Abbreviations, acronyms, and definitions. *Radiographics, 23*, 195–213.

Jablonski, S. (2005). *Dictionary of medical acronyms and abbreviations* (5th ed.). Philadelphia: Elsevier Saunders.

Johnson, A. H., & Jacobson, B. H. (Eds.). (2007). *Medical speech-language pathology: A practitioner's guide* (2nd ed.). New York: Thieme.

Jones, B. D. (2008). *Comprehensive medical terminology* (3rd ed.). Clifton Park, NY: Delmar Cengage Learning.

Keir, L., Wise, B., Krebs, C., & Kelley-Arney, C. (2008). *Medical assisting: Administrative and clinical competencies* (6th ed.). Clifton Park, NY: Delmar Cengage Learning.

Kirchner, J. A. (1987). The larynx-lung relationships. In M. Hirano, J. A. Kirchner, & D. M. Bless (Eds.), *Neurology* (pp. 160–166). San Diego, CA: Singular.

Lewis, L. W., & Trimby, B. K. (1988). *Fundamental skills and concepts in patient care* (4th ed.). Philadelphia: J. B. Lippincott.

Persons, C. G. (1987). *Critical care procedures and protocols.* Philadelphia: J. B. Lippincott.

Scott, A. S., & Fong, E. (2004). *Body structures and functions* (10th ed.). Clifton Park, NY: Delmar Cengage Learning.

Seikel, J. A., King, D. W., & Drumright, D. G. (2005). *Anatomy and physiology of speech, language, and hearing* (3rd ed.). Clifton Park, NY: Delmar Cengage Learning.

Tobin, M. J. (1989). *Essentials of critical care medicine.* New York: Churchill Livingstone.

CHAPTER 10

Neurologic and Psychiatric Disorders

Adults and children with neurologic and psychiatric disorders are of particular interest to speech-language pathologists (SLPs) in medical settings and are likely to make up the majority of referrals. Neurologic diseases and disorders can affect the sensory, motor, and cognitive-linguistic processes that underlie communication and swallowing. Psychiatric conditions may be revealed, in part, by the patient's verbal statements. Psychiatric status can confound and cloud the diagnostic workup or complicate communication and swallowing therapies. Thus, familiarity with these conditions and the terminology and abbreviations used to describe them are essential for SLPs who practice in a medical setting.

I. CHAPTER FOCUS

This chapter provides a brief descriptive outline of many of the more frequently encountered neurologic and psychiatric disorders and diseases. The goal is to provide definitions, descriptions, and explanations; thus, it includes both diseases (e.g., cerebrovascular diseases) and conditions resulting from or associated with those diseases (e.g., hemiparesis). It is beyond the intent of this chapter to describe the etiology, pathology, clinical features, or treatment of each of the disorders listed. Related terminology, abbreviations, descriptions of procedures, and the features of the mental status and neurologic examinations are found in Chapter 4. Infectious diseases and cardiovascular conditions that cause neurologic damage are discussed in Chapters 8 and 9, respectively, and some of the neurologic conditions likely to require intensive care are described in Chapter 11.

II. NEUROLOGIC DISORDERS

A. Mobility Disorders

In this section, disorders that affect mobility are listed under the broad headings "Paralysis and Paresis" and "Extrapyramidal Disorders." Disorders that cause paralysis and paresis include lesions in the motor cortex, pyramidal tract (corticospinal tract), corticobulbar tract, and bulbar and spinal motor nuclei. Paralysis refers to an absence of voluntary motor functions, and paresis refers to the partial presence of voluntary motor functions. **Extrapyramidal disorders** primarily include lesions and disorders involving the subcortical gray structures, or basal ganglia, and the cerebellum. Cerebellar disorders include lesions within the cerebellum itself and lesions involving cerebellar relay nuclei in the brain stem (midbrain, pons, and medulla). The cerebellum coordinates skilled movements and controls muscle tone, posture, and gait. Mobility disturbances associated with peripheral neuropathies, including neuromuscular diseases, are discussed later in this chapter.

I. *Paralysis and Paresis*

Flaccidity. Lower motor neuron paralysis results from destruction of the anterior horn cells and their axons, causing flaccidity. When muscle tone during passive movement and in response to myotactic, or stretch, reflexes is lacking, muscles are said to be flaccid, or hypotonic.

Hemiplegia. Paralysis of one side of the body. The location of a lesion producing hemiplegia may be anywhere along the corticospinal tract, and the level of the lesion is identified by the neurologic examination (see Chapter 4).

Monoparesis or monoplegia. Weakness or paralysis, respectively, of one limb.

Paraparesis or paraplegia. Weakness or paralysis, respectively, of both legs, usually following spinal cord injuries or diseases.

Quadriparesis or tetraparesis, quadriplegia or tetraplegia. Weakness or paralysis, respectively, of all four extremities.

Spasticity. Associated with upper motor neuron lesions and characterized by a state of heightened stretch reflexes and greater than normal muscular tone. Spasticity is more discrete following spinal cord lesions than lesions higher up the corticospinal tract. Following an acute lesion there is usually an *initial flaccidity and areflexia* (spinal shock), which evolves to hypertonicity and *exaggerated reflexes* for muscles innervated below the level of injury. Flaccidity followed by hypertonicity and exaggerated reflexes may also be seen acutely after cortical strokes. Evaluation of reflex functions is described in Chapter 4.

Spasticity results from the interruption of *descending inhibitory innervation* and *reticulospinal* and *vestibulospinal influences*. The effect of these combined influences is illustrated by the **clasp knife phenomenon**. A clasp knife reaction is seen when a hemiplegic limb is passively extended in a brisk manner, eliciting an abrupt catch followed by a degree of release, allowing further extension.

It is important to consider that **upper motor neuron (UMN)** paralysis is not absolute paralysis, as is the case with **lower motor neuron (LMN)** destruction (where the motor neuron is nonfunctional), and that upper motor paralysis involves muscle groups rather than individual muscles. Occasionally, hemiplegia with UMN lesions are described as flaccid with no discernible **electromyography (EMG)** activity, except in response to reflex testing. After UMN lesions there may be occasional involuntary activation of the "paralyzed" muscle, a phenomenon called **synkinesis**, in which movement of the weak limb occurs when the patient coughs, yawns, or moves the contralateral limb.

2. *Extrapyramidal Disorders*

Akathisia. Referring to motor unrest, such as that observed in patients receiving neuroleptic drugs, in which there is restlessness and a compulsion to move.

Asterixis. A disorder observed with hepatic encephalopathy and other metabolic and toxic conditions in which rhythmic, flexion movements of the hands are seen when the arms and hands are extended and dorsiflexed; sometimes referred to as a "liver flap."

Ataxias. Cerebellar ataxia is characterized by a wide-based gait with irregular steps, swaying of the trunk, and unsteadiness. **Sensory ataxia** indicates a disturbance in joint position sense. This disturbance can result from bilateral, parietal lobe lesions; posterior column damage in the spinal cord; or damage to the afferent fibers or posterior roots of peripheral nerves. During the neurologic examination, a "*positive Rhomberg*" sign may be reported (swaying and falling with the eyes closed but not with the eyes open). **Friedreich's ataxia** is an autosomal recessive trait associated with *spinocerebellar degeneration*. **Olivopontine cerebellar degeneration (OPCD)** is characterized by ataxia and dysmetria due to degeneration of the pontine cerebellar relay nuclei and inferior olives.

Ballism, ballismus. *Ballism* refers to a condition associated with an abrupt onset of flinging motions of the extremities. *Hemiballism* involves only one side of the body; *monoballism* involves only one limb. This condition seems to result from a lesion in the subthalamic nucleus or its connections.

Blepharospasm. A persistent tonic spasm occurring around the eyes during which the patient may be unable to maintain eye opening. The spasm may be limited to the muscles of the eyelids or may involve other facial musculature. Treatment can involve nerve sectioning or injection of a neurotoxin, such as botulinum toxin.

Cerebellar incoordination, intention tremor, and hypotonia. A complex of movement disorders associated with lesions to the cerebellar hemispheres or the middle and inferior cerebellar peduncles and brachium conjunctivum. Cerebellar signs are ipsilateral to the lesion, except for very rare lesions of the contralateral red nucleus (at the decussation of the superior cerebellar peduncle).

Choreas. Choreiform movements are abrupt, irregular, writhing movements of short duration. Various forms of chorea have been identified in association with basal ganglia lesions and degeneration. **Huntington's disease** (Huntington's chorea) is a hereditary, autosomal dominant disease characterized by a progressive onset of restlessness, choreiform movements, and dementia. Neurochemical deficiencies in Huntington's disease lead to atrophy of the caudate nucleus. **Rheumatic**, or **Sydenham's, chorea** has been associated with group A streptococcal infections. With this type of chorea, dysarthria has an explosive quality, due to sudden contractions of respiratory muscles.

Senile chorea is one of the movement disorders associated with basal ganglia degeneration in the elderly and in patients with known Alzheimer's disease. Patients with *hemichorea* exhibit unilateral choreiform movements. This condition has been seen following a unilateral, small vascular lesion (stroke) in the posterior ventrolateral nucleus of the thalamus.

Choreoathetosis, or paroxysmal kinesiogenic choreoathetosis, is a condition that begins in childhood and is characterized by sudden attacks of choreoathetoid movements, occurring frequently and without warning. These bizarre contortions are thought to be a variant of a seizure disorder, because they are diminished with anticonvulsant therapies.

Dyskinesias. Dyskinesias include a group of movement disorders of varying etiologies. *Involuntary dyskinesia* is associated with phenothiazine (tranquilizer) therapy. Patients who have long-term neuroleptic therapies may develop dystonias of the face and mouth, parkinsonian rigidity and tremors, tardive dyskinesia and dystonia, and akathisia. **Tardive dyskinesia** is a syndrome characterized by involuntary movements of the mouth, lips, and tongue and, in most cases, dystonic postures of the neck, trunk, and upper extremities. Tardive dyskinesias have occasionally been seen in both children and adults who are taking protein pump inhibitors for severe gastrointestinal reflux. The repetitive movements of the mouth and tongue usually include lip smacking or sucking motions. A condition termed "*rabbit syndrome*" has been associated with long-term neuroleptic use. This condition is diagnosed by eliciting fine, rhythmic contractions of the upper lip when the examiner taps his or her finger just above the patient's upper lip. Another complication of neuroleptic therapy is **malignant neuroleptic syndrome**, in which severe rigidity, high fever, and autonomic dysfunction result from high doses of neuroleptics.

Dystonia musculorum deformans, or torsion spasm. A dystonia involving limb and axial musculature on one or both sides of the body. This condition can be progressive, but in some cases, spontaneous remission occurs. Juvenile onset of this disorder has been described, and there may be hereditary factors in some cases. Lesions of the caudate nucleus, putamen, and globus pallidus have been associated with torsion spasms.

Gilles de la Tourette's syndrome. A syndrome associated with multiple tics, compulsive snorting, barking, sniffing, and involuntary **palilalia** (compulsive repetitions of the same words or phrases) and **coprolalia** (compulsive expressions of obscenities and scatologic utterances). Haloperidol can be an effective therapy.

Hepatolenticular degeneration, Wilson's disease. Wilson's disease is an autosomal recessive condition associated with accumulations of copper in tissues and in the urine, often occurring with an associated liver failure. Copper deposits in the basal ganglia damage the globus pallidus, thalamus, subthalamic nucleus, red nucleus, and claustrum. This disease presents with either choreiform or dystonic movements and behavioral disturbances. These patients are dysarthric and dysphagic and may become aphonic.

Meige syndrome, Breughel's syndrome, focal cranial dystonia, orolingual-facial-mandibular dystonia. These terms refer to dystonia syndromes involving the lingual and oromandibular musculature. These *action dystonias* (dystonia elicited by the initiation of movement and not present at rest) may occur in one or more muscle groups and there may be an associated blepharospasm (involuntary eye blinks) and writer's cramp.

Nothnagel syndrome. A brain stem syndrome associated with a tumor in the tectum, affecting the superior cerebellar peduncles, and associated with a gaze paralysis and cerebellar ataxia.

Palatal and facial myoclonus. A type of rhythmic myoclonus seen with lesions of the contralateral dentate nucleus or superior cerebellar peduncle, or the ipsilateral inferior olivary nucleus, and central segmental tract.

Parkinson's disease and parkinsonism. Parkinson's disease is a syndrome characterized by resting tremors, bradykinesia, and rigidity occurring in association with impaired or reduced activity of the neurotransmitter dopamine. Neuropathologic studies at autopsy of patients with Parkinson's disease have found multiple areas of neuronal loss in the cortex, basal ganglia, and thalamus and a notable focal neuronal loss in the substantia nigra. Parkinsonian signs may be found in association with infarctions in the basal ganglia, called **arteriosclerotic parkinsonism**. Other types of parkinsonism include **drug-induced parkinsonism** (resulting from the use of phenothiazine or butyrophenone); **toxic parkinsonism** (resulting from environmental toxins and gases); **postencephalitic parkinsonism** or **encephalitis lethargica** (possibly the result of a "slow virus" following viral encephalitis); parkinsonism **secondary to infectious disease** (symptoms co-occurring with conditions such as viral encephalitis and treated tuberculosis); and parkinsonism in **association with other degenerative neurologic diseases** (such as olivopontinecerebellar degeneration, Alzheimer's disease, Creutzfeldt-Jakob disease, Wilson's disease, and Huntington's disease).

Spasmodic laryngeal dystonia, spasmodic dysphonia. A dystonia limited to the laryngeal muscles, causing adductor or abductor spasms, and treated by sectioning or disrupting the recurrent laryngeal nerve; injection of a neurotoxin, such as botulinum toxin; and/or voice therapy.

Spasmodic torticollis. A dystonia limited to the shoulder and neck muscles treated by sectioning the spinal accessory nerve or by a neurotoxin (e.g., botulinum) injection.

Tremors. In general, tremors are regular, rhythmic movements of a body part. Parkinsonian tremors, or resting tremors, are localized tremors of one or both hands and, infrequently, involve the jaw, lips, or tongue. Parkinsonian hand tremors are rhythmic flexion-extension motions with "pill-rolling" adduction-abduction motions of the thumb. During voluntary movements, such as reaching for a cup, the tremor is absent or diminished. Conversely, intention tremors, ataxic tremors, or rubral tremors are not obvious at rest but occur during performance of fine, skilled actions. Action tremors resemble the tremors characteristic of intense fear or anxiety. Such tremors are seen with *hyperthyroidism, alcohol or drug abuse withdrawal*, and *toxic conditions*. Most action tremors are rapid and rhythmic; however, **kinetic tremors** are a coarser type of action tremor usually involving the hands, voice, or head. This coarser type of action tremor is sometimes described in association with *demyelinative polyneuropathy*.

Other action tremors include **essential tremors**, or benign familial tremors, which appear in adulthood and usually are limited to the upper extremities or the head. Essential vocal tremors, characterized by a tremulous phonation of no known cause, may be isolated to the voice or occur in association with head tremors. Head tremors are characterized by nodding or side-to-side movements. **Orthostatic tremor** refers to an essential tremor limited to the legs.

Writer's cramp. A type of focal dystonia occurring during fine motor activity, specifically writing, characterized by a cramping dystonia of the hand.

B. Seizure Disorders

Individuals who have more than a single seizure during their lifetime are usually diagnosed to have epilepsy, or a seizure disorder. When a seizure, or convulsion, occurs, it is proper to state that the patient is "**seizing**," not "seizuring." Seizures are abnormal, electrical discharges emanating from living cells in an area of the cortex. Diagnosis of the type of seizure disorder is made based on the time of onset, extent of loss of consciousness, and the characteristic motor pattern during the seizure. Seizures may occur with rare types of hereditary diseases and inborn errors of metabolism, such as *Sturge-Weber syndrome, trisomy D, tuberous sclerosis, leukodystrophies, lipidoses, aminoacidurias, phenylketonuria (PKU), maple syrup urine disease*, and *glucagon storage diseases.*

Prenatal and neonatal seizure disorders may be found in association with *teratogenic agents* (environmental agents damaging the developing fetus [see Chapter 6]). Infections such as cytomegalovirus, rubella, toxoplasmosis, and syphilis and exposure to substances such as alcohol or trimethadione are teratogens associated with neonatal seizures.

Atonic seizures. A form of generalized seizure characterized by a sudden onset of akinesis, "rag doll" muscle tone, with no loss of consciousness and rapid recovery.

Complex partial (partial complex) seizures. See "Partial Seizures" in Chapter 4.

Febrile convulsion. A grand mal, tonic-clonic-type seizure occurring in association with a fever, usually related to a viral illness.

Grand mal seizure. A generalized tonic-clonic seizure characterized by an initial loss of consciousness followed by rigidity (tonic phase), rhythmic jerking (clonic phase), sweating, and incontinence. Grand mal seizures usually are not life threatening unless they are prolonged. Grand mal seizures lasting 20 to 30 minutes require emergency medical assistance, because they are potentially life threatening (see "**Status Epilepticus**" in Chapter 11).

Infantile spasm. A type of seizure disorder most often associated with the early stages of inherited diseases affecting the nervous system. The spasm involves a series of sudden, "jack-knifing" contractions. This type of seizure disorder usually progresses to a grand mal type in association with progressive mental retardation when widespread nervous system damage has occurred.

Landau-Kleffner syndrome. A syndrome characterized by an acquired aphasia and bilateral temporal lobe epilepsy in childhood.

Lennox-Gastaut seizures. A form of absence seizures associated with motoric characteristics that may be varied (tonic-clonic, tonic only, or myoclonic). This type of seizure is seen in young children and is often associated with mental retardation syndromes and cerebral palsy.

Petit mal, or absence [pronounced /æb sAns/] **seizures.** Condition in which the affected individual momentarily loses consciousness and appears to be staring into space, often without loss of muscle tone or any tonic-clonic jerks.

C. Dysthymic Disorders

In psychiatry, the term *dysthymic disorder* generally refers to depression; in metabolism, a disorder in the thymus gland. Specific depression syndromes are discussed later in this chapter.

D. Syncope and Sleep Disorders

This section reviews several disorders related to alertness, disorders associated with sleep, and disorders occurring when the patient is reclining or attempting to sleep. Disorders affecting mental status are discussed later in this chapter and in Chapter 4.

Acroparesthesia. An unpleasant prickling or burning sensation present on awakening or after lying or sitting in one position for a prolonged period.

Bruxism. Referring to teeth grinding, especially during sleep.

Cardiac syncope. Referring to syncope of cardiac origin, including the Stokes-Adam type of cardiac syncope, dysfunction of the sinus node ("*sick sinus syndrome*"), syncope related to dysrythmias and myocardial infarction, and the cardioinhibitory syncope due to irritation of the vagus nerve (termed "vasovagal" faints).

Cataplexy. A sudden loss of muscle tone with temporary paralysis, often found in association with narcolepsy.

Insomnia. A chronic inability to sleep. The term *primary insomnia* is used to describe conditions where sleep is chronically disturbed despite a lack of medical or psychiatric problems. An inability to sleep due to conditions such as pain, anxiety, depression, or pharmacologic agents is called *secondary insomnia.*

Micturation syncope. Lightheadedness or loss of consciousness following urination seen mainly in the elderly.

Narcolepsy. A condition characterized by sudden attacks of irresistible sleepiness. Patients with narcolepsy may also have episodes of depressed consciousness while awake, during which they engage in automatic behaviors and will have no memory of the episodes.

Pickwickian syndrome. A condition characterized by obesity, somnolence, hypoventilation, tachycardia, and erythrocytosis; the syndrome name comes from the fat boy in Dickens' *Pickwick Papers.*

Primary autonomic insufficiency. Syncope related to degenerative diseases involving the brain stem autonomic structures or the peripheral autonomic nervous system.

Sleep apnea. A prolonged cessation of breathing during sleep that may be due to a disturbance of the respiratory centers (central apnea) or the result of airway obstruction (obstructive apnea) (see Chapter 4).

Syncope. A temporary loss of consciousness (fainting) due to diminished blood flow to the brain. The primary causes for syncope are circulatory and cardiac dysfunction, anemia, hypoxia, or emotional disturbances (hysterical fainting).

Syncope related to orthostatic (postural) hypotension. A type of syncope that occurs on standing up or when standing for long periods. This type of syncope is found in patients with chronic orthostatic hypotension, varicose veins of the legs, peripheral neuropathies, hypovolemia, primary autonomic insufficiency, and patients taking drugs such as sedatives, L-Dopa, or antihypertensive agents.

Vagoglossopharyngeal syncope. A reflexive type of syncope elicited by chewing or swallowing in a manner that causes pressure on the afferent pathways of the glossopharyngeal (CN IX) nerve, which then stimulates the vasomotor centers of the vagus (CN X) nerve.

Vasodepressor (vasovagal) syncope. Fainting in response to a painful or strong emotion; simple faint, also see cardiac syncope.

E. Disturbances in Cerebrospinal Fluid Circulation

Colpencephaly. Ventricular enlargement in underdeveloped brains.

Congenital hydrocephalus. Hydrocephalus occurring during fetal development as a feature of inherited conditions (such as Dandy-Walker syndrome or Arnold-Chiari malformation), defective nervous system development, or the result of fetal or neonatal infections or hemorrhages.

Hydrocephalus. Increased cerebrospinal fluid in the ventricles of the brain. (See "Communicating Hydrocephalus" and "Obstruction Hydrocephalus" in Chapter 7.)

Hydrocephalus *ex vacuo*. Ventricular enlargement subsequent to brain atrophy.

Normal pressure hydrocephalus. A condition of chronic hydrocephalus in adults associated with delayed absorption of cerebrospinal fluid and characterized by progressive neurologic deficits (gait disturbances, incontinence, and cognitive deficits). This condition, like other forms of hydrocephalus, may be treated with a **ventriculoatrial (V-A)** shunt, draining from the ventricles into the right atrium of the heart, or a **ventriculoperitoneal (V-P)** shunt, draining from the ventricle into the peritoneal cavity, usually near the liver.

Tension hydrocephalus. A condition in which there is increased pressure in cerebrospinal fluid (CSF) due to a disruption or obstruction of flow between the CSF production sites in the lateral ventricles and the subarachnoid space where it is absorbed. The forms of tension hydrocephalus include meningeal-obstructive, third ventricle-obstructive, and aqueductal-obstructive hydrocephalus.

F. Toxic, Nutritional, and Metabolic Disorders

This section reviews some of the conditions associated with toxic, nutritional, and metabolic disorders. The effects of hazardous chemicals or agents or neurologic complications associated with nonprescription drugs, "recreational" drugs, and prescribed drugs are not discussed. Discussions of the functions of various vitamins and minerals and effects of fluid and electrolyte imbalances are found in Chapter 5, Nutrition, Hydration, and Swallowing.

Alcoholic seizure disorder. Seizure disorders are frequent among alcoholics and are possibly related to repeated head injuries or a lowered threshold for seizures caused by the toxic effects of alcohol itself. Seizures may also be a prodromal symptom of alcohol withdrawal.

Diabetic neuropathy. A syndrome of polyneuropathies, focal asymmetric mono- or polymononeuropathies, and/or autonomic neuropathies.

Dialysis dementia. Progressive encephalopathy seen in patients who have undergone long-term hemodialysis for end-stage renal disease.

Disequilibrium syndrome. A syndrome characterized by nausea, vomiting, headache, and disorientation, usually due to a rapid change in the metabolic milieu.

Marchiafava-Bignami disease. A nervous system disease sometimes found in chronic alcoholics characterized by degeneration of the corpus callosum.

Nonmetastatic effects of carcinoma. Central nervous system (CNS) dysfunction can result from carcinoma remote from the brain without frank metastases. The causes of nonmetastatic effects of carcinoma, characterized by *gliosis* and/or *demyelination* in the CNS, are not known, although possible factors include an autoimmune dysfunction elicited by tumor antigen, viral infection, and metabolic or endocrinologic problems.

Protein-calorie malnutrition (PCM) syndrome. Two overlapping syndromes of malnourishment in children (diagnoses are sometimes used with adults) are included as forms of PCM: *kwashiorkor syndrome* and *marasmus*. Kwashiorkor syndrome refers to the severe protein deficiency with edema and ascites and stunted growth found in poorly nourished children; marasmus refers to the severe cachexia with growth deficiencies in children with inadequate diets (and a history of early weaning or lack of breastfeeding). Children with PCM are frequently found to have mental retardation, possibly as a result of decreased myelination. Chapter 5 contains related discussions.

Pseudotumor cerebri, benign intracranial hypertension. Referring to a syndrome of presumed toxic or metabolic etiology, causing increased intracranial pressure with papilledema and headache.

Thyroid-related dysfunction. Referring to the range of neurologic complications associated with hypo- and hyperthyroidism and hypo- and hyperparathyroidism, including weakness, seizures, mental status changes, paresthesia, and other neurologic problems.

Uremic encephalopathy. Encephalopathy associated with renal failure, characterized by asterixis, seizures, decreased alertness, and apathy and, in the later stages, hallucinations, and agitation.

Uremic neuropathy. The peripheral sensorineural deficits seen in association with renal disease include autonomic disturbances and motor disturbances (e.g., "restless legs syndrome").

Vitamin B_{12} deficiency. Patients with pernicious anemia as a result of vitamin B_{12} deficiency have a number of neurologic manifestations, including irritability, apathy, somnolence, progressive weakness, paresthesias, "pins and needles" tingling, and sensory losses, including visual deficits.

Wernicke's encephalopathy. Wernicke's encephalopathy is thought to be due to a thiamine (B_1) deficiency causing pathologic changes in the periaqueductal gray matter, including petechial hemorrhages, degeneration of neurons, and astrocyte formation. The classic syndrome includes ophthalmoplegia, ataxia, and dementia. If there is recent memory loss, poor retention of new information, and **confabulation** (**Korsakoff's amnestic syndrome**, or psychosis), the patient is diagnosed to have **Wernicke-Korsakoff syndrome**. (See alcohol-related dementia, discussed in Chapter 4.)

Whipple's disease. A disease thought to be the result of a bacterial infection involving the CNS, causing inflammation of the hypothalamus, thalamus, and mammillary bodies. Whipple's disease may be found in patients with HIV.

G. Cerebrovascular Disease and Cerebral and Brain Stem Syndromes

Brain stem syndromes are also discussed elsewhere in this chapter.

Aneurysms. Aneurysms of blood vessels usually occur at the bifurcations, presumably due to developmental defects. "Berry," or saccular, aneurysms are small blisters protruding from the artery walls. Giant aneurysms are defects large enough to cause pressure on surrounding structures.

Arteriovenous malformations (AVMs). Refer to abnormal blood vessel tangles in the cerebral arterial and venous systems.

Arvellis syndrome. A brain stem syndrome associated with malacia, hemorrhage, or tumor in the tegmentum of the medulla where the spinothalamic tract and pupillary fibers descend, resulting in an ipsilateral paralysis of the soft palate and larynx and contralateral hemianesthesia.

Atherosclerotic thrombotic strokes. Atherosclerosis is a vascular disorder caused by diseases affecting circulation as well as genetic factors and lifestyle factors. Risk factors include hypertension, diabetes, high (low-density lipoprotein [LDL]) blood cholesterol levels, smoking, and the extent of routine physical activity. **Atheromas**, which are small lipid deposits, form plaques along vessel linings that become fibrotic and calcified. These plaques can become ulcerated, leading to the formation of **mural thromboses**. Thromboses are blood clots made up of agglutinated platelets, white cells, and fibrin. **Atheroscleroic thrombotic strokes** are characterized by an abrupt onset of neurologic signs sometimes occurring in a *saltatory* (stepwise) manner over a period of several minutes, hours, or days.

Benedikt syndrome/paramedial midbrain syndrome. A brain stem syndrome associated with malacia, hemorrhage, or tumor in the area of the tegmentum, resulting in oculomotor palsy, cerebellar ataxia, contralateral intention tremor, and corticospinal tract signs.

Binswanger's disease, subcortical arteriosclerotic encephalopathy. Binswanger's disease, frequently listed as a cause for dementia, is associated with arteriosclerotic disease of the penetrating vessels of the cerebral hemispheres, causing multiple subcortical microinfarctions, particularly in the white matter.

Claude syndrome. A brain stem syndrome associated with vascular disease or tumors in the area of the brachium conjunctivum and red nucleus, resulting in oculomotor palsy, contralateral cerebral ataxia, and tremor.

Cranial arteritis. Temporal arteritis and giant cell arteritis are conditions characterized by severe focal headache and, if untreated, can result in blindness and multiple areas of focal neurologic damage. Giant cell arteritis refers to granulomatous microneuropathologic changes in artery walls. Arteritis is treated with corticosteroids.

Déjerine's syndrome, medial medullary syndrome. This syndrome, also called anterior spinal artery syndrome, is characterized by ipsilateral flaccid tongue weakness from

12th nerve involvement, contralateral hemiplegia from damage to the pyramidal tract, and contralateral loss of position and vibration resulting from damage to the medial lemniscus.

Embolic strokes. An embolic stroke occurs when a particle (air, fat, or thrombus) passes into a brain artery and occludes blood flow. Cerebrovascular diseases associated with embolic states are characterized by abrupt deficits that are at their peak at onset.

Foville's syndrome, inferior lateral pontine syndrome. A brain stem syndrome associated with malacia, hemorrhage, or tumor in the region of the anterior inferior cerebellar artery, causing an ipsilateral lower motor weakness (both upper and lower face are weak), loss of taste in the anterior two-thirds of the tongue, ipsilateral loss of pain and temperature sense over the face, ipsilateral loss of conjugate gaze, and an ipsilateral Horner's syndrome.

Hematologic disorders. A number of hematologic disorders are associated with cerebrovascular disease, including polycythemia, sickle cell disease, thrombotic thrombocytopenic purpura, thrombocytosis, and others.

Hemorrhages. There are several forms of intracranial hemorrhages, including hemorrhages occurring outside the brain's covering, called *extradural hemorrhage*; along the surface of the brain, called *subdural hemorrhage*; and within the substance of the brain, called *intracerebral hemorrhage*. Hematomas are "blood tumors," or hemorrhagic masses.

Hypertensive encephalopathy. Prolonged essential hypertension and hypertension secondary to other diseases can lead to multiple small hemorrhages (petechiae) and microinfarcts throughout the brain. Focal neurologic signs may be lacking unless a large vessel hemorrhage has occurred.

Jackson syndrome. A brain stem syndrome associated with malacia, hemorrhage, or tumor in the tegmentum of the medulla where the corticospinal tracts, spinothalamic tracts, and pupillary fibers descend, resulting in ipsilateral paralysis of the tongue, soft palate, and larynx, and contralateral hemianesthesia.

Lacunar syndrome. Refers to small cavities within the brain resulting when the small, penetrating branches of arteries are occluded. These lacunae usually are associated with focal neurologic damage. If a lacuna occurs in the internal capsule, then a pure motor hemiplegia or pure hemisensory loss may result. Lacunae in the pons may cause ataxic hemiparesis, characterized by the "dysarthria-clumsy hand syndrome."

Millard-Gubler syndrome, medial pontine syndrome. A brain stem syndrome associated with malacia, hemorrhage, or tumor located where the corticospinal tract passes through the base of the pons, resulting in facial and abducens palsies, a gaze palsy to the side of the lesion, a contralateral hemiparesis, and an ipsilateral loss of conjugate gaze.

Reduced cerebral perfusion. Refers to a general diminution in blood supply to the brain, usually the result of impairments in cardiac output or diseases involving the large vessels supplying the brain.

Reversible ischemic neurologic deficit (RIND). Ischemic events in which the neurologic deficits gradually resolve within a time frame of more than 24 hours up to 3 weeks postictus. Persistent neurologic deficits indicate a completed stroke.

Steal syndrome. Refers to disturbances in blood circulation that result in the diversion of (stealing) circulation away from one vessel into another, causing ischemia in the areas served by the vessel with diminished circulation.

Superior lateral pontine syndrome. Refers to a brain stem syndrome involving the superior cerebellar artery, producing ipsilateral intention tremor of the arm and leg due to infarction of the superior cerebellar peduncle, an **ipsilateral Horner's syndrome** caused by the loss of the descending sympathetic tract, and a contralateral loss of pain and temperature sense of the face and body due to destruction of the lateral spinothalamic end ventral ascending tract of the fifth cranial nerve.

Systemic lupus erythematosus (SLE). An autoimmune disease in which neuropathologic changes are associated with multiple strokes, resulting in multifocal neurologic signs and progressive dementia.

Transient ischemic attacks (TIAs). Episodes of temporary focal ischemia (reduced blood flow to neural tissues) with neurologic deficits lasting no longer than 24 hours. TIAs are considered to be "warning signs" or, more accurately, the first indication of an impending stroke and should prompt immediate medical attention.

Vertebral basilar artery insufficiency. Reduced blood flow in the vertebral basilar artery circulation results in deficits in the posterior areas of the brain, including visual deficits and neurologic signs indicative of brain stem and cerebellar ischemia.

Wallenberg's syndrome, lateral medullary syndrome. A brain stem syndrome associated with vascular (usually occlusive) disease of the posterior inferior cerebellar artery (PICA) in the lateral tegmentum of the medulla, resulting in an ipsilateral facial (CN VII), glossopharyngeal (CN IX), vagus (CN X), hypoglossal (CN XII), and spinal accessory (CN XI) involvement; Horner's syndrome; cerebellar ataxia; and a contralateral sensory loss for pain and temperature. Patients with a lateral medullary syndrome have ipsilateral laryngeal and pharyngeal paralysis (due to damage of the nucleus ambiguous) and a decreased gag response (due to infarction of the nucleus solitarius of the rootlets of CN IX).

Weber syndrome, medial midbrain syndrome. A brain stem syndrome associated with vascular causes or tumors at the base of the midbrain, resulting in an ipsilateral, complete oculomotor (CN III) palsy and contralateral hemiplegia with face and tongue involvement.

H. Degenerative Diseases

Many degenerative diseases are conditions that occur insidiously after a period of normal neurologic status. Some degenerative conditions are apparent during infancy or childhood and are considered hereditary. This section lists some of the more commonly encountered degenerative neurologic diseases, including selected hereditary diseases. Additional congenital diseases are listed later in this chapter. Additional degenerative diseases are found under "Extrapyramidal Disorders" in this chapter and elsewhere.

Amyotrophic lateral sclerosis (ALS), motor neuron disease. The cause of ALS is not known although a number of associated disorders and deficiencies have been reported (heavy metal intoxication, thyroid disorders, enzyme deficiencies, and metabolic disorders). ALS is associated with progressive degeneration of the motor neurons. The general forms of ALS are diagnosed depending on the primary area of motor destruction: *bulbar type, primary lateral sclerosis, progressive bulbar type, progressive muscular atrophy*, or a combined form.

Ataxia telangiectasia, Louis-Barr syndrome. See the discussion of congenital disorders in the next section.

Friedreich's ataxia. An autosomal recessive trait associated with progressive damage to the posterior columns, spinocerebellar tract, and corticospinal tract characterized by dysmetria, intention tremor, dysdiadochokinesia, and nystagmus. This condition typically emerges in adolescence or young adulthood. (Also see the discussion of "Ataxias" in this chapter.)

Frontotemporal dementia (FTD). Referring to a group of dementing diseases, including Pick's disease, frontotemporal lobar degeneration, progressive aphasia/primary progressive aphasia, and semantic dementia, that are commonly misdiagnosed as Alzheimer's disease (AD). Patients with FTD have a markedly different clinical course and set of behavioral manifestations from AD. Some of the early signs of FTD may be confused with psychiatric disorders. Early in the onset of FTD patients display a lack of inhibition and an array of inappropriate social behaviors. There may be repetitive or compulsive behaviors and changes in eating and personal hygiene. Of particular significance to the SLP is that these patients display difficulties with confrontational naming and progressively worsening word retrieval, reading, and writing disorders. Research has shown different areas of the brain to be associated with the different forms of FTD, principally the frontal lobes, anterior temporal lobes, and left perisylvian cortex.

Creutzfeldt-Jakob disease (CJD). A dementing disease presumably associated with a "slow virus," causing rapid progression of neuronal degeneration and astrocyte proliferation, termed *spongiform encephalopathy*, and characterized by a rapid onset of profound dementia.

Lewy body disease. A dementing condition sharing clinical features of parkinsonism and AD. Patients ultimately diagnosed with Lewy body disease initially will demonstrate visual hallucinations and psychotic delusions prior to showing evidence of Parkinson-like movement disorders, cognitive deficits, and fluctuations in autonomic regulation (with sleep disturbances). In postmortem pathologic assessment, these patients are found to have an abnormal aggregation of Lewy bodies in the CNS. Clinically, Lewy body disease can be confused with other disorders, such as AD or forms of what are now called **multiple system atrophy** (MSA), in which abnormal proteins accumulate in glia cells.

Olivopontinecerebellar degeneration (OPCD). A condition thought to be an autosomal dominant trait causing a metabolic dysfunction associated with progressive atrophic changes to the cerebellum characterized by ataxia, nystagmus, intention tremor, titubation of the head, and dysarthria.

Primary progressive dementias (PPD). The primary progressive dementias generally refer to AD, also called dementia of the Alzheimer's type (DAT) and senile dementia Alzheimer's type (SDAT); Pick's disease, and CJD, just discussed. The etiology of AD is not known, although there is speculation about abnormalities in the biosynthesis of neurotransmitters as well as viral, environmental, and genetic factors (see Chapter 6 for additional discussion). The appearance of senile plaques and neurofibrillary tangles (neuronal filament degeneration) and increased aluminum are reported in AD. In addition, aggregates of amyloid protein are found adjacent to and within cerebral blood vessels. Computerized tomography (CT) scans of patients with AD reveal ventricular enlargement with diffuse atrophy, depending on the advancement of the disease. CT scans of patients with Pick's disease reveal maximal atrophy in the frontal and temporal lobes.

Progressive supranuclear palsy (PSP), Steele-Richardson-Olszewski syndrome. A progressive disease associated with neuronal changes in the basal ganglia, cerebellum, locus ceruleus, substantia nigra, and brain stem and characterized by an initial loss in vertical and then horizontal gaze movements followed by the onset of a parkinsonian-like syndrome with dysarthria, dysphagia, and, occasionally, dystonias.

Shy-Drager syndrome. A syndrome with Parkinson-like features in combination with progressive autonomic neuronal degeneration associated with dry mouth, constipation, impotence, lightheadedness, and ataxia related to hypotension occurring with changes in posture. Currently, the preferred term for this condition is *multiple system atrophy (MSA)*. Other variants of MSA include **striatonigral degeneration** (where Parkinson-like features predominate) and sporadic *olivopontinecerebellar degeneration*, described earlier.

I. Hereditary, Teratogenic, and Other Congenital Disorders

This section lists syndromes and congenital conditions that have associated neurologic damage. Included in this list are conditions that have speech, language, hearing, and cognitive dysfunctions (mental retardation and developmental delays) as notable features of the syndrome complex. All of the teratogenic causes for *fetal dysmorphology* are not listed here, but it is recognized that exposure to drugs, alcohol, radiation, and infectious conditions (such as rubella and cytomegalovirus) will affect fetal development, depending on the embryologic timing and extent of the exposure. The basic principles of **Medical Genetics** are reviewed earlier in this text (also see Chapter 6), and a list of known teratogenic agents is provided there in Table 6–1. It is beyond the scope of this section and this text to list all of the hereditary conditions associated with profound mental retardation or the congenital disorders associated with hearing, speech, swallowing, and language impairment. These conditions are predominantly the autosomal recessive disorders that are characterized by inherited metabolic errors and enzyme deficiencies. Some of the more frequently encountered of these rare conditions are described here.

Alport syndrome. A hereditary condition (autosomal dominant or sex-linked) associated with nephritis and sensorineural hearing loss.

Anencephaly. An absence of the development of the forebrain and cranium.

Apert syndrome, acrocephalosyndactyly Type I. A congenital disorder thought to be the result of an autosomal dominant mutation and characterized by craniosynostosis, synostosis or syndactyly of the feet and hands, strabismus, midline hypoplasia, frontal bossing, speech impairment, and hearing loss.

Arnold-Chiari malformation (ACM). A condition often associated with fetal hydrocephalus in which there is an abnormal development of the cerebellum, skull, and upper cervical vertebra. In **Chiari Type I malformation**, there is a herniation of the cerebellum below the foramen magnum (see "Herniation").

Ataxia-telangiectasia. An autosomal recessive condition occurring relatively frequently in which there is a decrease in immunoglobulin (IgA); a progressive ataxia (dysarthria, grimacing, and choreoathetosis); and characteristic telangiectasias (dilatation of small capillaries forming a variety of angiomas) on the ears, neck, nose, cheeks, and wrists.

Ataxic static encephalopathy (ataxic cerebral palsy). A form of cerebral palsy (static encephalopathy) associated with congenital damage to the cerebellar motor system as a result of a vascular lesion or in association with cerebellar agenesis syndromes.

Athetotic, or extrapyramidal, static encephalopathy (athetotic cerebral palsy). A form of cerebral palsy characterized by choreoathetoid movements resulting from damage to the basal ganglia. Athetosis is a potentially unfortunate outcome from kernicterus deposits in the basal ganglia caused by high bilirubin levels postdelivery in Rh incompatibility.

Attention-deficit hyperactivity disorder (ADHD) or (hyperactivity) attention-deficit disorder (ADD-H). A symptom complex characterized by inattentiveness and specific learning disabilities. When ADD is present along with excessive physical activity, the term *attention-deficit disorder with hyperactivity* (ADHD or ADD-H) is applied. This symptom complex has been recognized by educators for many years; however, neuropathologic findings are notably inconsistent. Neurochemical disturbances, particularly for activities involving the reticular activating system's locus ceruleus, have been proposed. "Soft" neurologic signs are sometimes, but not invariably, present; a minority of ADHD/ADD-H children have abnormal electroencephalograms (EEGs).

Autism spectrum disorder (ASD), Aspergers. Autism is characterized by delayed speech and deviant language behavior (usually marked by high-pitched voice and echolalic utterances) and, in many cases, stereotypic behaviors and delayed pragmatic/social and mental development. Autistic children may exhibit ritualistic hand movements, self-injurious behaviors, and poor social skills, sometimes actively avoid contact with others. Research has suggested both environmental and genetic causal factors may be involved in autism. There is an exceptionally high incidence of autism in identical twins, and a gene generally associated with cancer appears more frequently in families who have more than one family member affected.

Cerebellar agenesis or dysgenesis. A lack of development of the cerebellum, resulting in cerebellar ataxic movement disorders.

Complex plegia, mixed cerebral palsy. A form of static encephalopathy (cerebral palsy) in which more than one motor system is involved (extrapyramidal, pyramidal, or cerebellar).

Congenital nystagmus. An inherited autosomal dominant or sex-linked condition in which nystagmus is present at birth.

Congenital seizure disorders. Referring to seizure disorders that are associated with certain chromosomal abnormalities, such as trisomy D, or disorders that accompany inherited metabolic disturbances, including hereditary hypoglycemias and inherited degenerative disorders such as Sturge-Weber disease, tuberous sclerosis, aminoacidurias, and leukodystrophies.

Craniocleidodysostosis. A rare condition in which there is a failure in the development of the membranous bones of the face and, usually, an associated mental retardation and a seizure disorder.

Dandy-Walker syndrome. A condition in which there is a malformation of the roof of the fourth ventricle, potentially causing hydrocephalus, and a lack of development of the cerebellum.

Diastematolomyelia. A rare condition in which there is a duplication of the spinal cord.

Down syndrome, trisomy 21. A chromosomal abnormality characterized by varied degrees of developmental delays and *mental retardation, hypotonicity, epicanthal* *folds, Brushfield spots in the iris, upslanted palpebral* (eyelid) *fissures, flat facial profile, brachycephaly, hyperextended joints, Simean crease of the palm, protruded tongue, small auricles, cardiac malformations*, and *duodenal atresia*, along with other gastrointestinal problems (see Chapter 5). The degree of mental retardation and dysmorphology may be less in the 1% to 2% of cases of **Down syndrome mosaics**, or incomplete expressions of the chromosomal abnormality (see Chapter 6 for further discussion).

Duane's syndrome. A congenital oculomotor disorder in which abductor movements are limited or lacking.

Duchenne's muscular dystrophy. An inherited, sex-linked, recessive disorder almost exclusively found in young males due to an inborn error of metabolism, resulting in failure of dystrophic synthesis and causing an excessive collagen formation. Duchenne's muscular dystrophy eventually leads to contractures, muscle wasting, and deformities.

Fetal alcohol syndrome (FAS). A condition found in the offspring of alcoholic mothers where the teratogen alcohol causes characteristic dysmorphology of the eyes, head, and face and alters the child's cognitive development (see Chapter 6 for additional discussion of teratogenic agents).

Fetal cytomegalovirus (CMV) syndrome. A condition associated with fetal exposure to CMV, a form of the herpes virus (HCMV) or **human herpesvirus 5** (HHV-5), resulting in congenital *neurologic damage, microencephaly, obstructive hydrocephalus, chorioretinitis*, and *profound bilateral sensorineural hearing impairment* (see Chapter 8). As with other **teratogenic agents**, the range and degree of fetal damage varies, depending on the time of exposure during development (see Chapter 6 for additional discussion of teratogenic agents).

Fragile X syndrome. A sex-linked hereditary condition (thus, more often found in males than females) characterized by mental retardation, large ears, macroorchidism, a prominent jaw, an asymmetric face, delayed speech and motor development, and, in some cases, autism (also see Chapter 6).

Hypertelorism. A condition characterized by a greater than normal distance between the orbits resulting from a disproportionately larger growth of the lesser wings of the splenoid compared to the greater wings of the splenoid. This condition is frequently, but not invariably, associated with mental retardation.

Klippel-Fiel syndrome. A condition in which there are cervical vertebral fusion(s) in association with other congenital abnormalities.

Laurence-Moon-Biedl syndrome. An autosomal recessive condition characterized by polydactyly, hypogonadism, obesity, retinitis pigmentosa, and mental retardation.

Lysosomal storage diseases. Referring to a group of genetic diseases in which storage of certain metabolites occurs within lysosomes due to a specific enzyme deficiency. Lysosomal storage diseases include *Niemann-Pick disease, Krabbe's disease, Fabry's disease, Gaucher's disease* (adult and child form), *Hurler-Scheie disease, Wolman's disease, mucopolysaccharidoses, Sanfilippo's syndrome, Marateaux-Lamy syndrome*, and other disorders.

Macroencephaly. An enlarged cranium usually associated with hydrocephalus or bony growth abnormalities, such as *osteogenesis imperfecta*.

Maple syrup urine disease and its variants. Conditions associated with autosomal recessive traits that have resulted in inborn metabolic errors in amino acid catabolism, often leading to seizures. With some of these conditions, restrictive diets allow normal neurologic development (see Chapter 5).

Microencephaly, microcephaly. Abnormally small cranium. A number of genetically linked conditions are associated with microencephaly, or microcephaly, as are intrauterine infections (including rubella, CMV, encephalitis and meningitis, and trauma).

Moebius syndrome. A congenital condition of heterogeneous etiology characterized by facial diplegia (weakness of the facial muscles) and bilateral inability to abduct the eyes.

Neural tube defects. Defects that result from incomplete closure of the neural tube during embryonic development. Such disorders include *anencephaly, spina bifida*, and certain forms of hydrocephalus. In spina bifida, there is a failure in the closure of the vertebral laminae, which could result in a *spinal meningocele*, or **myelomeningocele**. A fissure of the spinal column is sometimes referred to as a **rachischisis**.

Neurofibromatosis. An autosomal dominant disorder characterized by abnormal pigmentation (café au lait spots), freckling in the axilla, neurofibromas (dysplastic tumors), and, in some cases, acoustic neuromas.

Pendred syndrome. A congenital condition characterized by sensorineural hearing loss and goiter.

Peroneal muscular atrophy, Charcot-Marie-Tooth syndrome. An inherited condition in which there are chronic, symmetrical neuropathies with demyelination and neuronal loss of the anterior horn cells.

Phenylketonuria (PKU). Variants of an autosomal recessive disorder in which there is a fundamental biochemical deficiency of the hepatic enzyme phenylalanine hydroxylase. Early institution of low phenylalanine diets will, in the majority of cases, avert neurologic damage (see Chapters 5 and 6 for further discussion).

Pigmentary degeneration of the retina. Degeneration of the retina may occur as a feature of *Lawrence-Moon-Biedl syndrome, Refsum's disease*, and *Kearn-Sayre syndrome* (sometimes called **homocarcinosis**).

Prader-Willi syndrome. An inherited condition characterized by *hypotonicity, obesity, small hands and feet, almond-shaped palpebral* (eyelid) *fissures, hypogonadism, delayed speech development*, and *mental retardation* (see Chapter 6 for further discussion).

Refsum syndrome, phytanic acid storage disease. An autosomal recessive condition characterized by polyneuropathies, cerebellar ataxia, sensorineural hearing loss, retinitis pigmentosa, and chronic polyneuritis.

Rubella syndrome, congenital rubella, Gregg syndrome. A condition characterized by congenital heart defects, patent ductus arteriosus (see Chapter 9), hearing impairment, microcephaly, and central nervous system damage.

Sacrococcygeal dystrophy. A condition in which there is a defect in the development of the sacrum and coccyx along with other spinal abnormalities.

Spasmus nutans. This relatively rare condition is characterized by a *nystagmus* often accompanied by head bobbing or head tilting. Spontaneous resolution within a year of onset is common.

Spastic (pyramidal) diplegia, or quadriplegia, spastic cerebral palsy. A form of cerebral palsy (static encephalopathy) associated with bilateral damage to the corticobulbar or corticospinal tracts.

Spastic (pyramidal) hemiplegia. A form of cerebral palsy (static encephalopathy) resulting from unilateral damage to the motor cortex.

Tay-Sachs disease. An autosomal recessive disease mainly found in the offspring of Jewish parents of eastern European descent, associated with a basic enzymatic deficiency for *hexosaminidase A*. This metabolic deficiency leads to an accumulation of gangliosides, causing pervasive nervous system damage.

J. Cranial Nerve, Lower Motor Neuron Disorders, Neuromuscular Disorders, and Peripheral Neuropathies

Carpal tunnel syndrome. Pain, numbness, and paresthesia of the hand due to pressure on the median nerve in the wrist.

Cerebellopontine angle (CPA) tumors. Acoustic neuromas or meningiomas affecting the vestibulocochlear (CN VIII), facial (CN VII), and trigeminal (CN V) nerves or tracts, located at the cerebellopontine juncture.

Cranial nerve neuropathies. Cranial nerves may be damaged focally as a result of ischemic lesions, hemorrhage, neuromas, trauma, focal infections, and some viral inflammations that are prone to involve bulbar nerves. Bulbar palsy syndromes and multiple cranial nerve palsies refer to conditions where multiple nerves are affected. A number of specific brain stem syndromes and cranial nerve syndromes (several are listed separately in this section) result from medullary and pontine tumors, ischemia, or hemorrhages (discussed later in this chapter). Moreover, some viruses have a proclivity for damage to particular cranial nerves.

Neuropathies of cranial nerves III, IV, and VI cause *oculomotor palsies*, such at that found in Moebius syndrome (see earlier). *Trigeminal neuralgia*, or **tic douloureux**, is characterized by severe lancinating (stabbing) pain in the distribution of the trigeminal (CN V) nerve. Carbamazepine treatment has been used with some success. **Bell's palsy**, or seventh (facial) nerve palsy, is characterized by unilateral upper and lower facial paralysis resulting from a viral infection involving the geniculate ganglion. *Ageusia*, a loss of taste, is sometimes found in association with Bell's palsy. **Geniculate neuralgia** is associated with severe, spasmodic pain in the region of the external auditory canal and ear. **Facial myokymia** is a condition seen in some cases of multiple sclerosis, brain stem gliomas, and Guillain-Barré syndrome, in which fine, irregular contractions are observed on one or both sides of the face.

Neuropathies of the vestibulocochlear (CN VIII) nerve can result from the toxic effects of drugs, especially some of the "mycin," or "aminoglycoside," varieties. Streptomycin and gentamicin can affect the vestibular branch of the eighth nerve, and drugs such as vancomycin, neomycin, and streptomycin are known to have toxic effects on the auditory branch of the eighth nerve. Balance testing, magnetic resonance imaging (MRI), and brain stem auditory evoked response (BAER) (see Chapter 4) are used to diagnose the site of lesion with eighth nerve dysfunction. **Acoustic neuromas** are tumors of the *auditory branch* of the eighth nerve. A benign tumor on the *vestibular branch* of the eighth nerve is diagnosed as a Schwannoma, or a form of neurolemmoma/neurilemmoma. A tumor or aneurysm in this area may cause damage to or disruption of the seventh and eighth nerve functions and is referred to as a "*space-occupying lesion*" at the cerebellopontine angle area.

Glossopharyngeal nerve (CN IX) neuralgia is rarely described, except in association with vagus (CN X) and accessory (CN XI) nerve involvement. It usually results from ischemia or tumors located at the posterior fossa. Tumors and aneurysms in the posterior fossa may be referred to as **Vernet syndrome**.

Diphtheria. Neuropathy of the palatal musculature, dyspnea, aphonia, and dysphagia may be associated with diphtheria, an infectious disease and inflammatory toxicosis occurring in the presence of *Corynebacterium diphtheriae.*

Foix syndrome. Cranial nerve syndrome associated with sphenoid bone tumors, affecting the abducens (CN VI), trigeminal (CN V), trochlear (CN IV), and oculomotor (CN III) nerves.

Gradenigo syndrome. Cranial nerve syndrome associated with tumors of the petrous bone, affecting the trigeminal (CN V) and abducens (CN VI) nerves.

Guillain-Barré syndrome, postinfectious polyneuritis. Guillain-Barré syndrome is an ascending polyneuritis (with weakness progressing from the legs up to the bulbar muscles), occurring shortly (1–8 weeks) following a viral infection. When bulbar muscles become involved, patients become dysarthric, progressing to complete anarthria and an inability to eat by mouth. Guillain-Barré syndrome is thought to be due to lymphocytic sensitivity to peripheral nerve antigens that cause inflammation and demyelination of the peripheral nerves. (See Chapter 11 for additional discussion.)

Herpes zoster (shingles). Herpes zoster is a systemic illness involving the *varicella virus.* The viral activity is located predominantly in the sensory ganglia of the cranial nerves and spinal cord.

Jacod syndrome. Cranial nerve syndrome associated with tumors of the middle cranial fossa, affecting the optic (CN II), oculomotor (CN III), trochlear (CN IV), trigeminal (CN V), and abducens (CN VI) nerves.

Laryngeal neuralgia, which is associated with inflammation of the superior branch of the vagus (CN X) nerve, is characterized by lancinating pain on the side of the neck. Tumors, hematomas, or ischemic damage near the *jugular foremen* can cause ipsilateral damage to the areas innervated by the vagus (CN X), spinal accessory (CN XI), and hypoglossal (CN XII) nerves. Retroparotid space tumors may be referred to as **Villaret syndrome**, **MacKenzie syndrome**, or **Tapia syndrome**. Tumors of the posterior lateral condylar spaces are usually referred to as **Collet-Sicard syndrome**.

Mononeuropathy. Dysfunction of one peripheral nerve; a condition that can occur following trauma, infarction of peripheral nerves, or in association with diabetes mellitus.

Myasthenia gravis (MG). A mostly bulbar neuromuscular junction dysfunction characterized by a progressive weakening with exertion (also see Chapters 4 and 11). Patients with MG will display a lower motor neuron (flaccid) type of dysarthria that will improve along with other motor functions when treated with tensilon.

Nutritional neuropathies. Peripheral neuropathies are found with a number of nutritional deficiencies, including thiamin neuropathy (beriberi), caused by a chronic lack of vitamin B_1, and sometimes seen in vegetarians and alcoholics. (See Chapter 4; and see "Toxic, Nutritional, and Metabolic Disorders" in this chapter.)

Oculopharyngeal dystrophy. An inherited autosomal dominant trait that presents late in life (between age 40 and 50), characterized by a slowly progressive ptosis; dysphagia; and hoarse, weak phonation.

Parinaud syndrome. A brain stem syndrome associated with hydrocephalus, **pinealoma** (tumor of the pineal gland), or other lesions of the dorsal midbrain in the area of the periaqueductal gray matter, resulting in an upward gaze paralysis and fixed pupils.

Plexitis. Inflammation of a nerve plexus.

Poliomyelitis. An acute, viral infection characterized by headache, stiff neck, vomiting, and sore throat, which, in the major form, may result in CNS damage with atrophy of a muscle group (bulbar and/or spinal neurons may be affected).

Polyradiculitis. Inflammation of several nerve roots.

Restless legs syndrome. A condition with symptoms that include leg discomfort and prickling or burning dysesthesias. The cause is unknown in many cases, but in some patients it may be related with peripheral neuropathies.

Stiff-man syndrome. A syndrome of motor neuron dysfunction characterized by persistent muscle cramping, stiffness, and spasm that are relieved during sleep.

Viral or bacterial myositis. Inflammatory, neuromuscular disorder caused by infectious agents and resulting in weakness and tenderness.

K. Demyelinating Diseases

Acute disseminated encephalomyelitis. Referring to a group of allied demyelinating disorders, including postinfectious, postexantrem, and postvaccinal encephalomyelitis and acute perivascular myelinoclasis.

Acute necrotizing hemorrhagic encephalomyelitis. A condition almost invariably associated with a respiratory infection and characterized by abrupt onset of a fulminant variant of demyelinative disease.

Central demyelination of the corpus callosum, Marchiafava-Bignami disease. A condition almost exclusively found in chronic alcoholics and associated with central demyelination (revealed by MRI).

Central pontine myelinolysis (CPM). A loss of the myelin sheath covering nerve fibers in the pons usually due to a rapid, drastic change in sodium levels in the body when patients (usually alcoholics or women during childbearing age) are being treated for *hyponatremia* (low levels of sodium), causing sodium levels to rise too fast, or when there are high levels of sodium in the body, called *hypernatremia*, that are corrected too quickly (see Chapter 4). Patients with CPM are likely to have dysarthria, dysphagia, double vision, weakness, and movement disorders. If the lesion in the basis pontis is large, patients may have "*locked in syndrome*."

Multiple sclerosis (MS). A disease of unknown cause associated with a periodic autoimmune response directed at the oligodendrocytes and creating irregular patches of demyelination. MS is characterized by "waxing and waning" neurologic deficits. Restoration of myelin can occur, with a corresponding functional improvement, or the formation of gliosis can occur, leaving scars and destruction of white matter tracts (axons).

Progressive multifocal leukoencephalopathy (PML), Schilder's disease. A relatively rare demyelinating disease in which dementia is a prominent feature. PML is usually associated with an underlying malignancy, most often lymphoma.

L. Disorders Related to Mental Status

A review of the mental status examination and standardized instruments is found in Chapter 4; functional status assessments used in geriatrics and rehabilitation medicine are discussed in Chapter 14.

Acute confusional states. Referring to an inability to think with the normal degree of clarity, coherence, and speed. Confusional states in the intensive care unit (ICU) or following head injury may be rated with specific scales (see Chapters 4 and 11). Acute confusion reflects diffuse cortical dysfunction and can occur as a stage in the evolution of a number of metabolic disorders and CNS diseases or dysfunction, and stages can include descriptors such as *inattentive, confused, drowsy, somnolent*, and *stuporous.*

Amnestic states and syndromes. Impairments in memory may be present as a feature of **delirium** (as a result of faulty perceptions of the environment); **dementia** (related to damaged cognitive processes for interpreting, retrieving, or encoding information); or as a feature of specific amnestic states or an amnestic syndrome (Korsakoff's amnestic syndrome). **Korsakoff's amnestic syndrome** is diagnosed in the patient who is alert and responding appropriately to others but has a notable *anterograde* amnesia (impairment in learning new information) despite relatively intact immediate and remote, or *retrograde*, memory. Some patients with Korsakoff's psychosis are found to *confabulate*, which may be a compensation for faulty recollection of recent events (see Chapter 4).

Another amnestic disorder, **transient global amnesia**, is characterized by a period of confusion and bewilderment lasting for a few hours during which the patient is alert and shows no notable impairment in consciousness or lack of awareness of the environment.

Amnestic states are also found in association with bilateral hippocampal infarctions, infarctions of the basal forebrain, trauma, hypoxic states, herpes simplex encephalitis, spontaneous subarachnoid hemorrhage, and tumors involving the base and walls of the third ventricle and limbic system.

Coma. See Chapter 4.

Delirium. Sometimes referred to as a "*clouded sensorium*," in which patients may misinterpret their environment, experience hallucinations, and verbalize in an incoherent, nonsensical manner (see Chapter 4 and Chapter 11 for additional discussion of delirium).

Dementia. Dementia is a behavioral diagnosis indicative of a generalized intellectual deficit. Dementia is not a disease per se, rather it is a sign of pathology. Dementia may be irreversible or reversible; thus, the underlying cause needs to be diagnosed. Dementia can result from structural lesions, diffuse inflammatory processes, metabolic disturbances, progressive CNS diseases, chronic intoxications from drugs and/or alcohol, and as a related feature of psychiatric disorders (hysteria, hypomania, schizophrenia, or depression). (See "Degenerative Diseases," discussed earlier.)

Persistent vegetative state. A stabilized condition of incomplete recovery from coma in which responsiveness is limited to postural and reflexive movements of the extremities and eyes.

Pseudocoma. Refers to a neurologic state caused by lesions in the basis pontis, sparing somatosensory pathways and ascending neuronal pathways for arousal and wakefulness while interfering with corticobulbar and corticospinal pathways. Thus, the patient is motionless but fully awake and aware. This syndrome has been referred to as "locked in syndrome," coma vigil, or a de-efferented state.

M. Neurologic Tumors

Arachnoid cysts. Encapsulated cysts containing CSF in the arachnoid space.

Astrocytoma, Grade 1, 2. The most common form of brain neoplasms in children, these grades of astrocytomas are slow-growing tumors arising from the astrocytes. Cerebellar and pontine astrocytomes are the most common of the posterior fossa tumors. In adults astrocytomas are usually diagnosed in the third and fourth decades of life and are found more frequently in the frontal lobes than elsewhere. Once diagnosed, treatment may involve only excision or radiation, including brachytherapy (the temporary implantation of high-energy radiation) or combined radiation-chemotherapy (see Chapter 7).

Cerebellar astrocytoma. Histologically benign, slow-growing, cystic infratentorial tumors arising from astrocytes.

Chordoma. A congenital neoplasm arising from notochordal tissue in embryologic development.

Choroid plexus papilloma. A low-grade neoplasm arising from the choroid plexus and causing overproduction of CSF. Complete excision and reversal of the hydrocephalus is usually possible.

Craniopharyngioma. A benign tumor of congenital origin occurring in the suprasellar region potentially with extension into the hypothalamus, third ventricle, optic chasm, and circle of Willis, making total surgical removal of the mass difficult to achieve.

Ependymoma. Neoplasms arising from the ependymal lining of the ventricles, posterior fossa, or spinal cord; treated by surgical resection and radiation therapy.

Glioblastoma multiforme; astrocytoma Grade 3, 4; spongioblastoma multiforme. A malignant, invasive, and rapidly progressing neoplasm occurring most often in the fifth decade of life. Treatment may include surgical decompression and Decadron to reduce cerebral edema and chemotherapy.

Medulloblastoma. Highly malignant tumors more commonly found in children and usually developing in the *cerebellar vermis*. These tumors tend to "seed," leading to recurrence.

Meningioma. Benign, slow-growing tumors arising from the meninges; treated by surgical excision followed by radiation if complete excision is not possible.

Metastatic neoplasms. Tumors arising from distant extracranial neoplasms, usually through the arterial or lymphatic system.

Neurolemmomas/neurilemmomas. Slow-growing, benign tumors originating in the Schwann cells. These tumors may be found on any peripheral nerve but are most commonly found on the vestibular branch of the eighth cranial nerve; however, physicians sometimes refer to any benign eighth nerve, Schwann cell tumor as an *acoustic neuroma.*

Neuroblastomas. Tumors usually arising in the cerebral hemispheres and most often in the medial temporal lobes of children.

Neurofibromatosis, von Recklinghausen's disease. Condition characterized by multiple neurofibromas and cutaneous dark spots or patches (*café au lait* spots).

Oligodendroglioma. A slow-growing form of glioma arising from oligodendrocytes treated by surgical excision and radiation therapy.

Pineal region tumors. Tumors in the pineal region, or pinealomas, most frequently diagnosed in children (10–20 years of age).

N. Head Trauma

Axonal injury. An axonal shear, or diffuse axonal injury, occurs when rotational forces are associated with brain impact, causing stretching and tearing of the gray and white matter interfaces.

Basal fractures and CSF fistulae. Basal skull fractures refer to injuries to one or more of the five bones that make up the base of the skull, including the *orbital portion of the frontal bone, sphenoid bone, petrous squamous portion of the temporal bone, cribiform plate*, and *ethmoid bone.* A severe fracture of the brain's bony casing could cause a CSF fistula with drainage into the sinuses.

Cerebral contusion. Contusions range from small, largely reversible injuries, sometimes called a "cortical bruise," to a major brain lesion involving multiple cortical and subcortical areas. Contusions are the common post-traumatic brain lesion, consisting of varying amounts of necrosis, edema, and hemorrhage. Contusions are typically present at the site of primary injury and distant in the classic *contre coup* location; thus, most contusions are found in the frontal and temporal lobes.

Epidural, extradural hemorrhage. A collection of blood between the bony skull (or spine) and the dura is relatively rare and may reabsorb; consequently, epidural hemorrhages are not usually treated surgically unless they enlarge rapidly and/or cause compression on the brain.

Extracerebral subdural hematoma (SDH). A collection of blood within layers of the dura. *Acute subdural hematomas* may occur from a spontaneous rupture with an **arteriovenous malformation (AVM)**. Patients with an *acute SDH* usually have an underlying brain contusion. A subacute SDH is an injury that becomes evident or occurs several days (3–20) following a head injury. A *chronic SDH* is one that is present after more than 20 days. Chronic SDHs are occasionally found in the elderly during CT scanning when an SDH has gone clinically unrecognized at the time the injury occurred.

Herniation. Displacement of brain tissue through or across structural or dura openings or through a fracture or surgical craniotomy site (a **transcalvarial** or **external herniation**). **Uncal herniations** are the result of lesions of the temporal lobe in which its medial portion is forced medially and downward into the ipsilateral tentorial hiatus and the brain stem is then displaced contralaterally, resulting in an ipsilateral compression of CN

III. (Refer to Chapter 4.) **Central herniation** occurs when the brain is squeezed through a notch in the tentorium. **Tonsillar herniation (Chiari Type I Malformation)** occurs when the tonsils of the cerebellum are compressed through the foramen magnum. **Cingulate herniation** occurs when one hemisphere swells and its medial side is forced under the dura mater at the falx cerebri. Herniations are usually described as either *supratenorial* or *infratentorial* (above or below the dura "tent" separating the occipital lobes of the cerebrum and cerebellum at the brain stem).

Infarction from artery injuries. Injuries that cause compression on the major vessels of the brain can result in cerebral infarction, or tissue death. The regions affected depend on the vessels involved and their distribution. If the blood supply from the carotid artery, for example, is temporally diminished, upstream cortical damage may occur in the "watershed" areas of the parietal lobes (the border areas where the posterior and middle cerebral circulation overlap); in pericallosal regions; middle cerebral artery regions; or the occipital lobes. Injuries to the blood vessels following trauma can also produce "pseudoaneurysms," that require surgical correction.

Intracerebral hematomas. Well-defined hemorrhages within the brain parenchyma, usually located in white matter and typically the result of a rupture of a major perforating artery following a rapid acceleration and deceleration of the head.

Intracranial pressure and brain swelling. The balance and flow of CSF is intricately managed by fluid dynamic mechanisms within the cisterns, ventricles, and vascular system of the brain. Intracranial pressure is normally below a mean of 15 mmHg. Following brain trauma, these systems can be overwhelmed and disturbed, causing fluid accumulations and swelling within the substances of the brain itself. Increases in intracranial pressure can interfere with the mechanisms that allow intracranial blood flow; ultimately, brain death will occur. Swelling of the brain can occur with any type of head injury and can be difficult to control. On CT scans, the cisterns, ventricles, and cortical sulci will be diminished, and correction is initiated to avoid brain herniation and death. See Figure 11–1 for an illustration of intracranial monitoring in the ICU.

Subarachnoid hemorrhage (SAH). Small perforating vessel ruptures can cause hemorrhages to collect under the arachnoid covering of the brain and result in increased intracranial pressure.

Subdural hydroma. Collection of CSF in the subdural space can occur after trauma or rapid decompression of a ventricular system following shunting.

O. Brain Infections

Brain abscess. An encapsulated collection of pus in the brain.

Cerebritis. A regional infection and inflammation of brain tissue without necrosis (tissue death).

Encephalitis. Inflammation of the brain tissues, usually due to infection.

Meningitis. An inflammation of the meninges (arachnoid and pia) or CSF, usually due to infection.

Metastatic brain abscess. Chronic infections of the lungs or pleura, or dental infections can enter the bloodstream and be transferred to the brain.

Pyogenic infections. Pus-forming bacterial infections of the CSF.

Septic embolism. Sepsis refers to an infection within the blood. A thromboembolism can be transferred to the brain in conditions such as subacute bacterial endocarditis (SBE) and an infection or abscess in the brain may occur.

HIV-related infections. Neurologic complications with the human immunodeficiency virus (HIV) are often associated with various viral and bacterial infections. HIV is associated with subacute encephalitis, CMV, herpes simplex encephalitis, progressive multifocal leukoencephalopathy, and varicella-zoster encephalitis (see Chapter 8 for more detailed discussion).

III. PSYCHIATRIC DISORDERS

A. Psychiatric Classification and Diagnoses

1. DSM-IV Categories

Psychiatric diagnoses are based in large part on observations and reports of the patient's behavior. Thus, to achieve consistency in classification, the *Diagnostic and Statistical Manual of Mental Disorders* was published by the American Psychiatric Association in 1980 (see Chapter 4). This work was predicated on the *DSM-I* manual published in 1954 with revisions in 1968 and 1974. Its third edition was referred to as the *DSM-III-R (revised)*. The fourth version, *DSM-IV* (1995) is currently undergoing revision. The *DSM-IV* codes guide the categorization of psychiatric disorders in a manner compatible with the International Classification of Disease (ICD-9) codes. The *ICD-9* will soon be replaced with the *ICD-10* (see Chapter 2). Diagnoses using the *DSM-IV* diagnostic categories should be made only by professionals with extensive clinical experience and knowledge about psychiatric conditions and the *DSM-IV* categories and "decision trees" (e.g., psychiatrists, psychiatric social workers, psychiatric nurse practitioners). (Refer to Chapter 4.)

2. Psychoses and Neuroses

Descriptions of psychiatric disorders and conditions may be encountered in a patient's medical history, psychiatric consultation summaries, or elsewhere. Most, but not all, of these diagnoses are classified by *DSM-IV*. It is not unusual to find inaccurate and indiscriminate use of psychiatric labels in medical records. SLPs should avoid making psychiatric diagnoses and if a psychiatric diagnosis is included in Speech-Language Pathology reports, the date and source of that diagnosis should be stated. For example, "Patient was diagnosed to have a post-traumatic stress disorder by his attending psychiatrist (state name) during a Psychiatric admission at this Medical Center in August (specify exact date or year)."

Descriptions of psychiatric disorders, sometimes referred to as *organic* psychiatric conditions, are *personality disorders, neurotic disorders*, and *psychotic disorders*. These terms do not refer to exclusive categories of psychiatric problems. **Depression**, for example, may be discussed as a result of, or a response to, organic cerebral disease or as a preexisting disorder. Further, some individuals might be described as having a "depressive personality type," whereas others might be said to have a "neurotic depression." The psychiatrist and psychologist will apply the *DSM-IV* codes by using multiple axes to describe the emotional disorder, any related disorders, the etiology(ies) (including codes to indicate if the cause cannot be specified), related life stressors, and the level of functioning.

In psychiatry, it is generally felt that certain personality types are predictive of, or associated with, particular neurotic disorders and particular psychotic disorders. For example, an individual with an *obsessive-compulsive personality type* might also be said to have a related *major depressive episode.*

Neurotic disorders are usually discussed as either anxiety disorders (including phobias, panic states, etc.) or **somatiform disorders** (including hypochondriasis, hysterias, etc.). **Psychoses** can include conditions such as *schizophrenia, paranoia*, and *affective disorders with psychotic features* (manic-depressive disorder or bipolar states and major depressive syndrome). Psychiatrists may refer to *confusional-delirious states* and certain behaviors associated with focal and multifocal cerebral lesions (i.e., organically caused delusions, hallucinations, or major mood disorders) as types of psychoses. Several of the psychiatric labels and therapies encountered in medical reports are listed in the next section.

B. Psychiatric Terminology for Personality Disorders

Antisocial behavior. Referring to behaviors characterized by poor interpersonal relationships, frequent conflicts with others, impulsiveness, selfishness, low frustration tolerance, and tendencies to blame others.

Asthenic disorder. Referring to behaviors that indicate easy fatigability and chronic weakness.

Cyclothymic personality. Referring to personality characteristics that include periods of high energy, ambition, and optimism followed by periods of hopelessness, pessimism, and despair. When mood swings are extreme, ranging from severe depression to mania, a **bipolar disorder** may be diagnosed.

Dependent personality. Referring to personality characteristics that suggest excessive dependence on others, a lack of self-confidence, and a tendency to seek approval from others.

Explosive personality. Referring to individuals who display sudden outbursts of aggressive behavior usually followed by regret.

Histrionic personality. Referring to individuals with tendencies to be overly dramatic and displaying immaturity and dependency and engaging in sexualized relationships.

Immature personality. Referring to individuals with poor adaptation to social, psychological, and physical stressors.

Inadequate personality. Referring to individuals with a tendency toward dependency (on others or institutions) and with an inability to address the demands of everyday living.

Obsessive-compulsive personality. Referring to individuals who are overly meticulous, perfectionistic, and concerned about standards (as applied to themselves and others).

Paranoid personality. Referring to individuals with tendencies to be suspicious and wary of others and who display hypersensitivity and envy and have a heightened sense of self-importance.

Passive-aggressive personality. Referring to individuals who display obstructive and stubborn behaviors, particularly in response to authority.

Schizoid personality. Referring to individuals who are reclusive, secretive, and detached from others and who may demonstrate an inability to express feelings and ideas.

C. Psychiatric Terminology for Neurotic Disorders

Anxiety disorders. The term *anxiety* usually refers to a feeling of fearfulness and distress or panic in response to stress. Anxiety disorders include panic attacks and may be a related feature of phobias. Anxiety, or panic, states generally begin with a feeling of foreboding or a sense of unreality followed by autonomic disturbances, including palpitation, difficulty breathing, and diaphoresis (sweating).

Hypochondriasis. Hypochondriasis refers to an excessive preoccupation with health and an exaggerated concern for imagined illness(es). Hypochondriasis can be found in association with other psychiatric conditions; thus, psychiatrists might examine for conditions such as depression when treating hypochondriasis.

Hysterias. Hysterias include *conversion reactions* (in which there may be nonphysical symptoms of blindness, mutism, amnesia, weakness, etc.) and *hysterical neuroses. Briquet's disease* is a term used to refer to hysteria in females. Hysteria in males is sometimes termed *compensation neurosis*. Hysteria is typically polysymptomatic and can include hysterical pain, vomiting, seizures, paralysis, tremors, and amnesia. A condition called **globus hystericus** refers to an apparently nonorganic inability to swallow. A condition termed **Ganser's syndrome** refers to patients who pretend to be insane. When individuals are consciously and deliberately feigning illness or disability to attain a desired goal, they are said be **malingering**. Malingering may be seen in association with hysteria and sociopathic personality disorders. A form of sociopathic malingering increasingly recognized by the medical profession is called **Munchausen's syndrome**, a factitious disorder with physical symptoms. Such patients feign or embellish medical conditions for no obvious motive other than to obtain medical attention and receive medical or surgical treatment. Patients with Munchausen's syndrome can have an inordinate number of physician visits, hospitalizations, diagnostic procedures, and surgeries. Another, even more insidious disorder, is **Munchausen's-by-proxy**, which refers to *parentally induced illness* in children for the purpose of eliciting medical attention and sympathy for the parent (see in Chapter 1 "Factitious Illness, Functional Disorders" and "Conversion Disorders").

Neurotic depression. There is less than universal agreement about the use of this term; however, in general, neurotic depression refers to a depression occurring in patients who previously had symptoms of anxiety or other neuroses.

Obsessive-compulsive disorders. Obsessions refer to *thoughts* (not delusions) or impulses that intrude upon consciousness. Compulsions refer to *acts* that result from obsessions. These can be single acts or ritualized behaviors. A condition termed "*obsessional slowness*" refers to patients who exhibit extremely slow execution of everyday living tasks due to their time-consuming rituals, compulsions, and checking behaviors.

Phobias. Phobic neuroses are considered to be anxiety disorders that are characterized by obsessive fears. Phobias include panic states (see **anxiety neuroses**) and specific fears such as *agoraphobia* (fear of open spaces), *acrophobia* (fear of heights), *claustrophobia* (fear of enclosed places), *social phobia* (fear of eating in public, speaking in public, using public restrooms), and so forth. Phobic patients usually acknowledge that their fears are irrational but feel they are powerless to overcome them.

D. Psychiatric Terminology for Psychotic Disorders

Delusional or paranoid state. Paranoia refers to a psychosis characterized by persecutory delusions without hallucinations, dementia, or mood disorders. Delusional states are divided into *erotomanic type, grandiose type, jealous type, persecutory type, somatic type*, and unspecified type.

Depression (major). A major depressive episode refers to a prolonged state (at least 2 weeks' duration) of a depressed mood and apathy without delusions or hallucinations. A major depressive episode in the elderly is a frequent response to illness or bereavement and also may be a precursor or prodromal sign of dementia. Usually, major depressive episodes are characterized by weight changes, insomnia or hypersomnia, feelings of worthlessness, inability to concentrate, and recurrent thoughts of suicide.

Depression generally is described as having two forms: an **endogenous type** (having no apparent external cause) and an **exogenous type** (occurring as a reaction to loss or other forms of life stressors). Psychotic depression is characterized by faulty reality testing and impaired functioning. *Psychomotor retardation* and *agitation* may be present, and the patient may express delusional themes related to guilt, doom, or shame. **Neurotic depression**, **depressive neurosis**, and **dysthymic disorder** are terms sometimes used to refer to milder depressive states.

Reactive psychoses. A stress-induced psychotic condition characterized by a brief duration (a few hours to 1 month) of loose associations, incoherence, hallucinations, delusions, catatonia, or disorganized behavior.

Schizophrenia. Schizophrenia is categorized into subtypes, including *simple, undifferentiated schizophrenia* (the individual who exhibits a blunt affect, social withdrawal, and a thought disorder); *acute schizophrenia* (characterized by a rapid onset of schizophrenic psychosis, possibly related to toxic, metabolic, or endocrine causes); *hebephrenic schizophrenia* or *disorganized schizophrenia* (in which the individual has delusions, hallucinations, marked emotional swings, and, at times, stereotypic mannerisms); *catatonic schizophrenia* (a condition in which there is no response to the environment; some psychiatrists feel that catatonia may be a feature of manic-depressive disease rather than a form of schizophrenia); *paranoid schizophrenia* (a condition in which the delusions, hallucinations, and thought disorders have persecutory features); and *childhood schizophrenia* (psychosis diagnosed in childhood or adolescence characterized by hallucinations and thought disturbances).

E. Terminology Related to Other Psychiatric Disorders and Conditions

Anxiety disorders of childhood. Psychiatric disorders that include *separation anxiety* and *avoidant personality type* in childhood.

Disruptive behavior. Includes behavioral conduct disorders, such as oppositional, defiant behavior; aggressive behavior; and ADD-H in children.

Eating disorders. Include *anorexia nervosa, bulimia nervosa, pica* (eating nonnutritive substances, such as paste or paper), *food jags, oral sensory avoidances* (see Chapter 5), and *rumination eating disorder*. The latter refers to the tendency to regurgitate a portion of food immediately after swallowing.

Endocrine psychoses. Include psychotic behaviors associated with hyper- and hypothyroidism, *Cushing's syndrome, adrenal insufficiency*, or *psychosis in response to ACTH* and *cortisone therapy*.

Gender identity disorders. These conditions include *unresolved* adjustment related to transsexualism and gender identity issues that may occur in childhood, adolescence, and adulthood.

Impulse control disorders. Include *explosive disorder, pathologic gambling, kleptomania, pyromania, anger management issues*, and *trichotillomania* (impulse to pull out one's own hair).

Organic mental disorders. Include **primary degenerative dementia (PDD)**, **primary progressive dementia** (**PPD**) of the **Alzheimer type**; **multi-infarct dementia**; **frontotemporal dementia**; and dementias and other psychiatric impairments that are the result of cortical damage or dysfunction of a generalized nature (such as metabolic disorders) (see "Degenerative Diseases," discussed earlier).

Postpartum (puerperal) psychoses. Referring to the postpartum depression, delirium, or schizofreniform behavior observed in some new mothers occurring within hours to months following childbirth.

Sexual dysfunction. Includes *hypo-* and *hyperarousal disorders* and *paraphilias* (such as exhibitionism, pedophilia, masochism, sexual sadism, and fetishism).

Sleep disorders. Include *parasomnias* (e.g., sleepwalking, sleep eating), *insomnia*, and *hypersomnia*. (Also see "Syncope and Sleep Disorders" in this chapter and "Pain and Sleep" in Chapter 4.)

Substance-induced organic mental disorders. Include intoxication withdrawal delirium, alcohol-related amnestic disorder, alcohol-related dementia, and intoxication from other drugs (amphetamine, cannabis, cocaine, opiates, hallucinogens, sedatives, hypnotics, etc.).

F. Terminology Related to Psychiatric Therapies

Abreaction. A type of psychotherapy that involves reexperiencing a painful or repressed situation in a safe, therapeutic setting with the goal of gaining insight and a release of painful emotions.

Activity therapy. Treatment where the patient engages in activities that are directed toward a therapeutic goal, such as music therapy, recreational therapy, occupational therapy, bibliotherapy (providing written materials with a psychological benefit), and educational therapy.

Behavioral therapy. A therapeutic approach based on operant learning (behavioral conditioning) principles and manipulations, such as desensitization, administering or withdrawing the discriminating stimulus, providing positive and negative reinforcement, and applying a prescribed reinforcement schedule to elicit behavioral changes.

Biofeedback. A therapeutic approach in which the patient observes special monitors of his or her own biophysiologic functions (e.g., brainwave activity, blood pressure, nerve conduction activity in muscles) with the goal of learning to exert a conscious control over an autonomic or involuntary function, for example blood pressure.

Child Life Therapy. Refers to play therapy activities, for example, to help ill children cope with their illness and the medical setting.

Cognitive therapy. An approach to psychotherapy that attempts to identify and change disordered thought patterns, and to "break down" existing negative thoughts (cognitions) and replace them with positive and more functionally adaptable thoughts. Some therapists prefer to combine cognitive and behavioral therapies, taking the approach that how you behave depends on your thoughts, not the actions of other people or your life situation.

Dialetical therapy. In this approach the therapist applies contradictory facts and ideas, or "dialetics," to weigh against one another and ultimately come up with a balance between self-acceptance and the need for behavioral change.

Electroconvulsive therapy (ECT). ECT is considered an effective treatment for some patients with major depression and is usually used only when other forms of psychiatric therapy (talk therapy, medication) have been found to be ineffective. During ECT, electrodes are placed over each temple, and an alternating current is passed between them for 0.1 to 0.5 second. Usually, the patient receives a total course of 6 to 14 treatments administered every other day.

Eye Movement Desensitization and Reprocessing (EMDR). This is a fairly new therapeutic approach used with individuals diagnosed to have PTSD. The therapist uses hand movements, hand taps, snapping fingers, and other sounds to distract the patient and elicit specific eye movements while discussing traumatic memories. Although experts do not yet agree if or how EMDR works, and if eye movements are essential to the therapy, there is some evidence that PTSD symptoms are diminished.

Insight-directed therapy. An approach to psychotherapy that involves directing the patient toward recognizing and examining his or her motives and feelings.

Interpersonal therapy. An approach to psychotherapy that attempts to improve the quality of the patient's social and interpersonal functioning by enhancing the ability to cope with internal and external stressors.

Milieu therapy. The use of external, or environmental, adjustments and environmental controls to treat mental illness.

Pastoral or spiritual counseling. Counseling provided by a member of the clergy.

Pharmacologic therapy, biochemical therapy. The use of medications to treat psychiatric disorders or their symptoms. *Lithium carbonate* is used to treat bipolar conditions. Neuroleptic drugs, such as *haloperidol*, followed by a *tricyclic* and *monoamine oxidase inhibitors* (MAOIs) may be therapeutic for depression. Thyroid hormones may be used as an adjunct to tricyclic therapies to treat nonpsychotic depression.

Psychoanalytic and psychodynamic therapy. Several forms of psychotherapy techniques in which the fundamental concepts involve an increased awareness of unconscious emotional conflicts so that the patient can gain insight into motivations and resolve underlying conflicts.

Psychotherapy. Referring generally to treatment that uses explanation, encouragement, reassurance, education, support, and advice to allow the patient and significant others to understand and cope with stress, emotional states, and/or psychiatric disorders better.

Rational-emotive therapy. A cognitive and empirical type of psychotherapy directed toward improving controls on emotions by examining the relationship between beliefs about oneself and their influence on emotions and behaviors.

IV. CLINICAL COMPETENCIES

The learner outcomes, skills, and competencies gained from information contained in this chapter include the ability to:

- Read, interpret, and use terminology related to neurologic and psychiatric conditions and their management.
- List and describe pyramidal and extrapyramidal movement disorders.
- List and describe cerebrovascular diseases and disorders.
- List and describe cerebral and brain stem syndromes.
- List and describe the features of common neurodegenerative diseases.
- List and describe the features of common hereditary and congenital disorders that are associated with neurologic deficits in children.
- Describe how the *DSM-IV* multiple axes are applied in psychiatric diagnoses.
- Describe the difference between psychosis and neurosis.
- List the psychiatric terminology and characteristics of personality types.
- List the types of therapeutic approaches that may be used by psychiatrists and psychologists.

V. REFERENCES AND RESOURCES CONSULTED

American Psychiatric Association. (1987). *Diagnostic and statistical manual of mental disorders* (3rd ed., rev.). Washington, DC: Author.

American Psychiatric Association. (1994). *Quick reference to the diagnostic criteria from DSM-IV™*. Washington, DC: Author.

Andreoli, T. A., Carpenter, C., & Grigg, R. C. (Eds.). (2007). *Cecil essentials of medicine* (7th ed.). Philadelphia: W. B. Saunders.

Andreoli, T. A., Carpenter, C. J., Plum, F., & Smith, L. H. (1990). *Cecil essentials of medicine* (2nd ed.). Philadelphia: W. B. Saunders.

Berkow, R. (Ed.). (1990). *The Merck manual* (15th ed.). Trenton, NJ: Merck, Sharp, and Dohme.

Bonner, J. S., & Bonner, J. J. (Eds.). (1991). *The little black book of neurology* (2nd ed.). St. Louis, MO: Mosby Year Book.

Chenitz, W. C., Stone, J. T., & Salisbury, S. A. (1991). *Clinical gerontological nursing*. Philadelphia: W. B. Saunders.

Davies, J. J. (2008). *Essentials of medical terminology* (3rd ed.). Clifton Park, NY: Delmar Cengage Learning.

Flaherty, A.W. (2000). *The Massachusetts General Hospital handbook of neurology*. Philadelphia: Lippincott Williams & Wilkins.

Gelb, D. J. (Ed.). (2005). *Introduction to clinical neurology* (3rd ed.). Philadelphia: Elsevier Butterworth Heinemann.

Jacobs, J. W., Bernard, M. R., & Delgado, A. (1977). Screening for organic mental syndromes in the medically ill. *Annals of Internal Medicine, 86*, 40–46.

Jung, J. H. (1989). *Genetic syndromes in communication disorders*. Boston: College-Hill Press.

Leonard, P. C. (2007). *Quick and easy medical terminology* (5th ed.). St. Louis, MO: Saunders Elsevier.

Ocava, L. C. (2006). Antithrombotic and thrombolytic therapy for ischemic stroke. *Clinical Geriatric Medicine, 22*, 1, 135–154.

Weiner, W. J., & Goetz, C. G. (1999). *Neurology for the nonneurologist*. Philadelphia: Lippincott Williams & Wilkins.

CHAPTER

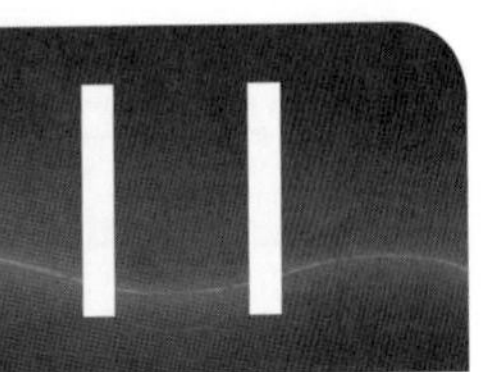

Acute and Critical Illnesses

Increasingly, speech-language pathologists (SLPs) are seeing sicker and more acutely ill patients. The assessment and management priorities in settings such as intensive care units (ICUs) and acute or critical care units (burn units, acute trauma, and stroke units) are focused on the most life-threatening and immediately critical problems. Issues and decisions faced by the SLP include determining the communication options for the tracheostomized or respirator-dependent patient, determining if by mouth versus enteral feeding options are preferable, and assessing the patient's level of responsiveness and comprehension for nursing instructions and informed consent. Acute care units and the various pediatric and adult ICUs are settings in which highly skilled clinical competency is expected from every member of the care team.

I. CHAPTER FOCUS

This chapter reviews several of the life-threatening acute and critical illnesses frequently found in pediatric and adult ICUs. The purpose of this review is to provide brief, descriptive information about catastrophic and life-threatening conditions, mainly cardiopulmonary; hematologic; gastrointestinal; fluid, electrolyte, and renal; metabolic, and related conditions. These conditions are likely to be encountered by clinicians who work in ICUs or will be a part of the medical histories of patients seen in postacute, extended care, or rehabilitation programs. Additional discussion of acute and life-threatening medical conditions is provided elsewhere, including the descriptions of levels of illness in Chapter 1; acute gastrointestinal disorders in children and adults in Chapter 5; infectious diseases in Chapter 8; cardiac, pulmonary, and hematologic disorders in Chapter 9; acute neurologic disorders in Chapter 10; and vital sign monitoring and physical examination of acute and critically ill patients in Chapter 3.

II. ACUTE AND CRITICAL CONDITIONS REQUIRING EMERGENT CARE OR ICU ADMISSIONS

A. Cardiac and Pulmonary Conditions (also see Chapter 10).

1. *Acute Myocardial Infarction (MI)*

An MI is a condition in which there has been death of heart tissue usually caused by an interruption in blood flow to the heart muscle due to atherosclerotic coronary artery disease (CAD). Typically, when an MI occurs, patients will have experienced acute, severe substernal chest pain radiating to the jaw, shoulders, and arms associated with shortness of breath, diaphoresis, nausea, vomiting, and syncope. The diagnosis is made by physical examination, electrocardiogram (EKG) findings, and laboratory analysis for the enzymes that are elevated in association with MI (additional discussion of MI is found in Chapter 3 and Chapter 9).

2. *Acute Pericarditis*

Acute pericarditis is a sudden inflammation of the lubricated sac encasing the heart. Pericarditis can be idiopathic (of unknown cause) or result from conditions such as infection, connective tissue disease (including scleroderma), uremia, myxedema, neoplasm, drugs, or a post-heart surgery or post-MI condition.

3. *Adult Respiratory Distress Syndrome (ARDS)*

ARDS is a clinical condition, not a specific disease, in which there is acute dyspnea, severe hypoxemia, decreased lung compliance, and diffuse infiltrates on chest x-ray. Conditions associated with ARDS include aspiration, sepsis, trauma, multiple blood transfusions, drug overdoses, near-drowning, head trauma, and lung contusions.

4. *Aortic Dissection*

An aortic dissection is a condition caused by an intimal (within layers) tear in the aorta, allowing a channel of blood (hematoma) to accumulate within the linings of the vessel. Hypertension and degenerative diseases may be predisposing factors. This condition is usually treated aggressively with antihypertensive and beta-blocking agents and, in some cases, surgery to avoid an aortic rupture. Arterial dissections can occur elsewhere, including the carotid arteries.

5. *Arrhythmias*

The basic principles of cardiac impulse initiation and conduction are described in Chapter 9. Cardiac arrhythmias, such as tachydysrhythmias (tachycardia) and bradydysrhythmias (atrial and ventricular bradycardias), may require conversion (with shock or drugs) in an acute cardiac care setting.

6. *Aspiration*

When a foreign body or substance enters the airway, respiratory status will be disrupted to varying degrees. If a foreign body occludes the airway, as might happen when choking on food ("café coronary"), sudden and extreme distress can occur, potentially leading to asphyxiation. Aspiration pneumonia can occur as a result of neurologic disorders (decreased level of consciousness, oropharyngeal weakness, or decreased sensation of the oropharynx), gastrointestinal disorders (esophageal disease, gastric disease, bowel obstruction), or pulmonary disorders (e.g., impaired mucociliary clearance and cellular defenses). (Also see Chapter 9 for additional discussion of pneumonia.)

7. Asthma, Reactive Airway Disease

A sudden onset of coughing and wheezing can occur in response to a variety of conditions and cause bronchial resistance. Asthma is sometimes referred to as "reversible obstructive pulmonary disease." *Acute severe asthma* may require emergent treatment with drugs (such as epinephrine, aminophylline, and sympathomimetic or parasympatholytic agents), oxygen support, and mechanical ventilation.

8. Bronchopleural Fistula (BPF)

A BPF is a condition usually associated with mechanical ventilation coupled with chest tube suction. These conditions contribute to a risk for air leaking into the pleural space. When the patient is asked to bear down or to exhale forcibly with the mouth and glottis closed and nose occluded (Valsalva maneuver), a "leak squeak" will be heard as air passes into the pleural space. Spontaneous BPF can occur in association with lung malignancies, suppurative pneumonia, and following a pneumonectomy (resection of the lung).

9. Cardiac Contusion

Nonpenetrating trauma to the heart can result in petechiae and ecchymoses of the myocardium (heart muscle). More extensive bleeding would be called a "localized cardiac hematoma." Dysrhythmias are common with myocardial contusions.

10. Chronic Obstructive Pulmonary Disease (COPD)

COPD is a condition associated with a chronic dyspnea (shortness of breath) and productive cough. Related conditions include emphysema, chronic bronchitis, and reversible obstructive pulmonary disease. Extreme conditions may require emergent endotracheal intubation, oxygen support, and/or mechanical ventilation.

11. Congestive Heart Failure (CHF)

CHF refers to a condition in which the heart is unable to pump blood sufficiently for the body's needs. CHF often follows diseases to the myocardium (such as MI and cardiomyopathy). Patients with CHF will be short of breath and unable to tolerate lying down in a flat, supine position. Patients with severe CHF will have **pulmonary edema**. Along with drugs acting on the heart itself, CHF is typically treated with diuretic therapies. Diuretic therapies can result in complications, including **azotemia** (a decrease in the glomerular filtration rate of the kidneys and increases in blood urea nitrogen (BUN) and creatinine serum concentrations), orthostatic hypotension, hyponatremia, hypokalemia, hypomagnesemia, contraction metabolic acidosis, and related mental status declines (see Chapter 3).

12. Endocarditis

Endocarditis refers to an inflammation due to infection of the linings in the chambers of the heart. Abnormal heart valves, as a consequence of congenital heart defects or valvular damage, are prone to infection. Vegetations form on the damaged valve and become surrounded by platelets and fibrin, making the normal immune responses ineffective. *Infectious endocarditis* is treated with the antibiotics appropriate to the culture findings.

13. Hemoptysis

Numerous disorders of the cardiorespiratory system can cause patients to cough up blood. The physician needs to determine if the patient has bleeding from the respiratory system (hemoptysis) or has *hematemesis* (spitting up or vomiting blood from the esophagus or stomach). Hemoptysis can occur in association with conditions such as tuberculosis, lung cancer, COPD, vascular disorders, pneumonia, bronchitis, bronchiectasis, infections, and trauma.

14. Hypertensive Crisis

A hypertensive crisis is a condition in which blood pressure reaches a level high enough to cause damage to vital organs, most notably, intracranial hemorrhages, MI, pulmonary edema, aortic dissection, and renal failure. The blood pressure level at which a hypertensive crisis might occur is not fixed; however, so-called *malignant hypertension* is clinically defined as a sustained diastolic pressure greater than 130 mmHg.

15. Pericardial Effusion

Fluid accumulating in the pericardial space is referred to as pericardial effusion. *Cardiac tamponade* refers to an accumulation of fluid in the pericardium that causes acute cardiac compression with pressure sufficient to diminish cardiac output.

16. Pneumothorax

A pneumothorax refers to air leaking into the pleural space. The cause can be spontaneous or the result of iatrogenic errors (e.g., an accidental lung puncture during a medical procedure). A pneumothorax also can occur with patients receiving mechanical ventilation, especially when they have aspiration or necrotizing pneumonia, ARDS, or obstructive lung disease (see Chapter 9).

17. Pulmonary Embolism (PE)

Pulmonary emboli are most often found in patients who have a history of *deep vein thromboses* (DVTs). When clots from the peripheral venous circulation are dislodged, they may be passed into the right side of the heart and occlude the pulmonary artery (which carries blood from the heart to the lungs to be oxygenated [see Figure 9–3]) and lead to tachycardia, pulmonary infarction, pleuritic pain, and pathologic lung changes (including atelectasis, pleural effusion, and localized infiltrates).

18. Unstable Angina

Cardiac angina is a condition in which there is pain related to a lack of oxygen perfusion to the heart muscle. *Exertional angina,* or effort angina, is a condition that occurs during effort, or exercise, when there is an increased demand for oxygen. *Unstable angina* can occur at rest, when there may be no extra demand on the heart, and is brought on by a vasospasm, hemorrhage, or thrombus of the heart vessel, causing an intermittent or transient loss of blood supply to the heart muscle.

19. Upper Airway Obstruction (UAO)

UAOs are life-threatening events. An upper respiratory obstruction produces extreme distress, stridor, cyanosis, and loss of consciousness. **Intrathoracic** causes of UAO include *tracheal stenosis, tracheomalacia, submucosal hemorrhage of the glottis or subglottis* (following intubation, biopsy studies, trauma), and *compression on the upper airway* (related to lymph node enlargement or tumors). **Extrathoracic** causes of airway obstruction include *aspiration of a foreign body, hypopharyngeal edema, hypopharyngeal hemorrhage, epiglottitis, acute angioedema, adenoidal hypertrophy, cricoarytenoid arthritis, hypertrophic thyroid disease*, and *bilateral vocal fold paralysis.*

B. Hematologic Conditions

1. Anticoagulation Disorders

Complications of anticoagulation therapies, chiefly *heparin* and *coumarin derivatives*, are often treated in the ICU. Bleeding is a major risk with heparin and coumarin derivative therapy because these drugs are intended to prevent the formation of thromboses. Anticoagulant therapies are routinely used with patients who have chronic *thrombotic disease.* Corrective management of anticoagulant complications involves administration of drugs that have a neutralizing effect with careful monitoring of coagulation parameters. Heparin therapy can cause **thrombocytopenia,** a condition in which there is a reduction in the number of blood platelets. Thrombocytopenia is a commonly acquired problem in the critically ill.

2. Antiplatelet Therapy

Unlike anticoagulant therapy, antiplatelet therapy has an effect on the prostaglandins in platelets and inhibits their aggregation. Aspirin is the antiplatelet drug most often prescribed as a prophylactic measure, especially following a **transient ischemic attack (TIA)** or thrombotic or thromboembolic stroke. Aspirin intake is usually discontinued before and immediately following a major surgery.

3. Disseminated Intravascular Coagulation (DIC)

DIC is a hemorrhagic condition in which there is gross intravascular clotting in association with profuse bleeding. DIC is one of several severe complications of **necrotizing enterocolitis** in premature infants (see Chapter 5).

4. Hemostatic Failure

Hemostatic failure refers to a disruption in the normal processes for blood clotting. Hemostatic failure occurs in association with drugs used for or known to affect bleeding, including coagulation therapies and drugs that cause platelet dysfunction (such as aspirin) and with hematologic diseases associated with blood clotting.

5. *Tumor Lysis Syndrome*

Tumor lysis syndrome occurs in response to large masses of tumor cells in association with conditions such as small cell lung cancer, widespread metastases, lymphocytic cancer, and myeloma. Widespread cell destruction causes the release of metabolites and intracellular ions, which overwhelms the kidney, requiring hemodialysis. Tumor lysis syndrome can occur following induction of chemotherapy.

C. Gastrointestinal Conditions

1. *Acute Hepatic Failure*

Hepatitis can occur when there is a deterioration of a preexisting liver disease or following sudden damage to liver cells due to disease, injury, or infection (see Chapter 8). *Icterus*, or *jaundice* (yellowed skin coloring), is associated with liver disease. **Hepatic encephalopathy** may result from hepatitis, in which an initial mental confusion can progress to stupor and coma. Other problems associated with acute hepatic failure include *respiratory alkalosis*; *hypoglycemia*; *renal failure*; and *hemorrhagic manifestations*, including **bleeding diathesis** (due to the loss of vitamin K stores).

2. *Acute Intestinal Ischemia*

Infarction of the bowel can result from occlusive vascular disease or hypoperfusion of the intestinal tissues. A commonly diagnosed acute intestinal obstruction in neonates is *intussusception*, in which a segment of the bowel telescopes into a more distal segment, usually at the junction of the terminal ileum and the ileocecal valve.

3. *Lower Gastrointestinal (LGI) Hemorrhaging*

LGI bleeding occurs with *inflammatory bowel disease*, *hemorrhoids*, *carcinoma*, *hemorrhagic diatheses*, *radiation colitis*, *angiodysplasia*, and *diverticulosis* (weakening of the intestinal wall). LGI bleeding from the rectum is usually described to be bright red blood, called **hematochezia**. Conversely, "black tarry stools" are usually found in association with *upper* gastrointestinal (UGI) bleeding, discussed later.

4. *Peritonitis*

Peritonitis is a condition in which bacteria have entered the peritoneal cavity. Peritonitis can occur in association with acute appendicitis, peptic ulcer perforation, diverticulitis, or postsurgical complications.

5. *Upper Gastrointestinal (UGI) Hemorrhaging*

Bleeding in the UGI tract can result from a variety of conditions, including *esophageal varices*, *Mallory-Weiss syndrome* (damage to the esophageal mucosa at the gastroesophageal juncture, which is most often found in alcoholics), *peptic ulcers*, *stress ulcers*, an *aortoenteric fistula*, and *UGI malignancy*. The diagnosis of UGI bleeding includes a **hemoccult test**. A hemoccult test is a stool study examining for a **guaiac reaction**, which is a test for the presence of occult (subtle) bleeding. Patients usually present with **hematemesis**, vomiting red blood or "coffee-ground" appearing blood, and **melena,** black tarry blood in the stool (feces).

D. Fluid, Electrolyte, and Renal Disorders

1. Acute Acid-Base Disturbances

Acid-base disturbances refer to imbalances in the **intracellular** or **extracellular fluids** that are either excessively alkaline or excessively acidic. Body systems vary as to their optimal acid-base balances, with the bloodstream being the most critically buffered system. These balances are quantified by the concentration of hydrogen ions, H^+, or pH (the negative logarithm of hydrogen ion concentration). A normal blood chemistry pH value is about 7.41 (7.35–7.45). The normal body pH level is maintained principally by the body's *carbonic acid buffering system.* The ratio between bicarbonate HCO_{3-} and partial pressures of carbon dioxide in the arterial blood, $PaCO_2$, determines the H^+ concentration. Regulation of these processes occurs with the interaction of alveolar ventilation, affecting $PaCO_2$, and kidney functions, affecting HCO_{3-}. The major forms of acid-base disturbances are **respiratory acidosis** (in which there will be an increase in $PaCO_2$ in blood gases), **metabolic acidosis** (in which there will be an increased HCO_{3-}), **respiratory alkalosis** (decreased $PaCO_2$), and **metabolic alkalosis** (decreased HCO_{3-}). The term **ketoacidosis** refers to metabolic acidosis associated with *diabetes mellitus, starvation,* and alcoholism.

2. Acute Kidney Injury (AKI)

AKI, or **acute renal failure (ARF)**, refers to a syndrome associated with a dramatic decrease in renal function, causing a reduction in the clearance of solutes (wastes) from the blood, which leads to an increase in the concentration of *creatinine* and *BUN* levels. Retention of water and solutes can cause uremia and fluid, electrolyte, and metabolite imbalances, producing neurologic changes (nausea, vomiting, and encephalopathy) and *metabolic acidosis.* ARF can result from diseases of other organs (e.g., CHF, liver disease); drugs; damage to the kidney itself; and obstructions to, from, or within the kidney.

3. Acute Fluid, Electrolyte, and Metabolites Disturbance

The proper function of the body's cells depends on maintaining a balance between the **volume of fluid** in the cells as well at the balance of salts and other metabolites in body fluids (see Chapter 5). The body is about 60% water. About two-thirds of that fluid is within cells; the rest is *extracellular.*

Water balances in the body, referred to as the balance between *fluid depletion* and *fluid expansion,* are monitored and controlled by renal (kidney) and extrarenal receptors and functions. Conditions associated with fluid expansion (hypervolemia) include *renal disorders, endocrine abnormalities,* and *conditions causing edema* (such as congestive heart disease). Patients who are **hypervolemic** are sometimes described as "wet," whereas patients who are **hypovolemic** are described as "dry." Conditions associated with fluid depletion (hypovolemia) include *vomiting; diarrhea; burns; sweating; hemorrhage; diabetes insipidus; chronic renal failure* and other renal diseases; and, commonly, the excessive use of *diuretics.* (See Chapter 5 for further discussion of fluid and electrolyte imbalances.)

E. Acute Metabolic and Endocrine Disorders

1. Adrenal Insufficiency

Acute adrenal insufficiency, or **Addisonian crisis**, usually occurs in patients who have some preexisting partial insufficiency. Total failure of the adrenal glands is usually fatal. There are numerous causes of damage to the adrenal glands, including *hemorrhagic destruction following anticoagulant use*, *tumors* and *metastases*, *tuberculosis*, and diseases associated with a *polyglandular autoimmune syndrome*. The adrenal glands are sometimes injured during kidney surgeries.

2. Diabetic Coma and Ketoacidosis

Diabetic coma may be referred to as **hyperosmolic nonketotic diabetic coma (HNDC)** in which acidosis is absent or, if present, is due to a coincidental lactate accumulation from poor circulation. **Diabetic ketoacidosis (DKA)** refers to a marked insulin deficiency in which there is *hyperglycemia*, *dehydration*, and *acidosis*. Patients with DKA have severe abdominal pain, hyperventilation, and tachycardia, and their breath may smell like *acetone*. HNDC is clinically less specific, and because a stuporous or obtunded mental state is part of the syndrome, it is sometimes initially confused with other conditions (such as stroke, polypharmacy, and excessive medication), especially in elder patients, until a blood glucose tolerance test is obtained.

3. Thyroid Dysfunction

Acute hyperthyroidism can cause a **thyrotoxic crisis** or so-called *thyroid storm*. Hyperthyroidism occasionally follows infection, trauma, surgery, and radioiodine therapy. Serious disease can be associated with hyper- or hypothyroidism. Late-stage chronic hypothyroidism in the elderly is usually referred to as a **myxedema crisis**, or **myxedema coma**. This state can follow infection, trauma, exposure to cold, and excessive medication.

F. Other Disorders

1. Severe Burns

Burns are classified as **moderate** or **major** according to the amount of the body affected, or the total body surface area (TBSA), and the depth of the burn. The TBSA is measured by an approximation based on the "rule of nines," in which the entire head makes up 9%, each arm makes up 9%, each leg makes up 18%, and the front and back of the body each make up 18%. Chapter 3 provides a discussion of burns in children and adults, and Figure 3–2 provides an illustration of the "rule of nines" in describing burn injuries with infants, children, adolescents, and adults.

The depth of burns is classified by degrees. A **first-degree burn** is the sort associated with sunburn and is superficial, characterized by erythema and dry or blistered, painful skin. A **second-degree burn**, or partial-thickness burn, is the sort associated with severe sunburn, scaldings, or flash burns (quick duration exposure to extreme heat) and involves the epidermis, extending into the dermis. Second-degree burns are painful and are characterized by blistering and weeping bullae. **Third-degree burns**, or full-thickness burns, result from prolonged contact with extreme heat and involve the epidermis and dermis. The skin is white, translucent, or charred, and touch sensation is lacking.

GI dysfunctions and hemolytic anemia are often associated with severe burns. Treatment of burn patients requires *fluid resuscitation, physiologic monitoring, topical antibiotics, analgesia and sedation, plastic surgeries, wound management, infection control*, and physical therapy. SLPs sometimes assist with oral-facial musculature exercises to improve functional recovery after facial burns. Infection prevention is extremely important when working with patients who have severe burns. **Sepsis** (infection in the bloodstream) can lead to **multiple organ systems failure (MOSF)**.

2. Coma

Coma refers to an extremely reduced state of consciousness associated with damage to or disruption of the cerebral hemispheres or the reticular activating system. Coma can result from structural or metabolic causes. Patients who are described to be in a "persistent vegetative state" may or may not be persistently comatose. Coma and its assessment are discussed at length in Chapter 4. Coma is a frequent complication of an acute head trauma. Figure 11–1 illustrates the array of tubes, drains, and monitors typically encountered in an adult coma patient with a traumatic brain injury and other injuries in the ICU. Methods for evaluating and rating coma states are discussed in Chapter 4.

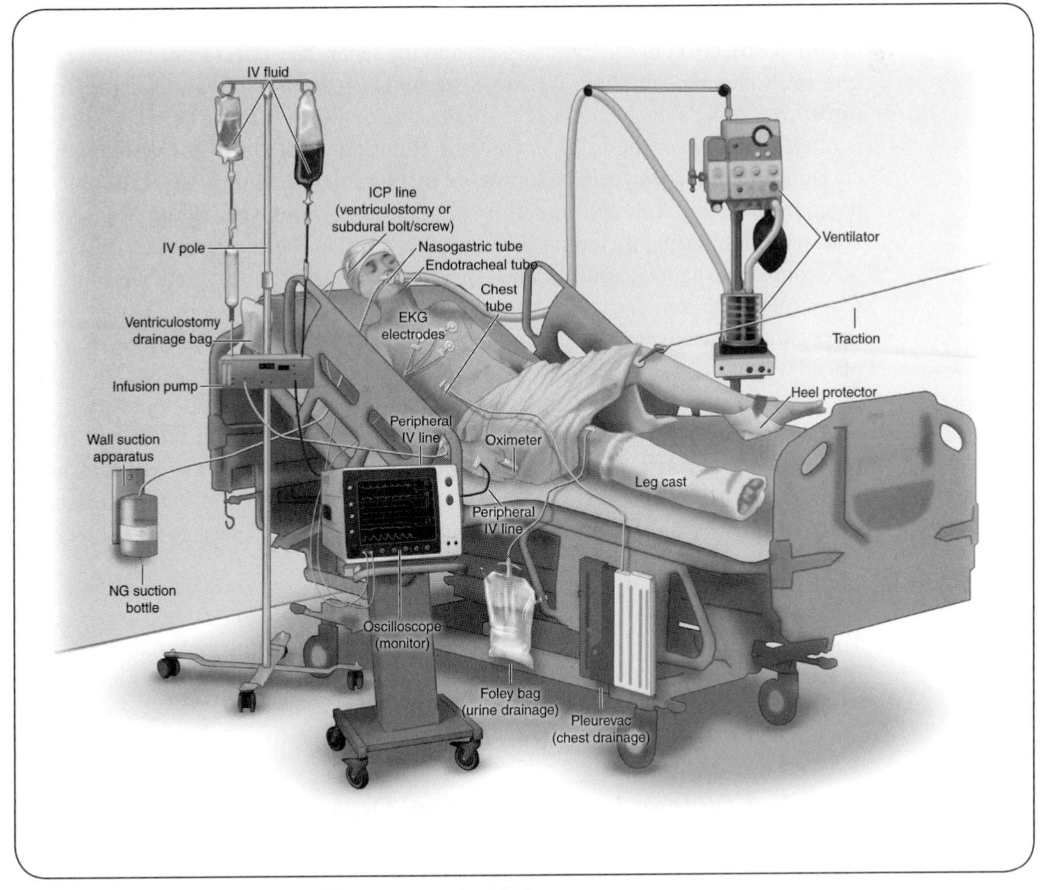

FIGURE 11–1 Illustration of TBI patient in the ICU. Source: Delmar/Cengage Learning

3. *Acute Eaton-Lambert Syndrome*

Eaton-Lambert syndrome has been associated with *small cell carcinoma* of the lung. This disorder causes thigh, shoulder, and pelvic weakness, sparing bulbar and ocular muscles. Unlike myasthenia gravis, anticholinergic drugs are not beneficial, whereas drugs that cause the release of acetylcholine are sometimes helpful and will be administered after an acute onset.

4. *Guillain-Barré Syndrome*

Guillain-Barré syndrome is characterized by an **acute polyradiculoneuropathy** occurring in association with immunologic stresses or challenges, such as a viral infection, immunization, or mycoplasma (bacterial) infections. Clinical features include progressive weakness of the extremities with *more proximal than distal* involvement, *paresthesias, areflexia, cranial nerve involvement, cramping limb pain*, and *autonomic disturbances.* **Plasmapheresis** has been demonstrated to benefit patients with Guillain-Barré syndrome by reducing the required number of days of intubation (see Chapters 4 and 10).

5. *Severe Head Injury*

The effects of a trauma to the head are usually discussed with reference to the **primary effects**, or **concussive effect** of the trauma itself, and the **secondary effects**, or resulting *edema, hemorrhage, hematoma, infection, hypoxia, hypercapnia, ischemia,* and *metabolic and cognitive disturbances.* Focal damage can result from the concussive blow to the brain. A "shearing effect" is often found when the brain encounters the rough surfaces of the frontal and temporal cranium and dural protrusions. **Increased intracranial pressure (ICP)** can cause additional damage; thus, this condition is carefully monitored in the ICU. Figure 11–1 illustrates the vital sign monitoring, including ICP, that is typical after a severe head trauma. The extent of secondary metabolic and vascular damage associated with traumatic brain injury plays a major role in the gradient and degree of recovery. Hemorrhaging around or within the brain is among the main concerns for intensive care management. When soft tissues are violently displaced within the cranium, blood vessel tears with hemorrhaging are likely. The types of pooling hemorrhages, or *hematomas*, associated with head injury include **epidural hematomas** (usually due to tears in the middle meningeal artery or vein), **subdural hematomas** (usually related to vessel tears as they pass the superior sagittal sinus), **subarachnoid hematomas** (bleeding between the layers covering the brain), and **intracerebral hematomas** (bleeding into the parenchyma of the brain). These conditions are also described in Chapter 10.

6. *ICU Syndrome*

The ICU syndrome refers to states of agitation and delirium reported in patients who remain in ICUs for extended periods. This syndrome is considered to reflect both physiologic factors and psychologic factors. Methods for standardized assessment of cognitive functions in the ICU are described in Chapter 4.

7. *Infectious Diseases Involving the Vital Organs*

Infectious processes can involve vital organs, causing life-threatening acute and critical illnesses. Examples include infections of the *heart valves* (endocarditis), the *lungs* (pneumonia), and the *brain* (encephalitis or meningitis). (See Chapter 8 for discussion of infectious diseases and their prevention and treatment.)

8. Late-Stage Myasthenia Gravis

Late-stage myasthenia gravis (MG) may require hospitalization, critical care, and ICU monitoring. MG is an *autoimmune, neuromuscular junction disease* in which antibodies to the receptor neurotransmitter acetylcholine are formed. Patients with MG have increased muscle weakness potentially requiring intensive care. An increase in muscle function typically follows administration of Tensilon®, an acetylcholinesterase inhibitor endorphonium chloride. Plasmapheresis has also been found to be therapeutic. Additional discussion of MG is found in Chapters 4 and 10.

9. Shock

Physiologically, shock is a state in which there is an acute circulatory failure leading to **hypoperfusion** of body tissues and damage to organs. The major forms of shock include **cardiogenic causes** (when there is an acute, severe diastolic function loss in the heart); **hypovolemic causes** (fluid loss due to hemorrhage, vomiting, diarrhea, burns, etc.); **distributive causes** (related to sepsis, anaphylaxis, spinal cord injury, adrenal insufficiency, etc.); and **extracardiac causes** (pericardial tamponade, constrictive pericarditis, pulmonary embolisms, or ventilator-related causes). Shock resulting from sepsis (disseminated infection in the blood or tissues) is called **septic shock**.

10. Status Epilepticus

This condition usually is defined as a seizure lasting approximately 20 to 30 minutes or a series of seizures lasting at least 30 minutes without a return to consciousness. Prolonged seizure activity can cause damage to neurologic substrate due to **cerebral hypermetabolism**. (Also see further discussion and description of related seizure disorders in Chapter 10.)

III. CLINICAL COMPETENCIES

The learner outcomes, skills, and competencies gained from information contained in this chapter include the ability to:

- Read, interpret, and use terminology related to life-threatening, acute, and critical medical conditions.
- List and describe common, critical cardiac, pulmonary, hematologic, renal, metabolic, and other conditions requiring admissions to intensive care units (ICUs).
- Describe the acute (primary and secondary), physical, and medical effects of head trauma.
- List and describe the purpose or function of the various monitors, tubes, lines, and life-support devices typically encountered with patients in ICUs.

IV. REFERENCES AND RESOURCES CONSULTED

Andreoli, T. A., Carpenter, C., & Grigg, R. C. (Eds.). (2007). *Cecil essentials of medicine* (7th ed.). Philadelphia: W. B. Saunders.

Ayres, S. M., Schlichtig, R., & Sterling, M. J. (1988). *Care of the critically ill* (3rd ed.). Chicago: Yearbook Medical.

Boggs, R. L., & Wooldridge-King, M. (1993). *AACN procedure manual for critical care* (3rd ed.). Philadelphia: W. B. Saunders.

D'Angelo, H. H., & Welsh, N. P. (1988). *The signs and symptoms handbook.* Springhouse, PA: Springhouse.

Davies, J. J. (2008). *Essentials of medical terminology* (3rd ed.). Clifton Park, NY: Delmar Cengage Learning.

Davis, M. A., Gruskin, K. D., Chiang, V. W., & Manzi, S. (Eds.). (2005). *Signs and symptoms in pediatrics: Urgent and emergent care.* Philadelphia: Elsevier Mosby.

DeGowin, R. L., LeBlond, R. F., & Brown, D. O. (2004). *DeGowin's diagnostic examination* (8th ed.). New York: McGraw-Hill Medical Publishing Division.

Fein, I. A., & Strasberg, M. A. (1987). *Managing the critical care unit.* Rockville, MD: Aspen.

Fuchs, A. (2007). *Pediatrics pocketcard set.* Hermosa Beach, CA: Börm Bruckmeier.

Kenner, C. A. (1992). *Nurse's clinical guide: Neonatal care.* Springhouse, PA: Springhouse.

Persons, C. G. (1987). *Critical care procedures and protocols.* Philadelphia: J. B. Lippincott.

Tobin, M. J. (1989). *Essentials of critical care medicine.* New York: Churchill Livingstone.

Willett, M. J., Patterson, M., & Steinbock, B. (1986). *Manual of neonatal care nursing.* Boston: Little, Brown.

Zschoche, D. A. (Ed.). (1980). *Mosby's comprehensive review of critical care* (2nd ed.). St. Louis, MO: C. V. Mosby.

CHAPTER 12

Oncology

Medical speech-language pathologists (SLPs) are frequently consulted to see adults and children with communication or swallowing deficits resulting from cancer or its treatment. Individuals with oral, laryngeal, or brain tumors are especially likely to come to the attention of SLPs. In some settings SLPs may participate with other health care providers on the Tumor Board, or Head and Neck Indications Team, and make recommendations regarding management plans. The medical management of cancer can include surgery, pharmacologic therapies, biological therapy, chemotherapy, radiation therapy, and bone marrow transplantation, along with experimental trials and complementary alternative medical therapies. At times the treatment itself may cause temporary or persistent swallowing problems or cognitive-communicative problems that require the expertise of an SLP.

I. CHAPTER FOCUS

This chapter defines terminology and abbreviations related to oncology and the treatment of malignancies. The categories of cancer and staging of selected tumor sites are outlined. Emphasis is placed on cancers of the nervous system, the head and neck, and the aerodigestive tract. A review of several of the **antineoplastic therapies** is provided. A discussion of cancer treatment by **radiation oncology** is discussed in Chapter 9.

II. TERMINOLOGY AND ABBREVIATIONS

A. Terminology

Acoustic neuroma, acoustic schwannoma. Referring to a neurilemmoma (Schwann cell tumor) of the eighth cranial nerve; a facial schwannoma involves the seventh cranial nerve. Schwannomas are neoplasms of the *nerve sheath.*

Adenocarcinoma. Malignant tumor of the glandular epithelium, particularly the breast, bronchi, digestive tract, and endocrine glands; characterized by anaplasia and metastases.

Adenoma. Benign neoplasm arising from glandular tissue.

Adequate margins. Surgical excision of tumors with edges that are (by histopathology) found to be free of tumor cells.

Adjuvant therapy. Usually refers to surgery followed by radiation or chemotherapy to help reduce the risk of recurrence of a tumor.

Alopecia. Hair loss.

Alpha-fetoprotein (AFP). An antigen tumor marker associated with testicular tumors, liver cancer, and stomach malignancies.

Anaplasia. Undifferentiated cells, often an indication of malignant growth.

Anemia. A condition characterized by a reduced number of erythrocytes and/or reduced hemoglobin in the circulating erythrocytes, resulting in a reduction in tissue oxygenation.

Angioma, hemangioma. Benign tumor of the blood vessels.

Angiosarcoma, hemangiosarcoma. Malignant tumor of the blood vessels.

Anorexia. Loss of appetite or desire for food.

Antiangiogenesis. Therapies aimed at reducing or starving a tumor by disrupting or interfering with *angiogenesis*, the body's natural repair mechanisms.

Antineoplastic. Anticancer.

Aspiration biopsy. The removal of suspect cells or tissue fragments by aspiration with a needle; a **needle biopsy** is similar but usually is placed into the core of the suspect tissue or lesion.

Astrocytoma. Tumor arising from the star-shaped neuroglia cells, or *astrocytes*. The "benign" form of astrocytoma (Grade 1, 2) is slow growing but can invade large areas. The malignant type of astrocytoma is called **glioblastoma multiforme**.

Basal cell carcinoma. Ulcerative, nodular, or scarlike neoplasm of the skin, especially facial skin.

Benign. Nonmalignant, nonrecurrent, slow-growing tumors that, by their location and histopathology, are not usually a threat to life.

Blasts. Referring to immature precursor leukocytes.

Blood-brain barrier. Neurophysiologic mechanism that prevents access of certain blood substances to brain tissue (see further discussion in Chapter 4).

Breast-cyst fluid proteins (BCFP). Antigens that may be associated with breast carcinoma.

Burkitt's lymphoma. A malignant tumor in children that causes gross swelling of the jaw.

Cancer. A group of malignant diseases characterized by abnormal cell growth.

Carcinoembryonic antigen (CEA). Antigens that may be associated with malignancies of the colon and gastrointestinal tract, lung, and breast cancer; the presence of CEA is also a tumor marker for recurrence following surgery.

Carcinogen. A substance that stimulates the formation of malignancies.

Carcinolysis. Destruction of cancer cells.

Carcinoma. A malignant tumor of epithelial tissues.

Cardiac tamponade. A condition characterized by an accumulation of excess fluid (pericardial effusion) with compression (tamponade) in the pericardium, often associated with lung cancer, affecting heart pumping.

Cellular immunity. A form of immunologic activity involving sensitized lymphocytes, or T-cells, which are produced in the thymus and stored in lymphoid tissue. After stimulation of an antigen, the sensitized lymphocytes are released into the blood to either destroy the antigen or prepare the antigen for destruction by macrophages.

Chalone. A glycoprotein that is thought to inhibit growth and proliferation of normal cells.

Chemodectoma, glomus jugulare tumors. Referring to tumors (composed of nests of epithelioid cells and nerve fibers in a highly vascular stroma) of the *chemoreceptors* located in the carotid body, aortic body, vagus nerve, glomus tympanicum, auricular and tympanic nerves, and the jugular bulb in the region of the jugular vein. Patients with these tumors are usually female in the fourth or fifth decade of life who present with deafness, tinnitus, vertigo, otorrhea, bleeding, otalgia, facial palsy, ear canal mass, and deficits of the 9th and 12th cranial nerves (illustrations of brain stem anatomy and locations of cranial nerves are provided in Appendix B). They may also present with *dysphagia* and a *pulsatile pharyngeal mass.*

Cholestoma. Although the suffix "oma" is used in the nomenclature, these are not tumors but rather an aggressive tissue growth (keratin and desquamated debris) that can invade bony structures in the middle ear.

Chondroma. Benign neoplasm of cartilaginous tissue.

Chondrosarcoma. Malignant tumor of the cartilage cells.

Chordoma. Tumors arising from remnants of the embryonic notochord (the structure giving rise to the spinal cord during fetal development).

Choriocarcinoma. Malignant tumor of the uterus.

Craniopharyngioma. A benign, congenital tumor that is cystic in nature, which appears in the midline, *suprasellar region* with involvement of the third ventricle, optic nerve, and pituitary gland.

Cystadenocarcinoma. Malignant, cystic growth of the glandular epithelium, especially the ovaries, salivary glands, breast, and thyroid.

Cystadenoma. Benign, cystic growth of the glandular epithelium.

Debulking. The surgical removal of the majority, but not all, of a tumor.

Dermoid cyst, cystic teratoma. A congenital tumor appearing commonly in the midline, suprasellar area and considered a benign tumor.

Diffuse malignancies. Widespread or systemic cancers, such as leukemia, multiple myeloma, and forms of lymphoma.

Distant metastases. Cancer spread outside the regional lymphatics.

Duke's criteria. A method for staging large bowel cancers.

Encapsulated. Enclosed in a sheath.

Ependymoma. Common childhood tumor that appears in the membranous lining of the posterior fossa and the cerebral ventricles. This tumor tends to be slow growing and may be benign or malignant.

Epidermoid carcinoma. Carcinoma of the skin and mucosa.

Erythroplakia. Velvety red patches. Erythroplakia, leukoplakia, and ulcerative lesions may be gross indicators or precursors of squamous cell carcinoma of the mucous membranes.

Ewing's sarcoma. Bone cancer involving the long bones or pelvis.

Excisional biopsy. Removal of the entire suspected tumor, with little or no surrounding margin, for diagnostic purposes. An **incisional biopsy** involves the removal of a wedge of tissue from a larger mass.

Family cancer syndrome. Referring to the genetic mutations occurring in families that are known to be linked to higher than normal risks for cancer (see Chapter 6 for additional discussion).

Fibrosarcoma. Cancerous tumor of the collagen-producing fibroblasts.

Functioning tumor. Referring to a neoplasm, usually of an endocrine gland, capable of synthesizing and releasing hormones into the blood.

Fungating. Growing rapidly in a fungus-like manner.

Ganglioneuroblastoma. Malignant ganglioneuroma.

Ganglioneuroma. Benign tumor of the ganglionic cells and neuroblasts.

Gastrinoma, Zollinger-Ellison syndrome. A syndrome characterized by hypersecretion of gastric acid due to a gastrin-producing tumor.

Glatosyl transferase isoenzyme II (GTI-II). An antigen thought to be a tumor marker for malignancies of the stomach, colon, and pancreas.

Glioblastoma multiforme. A highly invasive, destructive form of malignant tumor involving the glia (supportive cells) of the neurons; malignant astrocytoma.

Glioma. A family of tumors of the neuronal supportive cells (glia) of the brain.

Glucagonoma. Alpha cell tumors of the pancreas, which produce the hormone glucagon.

Growth factor. In general, referring to chemicals that promote growth. In tumor growth, referring to the ratio of proliferating to nonproliferating malignant cells.

Hairy cell leukemia. A form of lymphoid malignancy characterized by significant anemia, pancytopenia, and hairlike cytoplasmic projections in the blood and bone marrow.

Heavy chain disease. A plasmacytic-lymphocytic neoplasm that causes infiltration of tissues by malignant cells and deposition of pathologic proteins, especially into the small intestine and peripheral lymphoid tissues.

Hemangiosarcoma. Cancerous tumor of the blood vessels.

Hodgkin's disease. Lymphoma occurring in young adults characterized by a painless, progressive enlargement of lymph nodes, spleen, and general lymphoid tissues. **Non-Hodgkin's lymphoma** refers to a heterogeneous group of lymphoid malignancies, several of which are possibly related to viral or immunodeficiency causes. Non-Hodgkin's lymphomas occur uncommonly in children, and its average age of onset in adults is later than that of Hodgkin's disease (after young adulthood). Non-Hodgkin's lymphoma in children usually involves the mediastinum and abdomen, and the disease tends to be more diffuse and has more bone marrow spread than is typical for adults.

Hospice. A concept of care for terminally ill persons in which the notion of *intensive caring* (usually in the individual's home) replaces *intensive care*. In hospice care, the family is considered the primary caregiver, and medical treatment is palliative, directed toward optimizing the quality of life, alleviating pain, and reducing helplessness (see Chapter 14).

Human chorionic gonadotropin (HCG). A placental antigen known to be a tumor marker for choriocarcinoma and possibly a marker for testicular cancer.

Human T-cell leukemia-lymphoma virus (HTLV). Virus known to cause cancer in humans.

Hygroma. A sac, cyst, or bursa containing fluid.

Hyperkeratosis. Abnormal, horny, irregular growth that can be the result of noncancerous diseases or a premalignant condition.

Hypernephroma. Malignant tumor of the kidney.

Hyperplasia. Excessive growth of normal cells.

Induction therapy. Intensive chemotherapy directed at putting a malignancy into remission.

Infiltrative. Cancerous tumor growing or extending into normal tissue.

***In situ*.** At the site, not invading adjacent tissues.

Insulinoma. Beta cell tumors of the pancreas, producing the hormone insulin.

Interstitial. Between a space or between cells.

Invasive. Spreading.

Invasive procedure. Procedures, such as endoscopy or surgery, that allow internal access to areas of the body that are not easily accessible externally.

Kaposi's sarcoma. Malignant neoplasm characterized by soft, bluish nodules of the skin with hemorrhages and lymphadenopathy.

Karnowsky scale. The Karnowsky scale, or **Karnowsky Scale Placement**, is a scaled method for describing the condition and functional performance abilities of patients with cancer.

Leiomyoma. Benign neoplasm of smooth muscle.

Leiomyosarcoma. Malignant tumor of the smooth muscle.

Lesion. An injured or altered area of tissue.

Leukemias. Referring to cancers of the blood-forming bodies causing excessive formation of leukocytes.

Leukoplakia. Well-defined, white patches on mucous membranes that may be due to a fungus infection, lichen planus, or other oral disease, or may indicate early carcinoma.

Lipoma. Benign neoplasm of the adipose (fat) tissues.

Liposarcoma. Cancerous tumor of the adipose (fat) tissues.

Low-grade tumors. Referring to the histopathologic grades of tumor cells in which cells are well-differentiated, and thus graded to be at less advanced stages (Grade 1, Grade 2).

Lumpectomy. The surgical removal of a tumor mass and a small amount of surrounding tissue.

Lymphangioma. Benign tumor of the lymph vessels.

Lymphangiosarcoma. Malignant tumor of the lymph vessels.

Malignant. Bad; tumors that spread to adjacent tissues or to other areas and may ultimately be life threatening if untreated (see Table 12–1).

Medullary. Term referring to soft tissues, the medulla, or to bone marrow.

Medulloblastoma. Cancerous tumor arising in the fourth ventricle and base of the cerebellum. This malignant tumor of the posterior fossa is usually fast growing and more commonly occurs in children.

Melanoma. Malignant tumor usually arising from a *melanocytic nevus* (black mole).

Meningioma. Benign tumor arising from the arachnoid covering of the brain. These tumors tend to be slow growing and are usually encapsulated.

Metastasis. Process of cancer spreading to secondary sites.

Mohs' surgery. A technique named for Fredrick Mohs involving microscopically controlled, precise removal of skin cancers (and other forms of cancer) and sparing healthy tissues; also know as *chemosurgery.*

Moribund. Near death.

Mucositis. Mucosal inflammation associated with radiation therapy.

Myeloma, multiple myeloma. Cancer arising from plasma cells.

Natural killer (NK) immunity. A form of immunologic activity not mediated by B- or T-cells but probably a type of lymphocyte stimulated by viral injections (also see Chapter 8).

Necrosis, necrotic. Dead tissue.

Neoplasm. Abnormal new growth of tissue cells.

Neoplastic cardiac tamponade. A syndrome of pericardial constriction impeding normal expansion of the heart and venous blood return, due to malignant cell invasion of the pericardium.

Nerve block. Injection of neurolytic agents to achieve anesthesia.

Neurectomy. Neurosurgical sectioning of the peripheral nerve to produce anesthesia.

Neurilemmoma. Benign, encapsulated neoplasm arising from a peripheral nerve.

Neuroblastoma. A highly malignant tumor of the neuroblasts in the adrenal gland, sympathetic nerve chains, jaw, lip, and viscera; usually found in children.

Neurofibroma. Benign, non-Schwann cell, tumors of the peripheral nerve sheaths.

Neurofibrosarcoma. A malignant tumor of the peripheral nerve sheaths.

Nevus. Pigmented mole or malformation of the skin.

Oatcell carcinoma. Very malignant, undifferentiated small cell tumor of the lung.

Oligodendroglioma. An uncommon brain tumor with a slow growth rate arising from the oligodendrocytes.

Oncogenic. Causing the formation of a tumor.

Opsonin. A product that allows bacteria to become more susceptible to phagocyte destruction; opsonin enhances the recognition of nonself.

Optic gliomas. Referring to tumors arising from the optic nerve or optic chiasm.

Osteoid osteoma. Benign tumor arising from fibrous bone tissue.

Osteosarcoma. Malignant tumor arising from fibrous bone tissue.

Paget's disease. An inflammatory disease sometimes seen at the onset of the development of bone cancer. Paget's disease is characterized by local areas of bone destruction with development of porous bone and deformities. It is thought that Beethoven may have had this disease and that his deafness was the result of bony compression on the eighth nerves.

Pain trajectory. The direction or pattern of pain.

Palliative. Alleviating symptoms without curing the disease.

Pancreatic oncofetal antigen (POA). A fetal protein felt to be a marker for pancreatic cancer.

Pap smear. Named for the originator of the test, *Papanicolaou* smear test, a method for early detection of uterine and cervical cancer that involves swabbing cells from uterine and cervical mucosa for microscopic examination.

Pineal tumor. Rare brain tumors occurring mainly in males during adolescence through early adulthood. Pineal tumors are usually germ cell tumors categorized as germinal, parenchymal, or glial, depending on the cell type of origin. This tumor is difficult to approach surgically; thus radiotherapy and shunt procedures are used to relieve intracranial pressure.

Pituitary adenoma. Tumors involving the pituitary gland, occurring more often in young or middle-aged adults.

Pluripotent. In immunology, several cytokines are known to be pluripotent, in that they can potentially activate specific responses in certain cell types or inhibit responses in other cell types. *Interferon gamma* is an example of a pluripotent compound in that it can both inhibit growth and increase (upregulate) antigens in a general antiviral response.

Polyp. Nonspecific reference to tissue growth, usually on mucous membranes. *Sessile polyps* are fixed and attached with a broad base. **Pedunculated polyps** are attached with a narrow stalk and are mobile.

Primary tumor. Original tumor.

Proliferation. Rapid growth.

Prostatic acid phosphatase (PAP). An enzyme marker for prostate cancer.

Prostatic-specific antigen (PSA). A tumor marker for prostate cancer.

Reed-Sternberg cells. A type of malignant cell associated with Hodgkin's disease.

Remission. State in which no signs or symptoms of a disease are apparent.

Rescue technique. Term often applied to radiation therapy or chemotherapy when surgery has failed to eradicate a malignant tumor.

Retinoblastoma. A relatively rare, highly malignant tumor of the retina, more often found in children than adults.

Rhabdomyoma. Benign tumor arising from striated (skeletal) muscle tissue.

Rhabdosarcoma. Malignant tumor of the striated muscle tissue.

Rhizotomy. Neurosurgery on the nerve root to provide anesthesia.

Sarcoma. Highly malignant tumor composed of connective tissue, such as muscle, fat, bone, and blood vessels.

Scirrhus. Term used to designate a hard tumor.

Secondary tumor. Tumor that has metastasized from a primary site.

Seminoma. Malignant testicular neoplasm.

Sentinel node biopsy. Used to stage a tumor, such as melanoma, and nodes appear to be clinically negative. The method involves injection of an isotope near the lesion followed by a scan to detect the spread of the isotope and the nodal drainage pattern. Because tumors spread to the sentinel node first, that node will typically be removed as a precaution.

Squamous cell carcinoma. Malignant neoplasm of the squamous epithelial cells of the skin, mucosal linings, salivary glands, larynx, lungs, bladder, and elsewhere. Individuals who require laryngectomies often have late-stage tumors with this type of cell pathology.

Squamous papilloma. Benign neoplasm arising from squamous epithelia, characterized by a flat pavement-like appearance.

Staging. A method for classifying malignancies with reference to the size and location of the primary lesion, nodal involvement, and any metastases. **Surgical staging** refers to using a systematic surgical approach to determine the size of a primary tumor, the presence of lymph node involvement, and the extent of metastases.

Stomatitis. Inflammation of the mucosa of the mouth.

Substance P. A neuropeptide involved in the transmission of painful, noxious stimuli due to an alteration of the excitability of the pain responsive neurons, the dorsal horn ganglia.

Sympathectomy. Neurosurgery performed on the peripheral sympathetic ganglion chain.

Tennessee antigen (TennGen). A glycoprotein tumor marker felt to be associated with colorectal cancer.

Teratoma. A tumor containing types of embryonic tissues residues (vestiges of hair, teeth, bone, etc.).

Thanatology. The study of death and the dying process (see Chapter 14).

Thymoma. Tumor of the thymus gland.

Tractotomy. Neurosurgery performed through occipital craniotomy in which the spinothalamic tract is cut at the level of the mesencephalon for pain relief.

Trismus. Difficulty or pain with jaw opening; trismus is often a complaint following radiation therapy to the oral cavity; may be referred to as **trismus–pseudocamptodactyly syndrome**.

Tumor burden. Referring to the ratio of tumor cells to normal cells in a patient's body.

Tumor doubling time (TDT). An estimation procedure used to determine the preclinical stages of certain cancers, such as breast cancer.

Tumoricidal. Agents that are destructive to tumors.

Tumor marker. Biologic activities that indicate the presence and progression or regression of tumors.

Undifferentiated, dedifferentiated, differentiated. Histopathologic descriptors of the cellular state when there is an alteration of the specialization of cells due to neoplastic growth. In tumor grading, pathologists usually describe cellular states from tissue biopsies as *well-differentiated,* or *Grade 1* (indicating that the normal morphologic characteristics of malignant cells are maintained); *moderately differentiated,* or *Grade 2* (indicating that some morphologic changes have taken place); *poorly differentiated,* or *Grade 3* (indicating a near total lack of normal cell differentiation); and *undifferentiated,* or *Grade 4* (indicating that features of normal cell specialization from the tissues of origin cannot be determined).

Verrucous carcinoma. The clinical manifestation of slowly progressive, warty growths that are histopathologically well-differentiated (low-grade) squamous cell carcinoma.

Vesicant. A drug that causes extreme irritation if there is extravasation (spread outside the blood vessel) into surrounding tissues.

Wilms' tumor. Cancerous tumor of the kidney found mainly in children.

Wound seeding. Referring to the inadvertent spread of cancer from biopsy methods or tumor dissemination during surgery or other invasive procedures that might dislodge tumor cells into the blood or lymphatic circulation.

Xerostomia. Dry mouth.

Zinc glycinate marker (ZGM). An antigen thought to be associated with gastrointestinal malignancies.

B. Abbreviations

ACS. American Cancer Society; acute coronary syndrome

ACTH. Adrenocorticotropic hormone

Adeno CA. Adenocarcinoma

ADH. Antidiuretic hormone

AFP. Alpha fetoprotein

AJCC. American Joint Committee on Cancer

ALL. Acute lymphocytic leukemia

AML. Acute myelogenous leukemia

ANLL. Acute nonlymphytic leukemia

Astro. Astrocyte (star-shaped cell)

BhCG. Beta human chorionic gonadotropin

BMT. Bone marrow transplant

Bx. Biopsy

CA. Cancer, carcinoma

chemo. Chemotherapy

CI. Continuous infusion

Cis. Carcinoma *in situ*

CML. Chronic myelogenous leukemia

CR. Complete remission

CS. Clinical stage

DNA. Deoxyribonucleic acid

5-FU. 5-fluorouracil

G. Grade

GVHD. Graft versus host disease

HD. Hodgkin's disease

HLA. Human leukocyte antigen

HTLV. Human T-cell leukemia-lymphoma virus

IL-2. Interleukin-2

IUAC. International Union Against Cancer

LAK. Lymphokine-activated killer (cells)

MEN. Multiple endocrine neoplasia

Mets. Metastases

MUGA. *MU*ltiple *G*ated *A*cquisition (scan)

MUO. Metastasis of unknown origin

N. Node

NED. No evidence of disease

NGF. Nerve growth factor

TABLE 12–1 Tumor Growth Terminology

TERMINOLOGY	DESCRIPTION
Hyperplasia	Excessive proliferation of cells with normal pathology
Dysplasia	Excessive proliferation of cells that have undergone some physical change (shape, size, or structure)
Benign	Tumors that do not invade local tissues or spread to other locations
Carcinoma *in situ*	Severe dysplasia at a particular location
Malignant	Tumors that have invaded surrounding tissues and/or have spread to other locations

NSD. Nominal single dose

PS. Pathologic state

RNA. Ribonucleic acid

SCCA. Squamous cell carcinoma

SI, SII, SIII, and so on. Stage one, two, three (etc.)

SIADH. Syndrome of inappropriate antidiuretic hormone secretion

TAA. Tumor associated antigens

Tis. Tumor *in situ*

TNF. Tumor necrosis factor

TNJ. Tongue, neck, jaw

TNM. Tumor, node, metastases

T0. No evidence of primary tumor

TX. Primary tumor cannot be assessed

III. CLASSIFICATION AND STAGING OF CANCER

The American Joint Committee on Cancer (AJCC) and the International Union Against Cancer (IUAC) have jointly developed a system for classifying and staging cancers that is internationally endorsed and applied in the field of oncology. The most recent manual for staging was published in 2002 by the AJCC (Greene et al., 2002). This version sought to bring head and neck tumors to uniformity for all sites, including paranasal sinuses, salivary tumors, and thyroid tumors. A more uniform staging of advanced tumors was also implemented, with **T4 lesions** divided into *T4a (resectable)* and *T4b (nonresectable)*. This system has allowed for a better description of advanced stage disease: *Stage IVA (advanced, resectable)*, *Stage IV B (advanced, nonresectable)*, and *Stage IVC (advanced, distant metastatic disease)*. Descriptors for nodal metastases of the neck were added, with *U* for the upper neck and *L* for the lower neck. These classifications and stages are specific to particular region or organ sites and malignancy types. For example, there is no staging system for some cancers, such as cancer of the pinna, external auditory canal, middle ear, and inner ear, and lymph node classifications do not apply to staging of brain tumors.

Certain types (solid tumors and lymphomas) and sites of cancer are staged based on **TNM**, or *tumor, node,* and *metastasis* status categories. Various qualifiers are applied to refine the TNM categories further. These include lowercase letter qualifiers applied to the TNM staging numbers. For example, *clinical* diagnostic staging of patients who have had biopsies but no treatment is designated as *cTNM*. Postoperative staging is designated as *pTNM*. Staging at the time of repeated treatment for recurrent cancer is designated as *rTNM*, and staging at the time of autopsy is designated as *aTNM*. Pathologic classification of regional nodes, which is done from resected tissue samples, is indicated as *pN*, and additional qualifiers (pNa, pNb, pNbi, pNbii, etc.) are used to denote the size of the nodal metastases. The TNM classification scores are made in order to determine the stages of cancer for a given tumor type and site; these scores are critical in determining the prognosis and treatment choices. Lesion *size* is usually discussed as the most critical factor; however, for some sites and types of tumors the categorization and staging of the primary tumor depend on the extent of involvement of particular structures rather than the size of the lesion per se. The following section describes the staging methods with head and neck cancer. Consult the ***AJCC Manual on Cancer Staging*** (6th edition) (Greene et al., 2002) for further elaboration and criteria for staging other sites.

A. Lymph Node Classification

N0. No regional lymph node metastasis.

N1. Metastasis in a single ipsilateral lymph node, 3 cm or less in dimension.

N2a. Metastasis in a single ipsilateral lymph node, more than 3 cm but not more than 6 cm in greatest dimension.

N2b. Metastases in multiple ipsilateral lymph nodes, none more than 6 cm in greatest dimension.

N2c. Metastases in bilateral or contralateral lymph nodes, none more than 6 cm in greatest dimension.

N3. Metastasis in a lymph node, more than 6 cm in greatest dimension.

B. Distant Metastases

M0. No known distant metastasis.

M1. Distant metastasis present.

C. Lymphoma (Hodgkin's and Non-Hodgkin's) Classification

Stage I. Limited to one area.

Stage II. Involvement of two or more areas on the same side of the diaphragm.

Stage III. Involvement of two or more areas on both sides of the diaphragm.

D. Primary Laryngeal Tumors

1. Supraglottal

TX. Primary tumor cannot be assessed.

Tis. Tumor *in situ*.

T0. No evidence of tumor.

T1. Normal cord movement, tumor is limited to the supraglottal larynx.

T2. Tumor involves the adjacent supraglottic sites without glottic fixation.

T3. Tumor is limited to the larynx with fixation or extension to the precricoid area, medial wall of the pyriform sinus, or pre-epiglottic space.

T4. Massive tumor extends beyond the larynx to involve the oropharynx, soft tissues of the neck, or destruction of the thyroid cartilage.

2. *Glottal*

TX. Primary tumor cannot be assessed.

Tis. Tumor *in situ.*

T0. No evidence of tumor.

T1. Tumor is confined to the vocal fold with mobility preserved at the anterior and posterior commissures.

T2. Supraglottic and/or subglottic extension of tumor, with normal or impaired cord mobility.

T3. Tumor is confined to the larynx with fixation of the cords.

T4. Massive tumor with thyroid cartilage destruction or extension beyond the laryngeal confines.

3. *Subglottal*

TX. Primary tumor cannot be assessed.

Tis. Tumor *in situ.*

T0. No evidence of tumor.

T1. Tumor is confined to the subglottic region.

T2. Tumor extends to the vocal folds with normal or impaired movement.

T3. Tumor is confined to the larynx with vocal fold fixation.

T4. Massive tumor with cartilage destruction or extension beyond the laryngeal confines, or both.

E. Primary Oropharyngeal Tumors

TX. Primary tumor cannot be assessed.

Tis. Tumor *in situ.*

T0. No evidence of tumor.

T1. Tumor is 2 cm or less in greatest dimension.

T2. Tumor is more than 2 cm but not more than 4 cm in greatest dimension.

T3. Tumor is more than 4 cm in greatest dimension.

T4. Massive tumor invading the adjacent structures (cortical bone, extrinsic tongue muscles, maxillary sinus, skin).

F. Staging

Tis. Tumor *in situ.*

Stage I. Tl, N0, M0.

Stage II. T2, N0, M0.

Stage III. T3, N0, M0; Tl, T2 or T3, N1, M0.

Stage IV. T4, N0 or N1, M0; any T, N2 or N3, M0; any T, any N, M1.

IV. STAGING BRAIN TUMORS

A. Primary Tumors

Tx. Primary tumor cannot be assessed.

T0. No evidence of primary tumor.

1. Supratentorial Tumor

T1. Tumor is 5 cm or less in greatest dimension and limited to one side.

T2. Tumor is more than 5 cm in greatest dimension and limited to one side.

T3. Tumor invades or encroaches on the ventricular system.

T4. Tumor crosses the midline and invades the opposite side or invades infratentorially.

2. Infratentorial Tumors

T1. Tumor is 3 cm or less in greatest dimension.

T2. Tumor is more than 3 cm in greatest dimension and limited to one side.

T3. Tumor invades or encroaches on the ventricular system.

T4. Tumor crosses the midline, invades the opposite side, or invades supratentorially.

B. Distant Metastases

MX. Presence of distant metastasis cannot be assessed.

M0. No evidence of distant metastasis.

M1. Distant metastasis is present.

C. Histopathologic Grade

(Roman numerals are also used [e.g., **G I**].)

GX. Grade cannot be assessed.

G1. Well-differentiated.

G2. Moderately well-differentiated.

G3. Poorly differentiated.

G4. Undifferentiated.

D. Staging

Stage IA. Gl, Tl, M0.

Stage IB. Gl, T2, M0; Gl, T2, M0.

Stage IIA. G2, Tl, M0.

Stage IIB. G2, Tl, M0; G2, T3, M0.

Stage IIIA. G3, Tl, M0.

Stage IIIB. G3, T2, M0; G3, T3, M0.

Stage IV. Gl, 2, 3, T4, M0; G4, any T, M0; any G, any T, M1.

V. CANCER THERAPIES

Most of the time surgery is required for complete removal of malignant tissues and tumors or for "debulking" tumors. Descriptions of common surgeries, including those to manage cancer, are discussed in Chapter 13. Radiation oncology is discussed in Chapter 7. Some of the primary medical therapies for cancer treatment are outlined in the next sections.

A. Chemotherapy

Chemotherapy uses *chemical agents* and *drugs* (including hormonal manipulation) to combat disease in anticancer therapies. At this time, there are approximately 40 drugs that have been approved as anticancer agents in the United States. These agents are selected to direct *antineoplastic effects* on certain malignant cells, but there are typically toxic effects on normal cells as well. The normal tissues that are most susceptible to the toxic effects of antineoplastic agents are those that reproduce rapidly, such as hair follicles, cells lining the gastrointestinal tract, and cells in the bone marrow, which is why people lose hair, feel nauseated, and are susceptible to infection while undergoing chemotherapy. Another complication of the induction of chemotherapy is *tumor lysis syndrome,* discussed in Chapter 11.

Cell-cycle dependent chemotherapy refers to antineoplastic drugs that have an effect on cells only at a particular stage of reproduction. Cell-cycle independent chemotherapy refers to antineoplastic drugs that exert anticancer effects at any stage of cellular reproduction. Chemotherapy is the treatment of choice in disseminated malignancies, such as leukemia. The advent of antineoplastic agents has dramatically changed cancer survival rates for a number of malignancy types.

Chemotherapy is used in conjunction with other therapies and as a **palliative therapy** for certain localized tumors that cannot be adequately treated with surgery or radiation therapy. Combined-modality therapy, or **adjuvant therapy**, refers to the use of chemotherapy following the completion of local therapy (surgery or radiation therapy). **Combination chemotherapy** refers to the simultaneous or sequenced use of two or more drugs to treat a particular cancer. Forms of chemotherapy include *antimetabolites, hormone and hormone antagonists, alkylating agents, vinca alkaloids*, and *antibiotics.*

Patients receiving certain types of chemotherapies, for example, **doxorubicin** (whose trade name is **Adriamycin**), may have their heart functions monitored with **Multiple Gated Acquisition (MUGA) scans**, discussed in Chapter 9. Before a patient receives his or her first dose of Adriamycin a MUGA scan is usually performed, both to establish a baseline for heart functions and to rule out preexisting cardiac disease.

1. *Antimetabolites*

Antimetabolites are substances that interfere with the metabolic processes for manufacturing protein in the cells. Antimetabolite drugs include 5-fluorouracil (5-FU); methotrexate (MTX); 6-mercaptopurine; cytosine arabinoside (Cytarabine, Ara-C, Cytosar); and 6-thioguanine (6-TG).

2. *Hormone and Hormone Antagonists*

Endocrine manipulation with hormones may be used as a therapy for neoplastic disease by influencing RNA-to-protein synthesis. *Androgens* are used to treat breast cancer, depending on the pathology. Tamoxifen is a drug used in recurrence prevention therapy that may be prescribed after mastectomy for breast cancers, especially in the familial form of breast cancer due to mutations of *BRCA1/BRCA2* (see Chapter 6). Estrogen manipulation also is used to treat prostate cancer. Adrenocortical hormones are used to treat leukemia, and progestins are used to treat endometrial, renal, breast, and prostatic cancers. Antiestrogens, such as tamoxifen citrate (Novadex), are used for metastatic breast carcinoma.

3. *Alkylating Agents*

Alkylating agents are compounds that have the ability to produce breaks in DNA as well as cross-linking the strands to interfere with reduplication of DNA and transcription of RNA effectively (see Chapter 6). Such agents are a class of cell-cycle nonspecific antineoplastic drugs. Alkylating agents, such as cis-platinum (Platinol), nitrogen mustard, chlorambucil (Leukeran), busulfan (Myeleran), thio-TEPA (Triethylene Thiophosphoramide), melphalan, and cyclophosphamide (Cytoxan) are used in the treatment of leukemia, lymphomas, and other disseminated malignancies. Semustine (methyl-CCNU) is an oral alkylating agent that crosses the blood-brain barrier and may be used to treat brain tumors.

4. *Vinca Alkaloid Antineoplastic Drugs*

Substances in the periwinkle plant that inhibit the formation of protein structures necessary for DNA activity and interfere with cell division, reducing cancers, are called vinca alkaloid antineoplastic drugs. These agents may be used in the treatment of Hodgkin's disease, neuroblastoma, Wilms' tumor, sarcomas, and acute lymphoblastic leukemia. Vinca alkaloid agents include vincristine (Oncovin), vinblastine (Velban), and vindesine.

5. *Antibiotics*

Certain antibiotics may be used in cancer therapy to stimulate the natural processes that interfere with DNA and RNA synthesis. These drugs include streptozotocin, mitomycin-C (Mutamycin), mithramycin (Mithracin), bleomucin (Blenoxane), dactinomycin (Actinomycin-D), doxorubicin (Adriamycin), and daunorubicin (Daunomycin).

B. Biological Therapies

1. *Biological Immunotherapy*

Biological immunotherapy uses certain antigens to *stimulate, augment,* or *suppress* the host's immune response and enhance the reduction of tumors and resistance to specific cancers. The technology for this treatment was made possible through advancements in the 1970s in developing **recombinant DNA** (see Chapter 6). Immunotherapy is usually described as *active specific* (the use of agents to produce a specific host-immune response), *nonspecific* (the use of agents to produce a generalized immune reaction), and *passive* (the use of agents from an immunocompetent donor to elicit an immune response in the recipient). The rationale for this therapy developed out of the discovery of *tumor-surface* (tumor-specific) antigens and *tumor-associated* antigens that can stimulate an immune response in the host. When cells are exposed to environmental carcinogens or undergo a transformation due to the malignancy, normally the **immune surveillance system** will attack the neoplastic cells. However, individuals who have an impaired immune system lack the ability to suppress cell proliferation, so biologic immunotherapies are employed. The biological agents that are used in antitumor biotherapies include *cytokines* (interferons, interleukins), *vaccines* specifically engineered to destroy certain tumor antigens, and *monoclonal antibodies* (Campath, Mylotarg, Rituxan, Herceptin). *Interleukin-2 (IL-2)* stimulates an immune system to produce *lymphokine-activated killer* (LAK) cells. *Recombinant interferon* is felt to strengthen the immune system and has been used efficaciously with hairy cell leukemia. These drugs are also known to produce behavioral and cognitive changes, delusion, and hallucinations.

2. *Antiangiogenesis Agents*

Angiogenesis refers to the body's mechanisms that help to repair and keep tissues healthy, such as the development of a new vascular supply for injured tissues. Scientists have long understood that both healthy tissues and tumors naturally produce proteins and molecules that either promote or inhibit angiogenesis. Experiments on mice have proved that tumors initiate angiogenesis by releasing growth factors into the surrounding tissue, which essentially orders the tissue to start making blood vessels to support the neoplasm. For a tumor to grow, it must release more angiogenesis-promoting factors than inhibiting factors into the surrounding tissue, which helps to explain the mechanisms for metastasis. Different approaches to antiangiogenesis therapy are being examined by researchers, including the use of agents targeting interference with the development of a vascular supply to the tumor or targeting the development of endothelial cells specifically.

C. Bone Marrow and Peripheral Blood Stem Cell Transplants

Bone marrow transplantation (BMT) has been an available therapy for certain cancers for several decades and known to be an effective treatment for certain types of malignancies. BMTs allow other therapies to be escalated to more effective levels and can, thus, increase sensitivity to other therapies. The three major categories of BMT are *syngeneic transplants* (between genetically identical twins), *allogenic transplants* (from a non-twin donor), and *autologous transplants* (from the patient's own harvested bone marrow). The outcomes and alternatives to BMT have been greatly enhanced by advances in medical genetics (see Chapter 6) and other technologies and therapies (such as plasmapheresis). For example, the development of immunosuppression therapies has allowed for better tolerance and success of BMT by diminishing the **graft versus host disease (GVHD)** complications. The application of plasmapheresis has allowed for the collection of **peripheral blood stem cells (PBSCs)**, which then provide an alternative source for **stem cell transplantion (SCT)** and eliminates the need for painful cell harvesting through *bone marrow aspiration*. More recently, the use of **cell banking** from **umbilical cord blood (UCB)** has given oncologists a rich source for **hemotopoietic stem cells (HSCs)**. HSCs are stem cells that are capable of developing into blood cell types, including monocytes and macrophages, neutrophils, basophils, eosinophils, erythrocytes, megakaryocytes/platelets, dendritic cells, and lymphoid cells (T-cells, B-cells, NK-cells). BMT involves replacement of HSCs in the affected patient following high-dose chemotherapy and sometimes immunosuppression therapy and radiation. Patients undergo a transplantation of bone marrow cells or stem cells through infusion into the bloodstream. During the recovery phase patients must be careful to avoid infections because full recovery of immune functions can take many months. Patients will be required to undergo repeated immunizations for childhood diseases, because all of their previously acquired immunities will be lost as an effect of the treatment. The conditions treated by BMT and PBSC therapy include malignant conditions such as multiple myeloma, lymphomas, Hodgkin's disease, neuroblastoma, sarcomas, ovarian cancer, leukemias, testicular cancer, and nonmalignant conditions such as sickle cell anemia, mucocopolysaccharidoses, and thalassemia. Bone marrow transplants may also have some benefit for oat cell carcinoma, breast carcinoma, Ewing's sarcoma, and glioblastoma multiforme.

D. Hyperthermia

A treatment termed "selective tumor heating," or hyperthermia, uses ultrasound, microwaves, radio frequency waves, induction coils, and magnet loops for direct tumoricidal therapy. Regional hyperthermia is sometimes used to treat cancers in the extremities by perfusion with prewarmed blood. Whole body hyperthermia (raising the body temperature to 108°F) is felt to enhance the effect of other therapies. Hyperthermia is nearly always combined with another cancer therapy, usually chemotherapy.

E. Photodynamic Therapy

The systemic administration of *hematoporphyrin dye* followed by red laser light exposure to specific sites has been used for treatment of certain cancers, such as recurrent breast cancer and certain skin cancers.

F. Complementary Alternative Medicine

Patients may choose to pursue complementary alternative medicine (CAM) or complementary alternative therapy in cancer intervention. There are many forms of CAM, generally grouped as: **mind-body intervention** (homeopathy, holistic medicine, faith healing, psychotherapy); **biology-based interventions** (ingesting garlic, ginger, flaxseed, evening primrose, ginkgo, goldenseal, green tea, omega-3 fatty acids, saw palmetto, phytochemicals, vitamin B complex, and the like); and **manipulative methods** (acupuncture, heat therapy, chiropractic, hyperbaric oxygen therapy, massage, Reiki, therapeutic touch, and so forth).

VI. TYPES OF TUMORS

The name of the tumor type indicates the characteristics of the tissue pathology. **Carcinoma** refers to epithelial tissue (adeno or squamous); for example, adenocarcinoma of the lung and breast and colorectal cancer or squamous cell carcinoma of the larynx. **Sarcoma** refers to connective tissue cancers. Examples include osteosarcoma (bone), liposarcoma (fat), and rhabdomyosarcoma (skeletal muscle). **Lymphoma** refers to cancer of lymphatic tissue, as found in Hodgkin's disease and non-Hodgkin's lymphoma (Shelton, Ziegfeld, & Olsen, 2004).

VII. CLINICAL COMPETENCIES

The learner outcomes, skills, and competencies gained from information contained in this chapter include the ability to:

- Read, interpret, and use terminology and abbreviations encountered in oncology.
- List the most common forms of cancer.
- Describe the various types of malignancies and tumors.
- Describe the AJCC's system for cancer staging in head, neck, and brain tumors.
- Discuss the array and basic mechanisms of current therapies for various forms of cancer.
- List the major broad types of tumors relative to their tissue pathology.

VIII. REFERENCES AND RESOURCES CONSULTED

Beahrs, O. H., Henson, D. E., Hutter, R. V. P., & Myers, M. H. (Eds.). (1988). *Manual for staging of cancer* (3rd ed.). Philadelphia: J. B. Lippincott.

Friedman, M. (Ed.). (1986). Nonsquamous tumors of the head and neck: I. *The Otolaryngologic Clinics of North America* (Vol. 19). Philadelphia: W. B. Saunders.

Gomella, L. G. (Ed.). (1993). *Clinician's pocket reference* (7th ed.). Norwalk, CT: Appleton & Lange.

Greene, F. L., Fritz, A. G., Page, D. L., Fleming, I. D., Haller, D. G., & Morrow, M. (2002). *AJCC manual on cancer staging* (6th ed.). New York: Springer-Verlag.

Jemal, A., Murray, T., Samuels., A., Ghafoor, A., Ward, E., & Thun, M. J. (2003). Cancer statistics. *CA: Cancer Journal, 53*, 5–26.

Layland, M. K. (Ed.). (2004). *Otolaryngology survival guide.* Philadelphia: Lippincott Williams & Wilkins.

McIntire, S. N., & Cioppa, A. L. (Eds.). (1984). *Cancer nursing.* NewYork: John Wiley & Sons.

Rice, D. H., & Spiro, R. H. (1989). *Current concepts in head and neck cancer.* New York: The American Cancer Society.

Shapshay, S. M., & Ossoff, R. H. (Eds.). (1985). Squamous cell cancer of the head and neck. *The Otolaryngologic Clinics of North America* (Vol. 18). Philadelphia: W. B. Saunders.

Shelton, B. K., Ziegfeld, C. R., & Olsen, M. M. (2004). *Manual of cancer nursing* (6th ed.). Philadelphia: Lippincott Williams & Wilkins.

Snyder, C. C. (1986). *Oncology nursing.* Boston: Little, Brown.

CHAPTER 13

Surgeries and Other Procedures

Surgeries involving the oral, pharyngeal, and laryngeal structures are likely to result in changes in speech or swallowing, which require attention from a speech-language pathologist (SLP). Neurologic, cardiothoracic, gastric, and vascular surgeries are frequent features in the histories of patients with neurogenic speech, language, and swallowing disorders. Thus, SLPs often cross paths with children and adult patients who have had surgeries as a part of their history, or who have swallowing and communication disorders directly linked to surgical management.

I. CHAPTER FOCUS

This chapter provides brief descriptions of some of the surgeries that SLPs are most likely to encounter in medically based practice, as well as other procedures usually performed by surgeons. Terminology and abbreviations that may be encountered as part of the patient's surgical history or in summary reports of an operation procedure ("op. reports") and "postop" care are provided. This chapter emphasizes surgeries involving the nervous system; oral and laryngeal structures; gastrointestinal tract; and those commonly performed in childhood with normally developing and disabled children. Several gastrointestinal surgeries in both adults and children are discussed in some detail in Chapter 5, and Chapter 10 references neurologic conditions requiring surgical intervention. Although surgery is frequently a part of the treatment for cancer, particularly with malignant tumors, Chapter 12, Oncology, mainly focuses on the biological and chemotherapies for cancer management; thus, brief descriptions of oral, pharyngeal, and laryngeal surgeries and procedures are provided here.

II. SURGICAL TERMINOLOGY

Abdominal pad. Drainage dressing used over large abdominal suture sites.

Abdominal tray. Instruments and supplies for abdominal surgeries.

Abscess. Localized area of pus.

Absorbable suture. Temporary suture (surgical "thread") that is absorbed in the body.

Administration set. Devices and materials used to deliver or dispense fluids (e.g., intravenous fluid administration set).

Amputation. Removal of a limb or body appendage.

Anastomosis. Joining two tubular or hollow organs; for example, *coronary artery bypass grafts* involve anastomoses of heart vessels.

Anesthesia. Complete or partial loss of feeling and/or consciousness resulting from administration of an anesthetic agent or from disease or injury.

Approach. Referring to the method used and the route taken to reach a body structure in surgery.

Approximate. Bringing tissues together by suturing or other means.

Arthroplasty. Generic term for any joint surgery, including joint replacements.

Atraumatic. In surgery, techniques causing little tissue trauma.

Bed specs. Graduated plastic or metal containers for measuring urine output.

Bifurcated. Y-shaped.

Biopsy needle. Hollow needle used to extract tissue samples.

Bistoury. A slender surgical knife used most frequently to open an abscess.

Bladder irrigation. Washing of the urinary bladder with a solution.

Bleeder. Severed blood vessel.

Blood administration set. Tubing and devices used to dispense whole blood to the patient.

Blood gas tray. Equipment used to measure oxygen and carbon dioxide levels in the blood.

Blowout fracture. Fractures of the orbital walls or orbital floor in association with other facial trauma.

Blunt dissection. Use of a sponge or blunt instrument to separate tissues.

Body restraint. Belts, bands, or vests used to immobilize a patient.

Bougienage dilation. Stretching and expanding a tubular structure with **bougies** (flexible tubes of increasing sizes), done often in cases of esophageal stricture.

Brown and Sharp (B & S) sizing. System for sizing stainless steel suture.

Brushing. Removing debris from a hollow organ or tube by means of a brush and basket.

Burr. A round instrument used for cutting holes into bone.

Butterfly Band-Aids. Adhesive bandages cut in a butterfly shape.

Butterfly infusion set. Scalp vein set with an intravenous catheter and tubing used for intravenous fluid administration with children and infants.

Cadaver. Referring to a dead body or the tissues and organs harvested from a dead body.

Cannula. Inner lining within a hollow tube, such as a tracheostomy tube; tube used to aid in insertion of a drain or to inject medication.

Catgut. Suture material made from the intestines of sheep; it is eventually absorbed into the body.

Catheterization. Introduction of a flexible tube to inject fluids into or drain fluids from the body.

Cautery. Destroying tissue by heat, electricity, or caustic chemicals.

Cavitron. A motorized scalpel that cuts through delicate flesh but leaves blood vessels and ductal tissues intact; used in brain and liver surgeries.

Chest stripper. Instrument used to remove tissues from ribs.

Chest trocar, thoracic trocar. Large-handled sharp instrument with a triangular tip.

Chux. Absorbent underpads used with incontinent patients.

Cisternal puncture. Spinal puncture of the cervical vertebrae.

Clip remover. Instrument used to remove surgical staples from wounds.

Closure. The suturing of a wound.

Clyster. An enema.

Compound F tray. Instruments and supplies used to remove fluid from a joint.

Connecting tube. Plastic or rubber devices used to connect drainage tubes, catheters, pumps, and air supplies.

Conscious sedation. A minimally depressed level of consciousness in which the patient retains the ability to respond to physical or verbal stimulation and maintains protective (swallow, cough) reflexes.

Cryosurgery. Surgery using methods to destroy tissue by extreme cold.

Currette. A spoon-like instrument used to scrape away diseased tissues and growths.

Cutdown. Surgery to expose a vein.

Cutdown tray. Instruments and supplies used to perform a venous cutdown.

Cystectomy. Removal of a cyst.

Debridement. Removal of dead or diseased tissue.

Deep sedation. A controlled state of depressed consciousness or unconsciousness in which there may be a partial or complete loss of protective reflexes and purposeful response to physical or verbal stimulation and from which the patient is not easily aroused.

Dehiscence. Splitting or opening wound.

Desiccation. Drying out (of tissues).

Detritus. Dead epithelial tissue, such as that sloughed from the surface of the skin.

Dilator. Instrument used to expand a hollow organ.

Dissection. Separating tissues.

Divinyl ether. An inhaled anesthetic agent.

Drainage bag. Plastic bag with tubing connectors used to collect fluids, such as urine from indwelling catheters or drains from wounds.

Dressing. External covering or bandage for a wound.

Electrocoagulation. The use of electrical current to produce coagulation and wound closure.

Emerson suction pump. Three bottle suction apparatus used for withdrawing fluid from the chest.

Emesis basin. Kidney-shaped container for collecting vomitus or other secretions.

Epistaxis tray. Instruments and supplies to control nasal hemorrhages.

Ethyl chloride. A local anesthesia that freezes the tissues it contacts.

Evacuation. Removal of drainage from a natural passage.

Eviscerate. In surgery, splitting open a (surgical) wound and to remove contents. The term *evisceration* can also refer to opening of the abdomen to remove or expose the intestines.

Excision. Removal of a piece of tissue.

Exploration. Surgical opening to examine internal organs.

Fenestrated. Having openings.

Finger cot. Small rubber or plastic shield used to protect a finger from soil or infection.

Fistula. An abnormal opening or communication between cavities, or vessels; fistulae may be surgically created, for example, a tracheoesophageal fistula (TEF) is created to accommodate a voice prosthesis after laryngectomy, or it may occur spontaneously, for example, an unwanted fistula may develop following wound closures in surgery.

Flatus bag. Plastic tubing attached to a bag inserted to expel gas from the colon.

Fluffs. Pressure dressings for postoperative wound coverings with certain surgeries, such as hemorrhoidectomies and thyroidectomies.

Fowler's position. Position in which the patient is sitting in a reclined posture with the head raised by about 20 inches to aid in draining fluids from the peritoneum or as a preferred positioning for endotracheal suctioning.

Fracture. Broken bone. A **compound fracture** refers to a fracture that penetrates adjacent soft tissue; **open fractures** penetrate the skin; **greenstick fractures** are partial breaks in bone; **comminuted fractures** refer to a bone splintered into many fragments; **impacted fractures** refer to bones that have penetrated other bones; **spiral fractures** are bones twisted apart in a spiral pattern; **transverse fractures** have fracture lines perpendicular to the length of the bone; and **pathologic fractures** are bone breaks caused by disease rather than injury.

French catheter scale. A scaled method of measurement in which "1" equals ⅓ mm diameter and each incremental size increase is increased by ⅓ mm (e.g., #2 French equals ⅔ mm diameter, #3 French equals 1 mm, etc.).

Friable. Tissue that is easily torn.

Frozen section. Process by which a piece of tissue is frozen for microscopic examination; tissue analysis is conducted during the surgery to provide a diagnosis before closure.

Furacin pads. Gauze dressings soaked in antibacterial ointment.

Gastric connecting tubing. Flexible tubing used to connect nasogastric tubing with a suction machine.

Gelfilm™. Trademarked name for a gelatin film used to stop local bleeding.

Gelfoam™. Trademarked name for a foam product used to stop bleeding.

General anesthesia. A controlled state of unconsciousness accompanied by a loss of protective reflexes and purposeful response to physical or verbal stimulation.

Graduate. Container with graduated markings used for liquid measurements.

Graft. Transplanting tissue from a donor or from one part of the body to another.

Hagedorn needle. A surgical needle with a cutting edge, used to sew up skin, and as a finger-pricking needle used to draw blood.

Halo brace. Halo ring with a brace suprastructure used to immobilize the neck of a patient with a high spinal cord injury.

Head halter. Device made of foam rubber and cotton used to secure head positioning for cervical traction.

Hemostat. A device or agent that stops the flow of blood.

Hot pack. Moist, hot dressing.

Huck towels. Specially woven towels used to dry hands after a surgical scrub or for surgical draping and to absorb fluids during surgery.

Hypodermic. Below the skin.

Incision. A cut into soft tissue with a sharp instrument.

Infusion. Introduction of fluid into a vein.

Intracatheter. Narrow tubing inserted into a vein for infusion of fluids, injection, or venous pressure monitoring.

Iodoform. Iodine compound used as an antiseptic.

Irrigation. Cleansing of a body cavity, surface, or wound with a stream of fluid solution or water.

Jackson tracheostomy tubes. Variable-sized stainless steel or silver-plated tracheostomy tubes.

Javid shunt™. Trademarked name for a type of plastic tubing used to temporarily bypass the carotid artery during carotid endarterectomy.

Kelly forceps. Forceps with scissors-like handles used as hemostats to stop blood flow.

Kerlix bandage. A soft, woven rolled bandage.

Lancet. A surgical knife used for puncturing.

Laparotomy. Opening used for freeing adhesions and/or exploring the abdomen.

Leg bag. Drainage bag for a urinary catheter that is attached to the leg with two rubber straps.

Lidocaine. A local anesthesic agent.

Ligate. To tie something together.

Ligation clips. Special metal clips placed around a structure to ligate vessels, nerves, or ducts.

Local anesthesia. A limited loss of sensation around a particular site.

Logan bow. External metal loop used to close skin and reduce tension on deep muscles and fascia.

Loupes. In surgery, magnifying lenses used by the surgeon during microsurgery; loupes may be fitted to glasses; other physicians as well as dentists and others (e.g., jewelers and other individuals who do fine assembly work) also use loupes for close visual inspection.

Lumen. The channel or opening into a tubular or other hollow structure.

Lumpectomy. Removal of a tumor or other mass.

Malecot catheter. Wing-tipped catheter used for fluid drainage from the body cavities.

Mask. Facial covering.

Microtome. A laboratory device used to slice thin sections of tissue for examination under a microscope.

Nasal cannula. Plastic tubing with a nosepiece used to administer oxygen through the nose.

Nasal speculum. Instrument used to expand or dilate the nares.

Necrotic. Dead tissue.

Nidus. Point where a pathologic lesion has developed.

Nitrous oxide. The anesthetic gas used for light anesthesia, known as "laughing gas."

Operative monitoring. During surgeries, there is continuous monitoring of heart rate, respiratory rate, and blood pressure as well as visual monitoring of the patient's color every five minutes.

Osteoclasis. The deliberate rebreaking of a bone to reset alignment more adequately.

Osteophyte. Bony outgrowth.

Osteotome. A surgical bone chisel.

Paracentesis. Puncture and drainage of a body cavity.

Penrose drain. A rubber tube with a gauze center inserted into a wound to drain fluids; also called a *cigarette drain.*

Pentothal. An intravenous anesthetic agent.

Percutaneous needle biopsy. A procedure usually done under fluoroscopy in which a biopsy needle is inserted through a small incision and cells are aspirated for analysis.

Phantom limb pain. Sensation sometimes following amputations in which pain is felt to be emanating from the missing limb as if the limb were still there.

Pipette. A calibrated, open-ended glass tube used to measure or transfer small volumes of fluids.

Pledget. Small compress of gauze, such as a "2 × 2" or "4 × 4" gauze square.

Politzer's bag. A device used to inflate the middle ear.

Prosthesis. An artificial body part.

Radiosurgery. Using radium in surgical treatment.

Ratchets. Interlocking clasps that hold the finger rings of an instrument together (such as the clasps found on a hemostat).

Resection. Removal of all or part of an organ or structure.

Robinson catheter. A round-tipped, double-ported plastic or rubber tube used for wound drainage or aspirating fluids.

Rongeur. A pliers-like instrument with sharp edges.

Salvage procedure. A surgical repair procedure usually performed after other procedures have failed or resulted in complications.

Scalpel blade. A thin, disposable blade that attaches to a scalpel handle.

Scalp vein needle. An intravenous catheter used to administer fluids to infants.

Section. Cutting through a structure.

Serrated. Referring to a notched or saw-toothed margin.

Sheepskin. Fleece pad used to reduce risks for pressure sores in immobile patients.

Shunt. A congenital, acquired, or surgically placed hole or passage to move or allow movement of fluid from one location or body part to another; examples include *portacaval shunts* for treatment of hypertension in the liver; *cardiac shunts*; *cerebrospinal fluid* (CSF) *shunts*; *pulmonary shunts*; *portosystemic shunts*; and *dialysis access shunts.* Types of CSF shunts are listed later in this chapter, under "Neurosurgeries and Procedures."

Skin bond cement. Adhesive paste used to attach prostheses or stomal bags to the skin.

Snare. An instrument fitted with a wire loop used to snare and sever a tumor or polyp.

Sponge. Gauze pad.

Staples. Fine stainless steel surgical wires formed into a "B" shape when inserted through the skin; used to approximate (close) surfaces or wound edges.

Stents and keels. Silastic or Teflon devices used to fix tissues into place to prevent closures. Stents may be used to keep a fistula or vessel open when desirable, and keels may be used, for example, to prevent re-formation of webs after glottic webs have been sectioned or excised.

Stereotaxis. The use of a three-dimensional apparatus to precisely locate structures.

Sterile tape. Paper tapes that are adhesive on one side; used to approximate edges of skin wounds.

Stilet, stylet. Sharp instrument used to probe or to guide catheters during insertion.

Stryker frame™. Positioning frame; trademarked name for an apparatus used to move and position patients.

Suppuration. Pus formation in infected tissue.

Suture. To sew up a wound; also the thread or wire used to sew up a wound.

Swab. Small pledget, or gauze pad.

Tamponade. Stopping blood flow by pressure.

T.B.C. syringe. Referring to a tuberculin calibrated syringe.

T-drain. Small tubing used especially for bile drainage following gallbladder surgery.

Telfa™. Trademarked name for absorbent, nonadherent dressings used on burns and superficial wounds.

Tenaculum. A tongs-like instrument used to hold a body part during surgery.

Tissue forceps. Fine-tipped, tweezer-like instrument used to grasp tissue.

Tracheostomy ties. Twill tape used to secure tracheostomy tubes.

Triage. System used to classify emergencies by the severity of the injury or illness.

III. SURGERIES AND PROCEDURES IN CHILDREN AND ADULTS

A. Otolaryngology and Head and Neck Surgeries and Procedures

Adenectomy. Removal of a gland.

Adenotonsillectomy. Removal of the pharyngeal lymphatic tissue (adenoids) and the lymphatic tissue of the fauces (palatine and lingual tonsils).

Arytenoidectomy. Removal of an arytenoid.

Arytenoid-epiglottic flap. Procedure to close off the entrance to the larynx by folding the epiglottis posteriorly and suturing it to the arytenoid cartilage to prevent aspiration.

Arytenoid rotation. Repositioning of the arytenoid, usually following traumatic dislocation.

Atticotomy. Surgical opening into the attic of the middle ear.

Aural toilette. Cleaning the external ear with a Frazier suction tip under microscopic visualization.

***Botulinum* toxin injection.** Needle injection of botulism (Botox), a neurotoxin, into muscles usually under electromyographic guidance; Botox is used in treatment for a variety of disorders, chiefly the treatment of certain facial, neck, and laryngeal dystonias and or as an aesthetic procedure to reduce wrinkles.

Cheiloplasty. Plastic surgical repair of the lip.

Cheilostomatoplasty. Plastic surgical repair of the lip and mouth, as in cleft lip repairs.

Cochlear implantation. A surgical technique in which a hole is drilled into the mastoid bone (specific approach is called a *facial recess approach)* into the middle ear space to get access to the round window. Electrodes are then threaded into the round window opening to provide direct stimulation of the cochlea from a receiver that has been secured to the temporal (mastoid) bone.

Cordectomy. Removal of a vocal fold.

Cricopharyngeal myotomy. Surgical dissection of the cricopharyngeous muscle to cause a relaxation of the upper esophageal sphincter in an effort to discourage recurrence of a Zenker's diverticulum, to treat chronic aspiration and vocal fold paralysis, or to improve alaryngeal voice with the tracheoesophageal (TEP) fistula voice prostheses.

Cyst, mass, and tumor excisions. Children and adults can have infectious, autoimmune, benign and malignant cysts, masses, and tumors. Cysts, masses, and tumors may be congenital or develop late in life, and many require excision by a surgeon, particularly if the pathology findings indicate malignancies or if their presence is compromising vital organs and breathing. Examples of common head and neck masses in children include *branchial cleft masses*; *dermoid cysts*, *thymic cysts*; *lymphangiomas*; *laryngoceles; hemangiomas;* and *teratomas* (congenital masses that contain one to three germ layers, and typically have remnants of hair, teeth, or bone). Both children and adults may be diagnosed with any of the range of malignant tumor types discussed in Chapter 12, requiring surgical removal or tumor "debulking" (removal of a part of the mass or tumor).

Dilatation of the larynx. Stretching the laryngeal structures with instruments.

Epiglottectomy. Removal of the epiglottis.

Fat patch. Repair of a tympanic membrane perforation with a small amount of fat tissues taken from the retroauricular tissue of the earlobe.

Frenulum clipping. Surgically cutting a shortened frenulum to relieve restricted tongue movement, "tongue tie."

Full mouth extraction. Removal of all of the patient's teeth.

Gingivectomy. The surgical removal of part of the gums.

Glossectomy, hemi- or partial glossectomy. Removal of all or part of the tongue.

Hemilaryngectomy. Removal of one-half of the structures of the larynx in the vertical plane; **vertical laryngectomy** is synonymous.

Hemimandibulectomy. Removal of up to half of the mandible.

Laryngectomy. Removal of the larynx, hyoid bone, and strap muscles along with creating a permanent tracheostomy and closing any communication between the trachea and the oropharynx (see Figure 13–1 for a comparison of the anatomical changes pre- and postlaryngectomy).

Laryngofissure. Surgical incision to create a "wide window" with medial opening into the thyroid cartilage, usually done to remove a cancerous tumor.

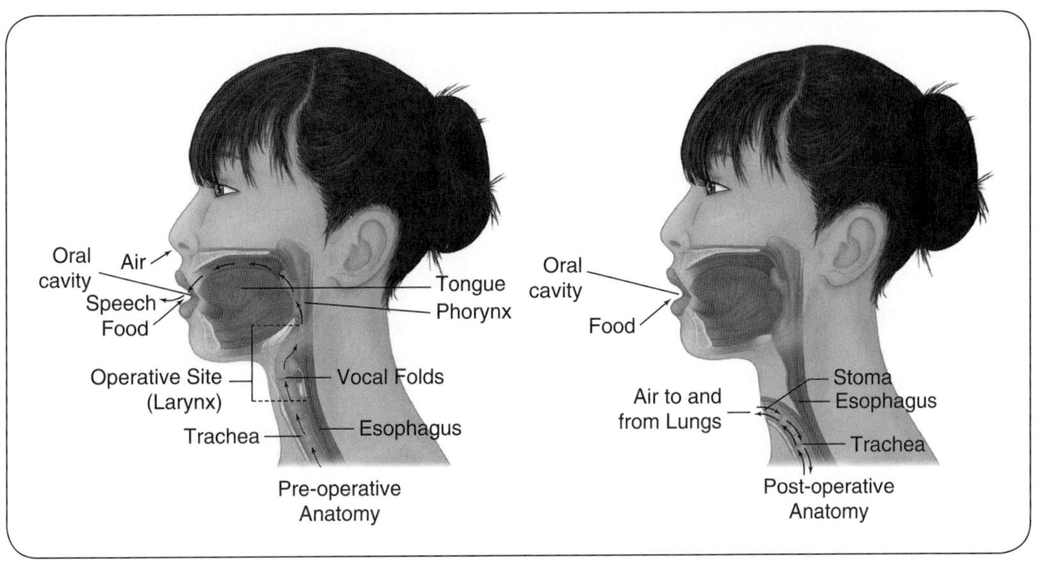

FIGURE 13–1 Laryngectomy: (A) Preoperative anatomy. (B) Postoperative anatomy. Source: Delmar/Cengage Learning

Laryngostomy. Opening into the larynx.

Mandibulectomy. Removal of all or most of the mandible.

Near-total laryngectomy. An operation designed to ablate (remove) all of a laryngeal tumor but not all of the larynx. Most near-total techniques leave a mucosal bridge over the uninvolved arytenoid, and the recurrent laryngeal nerve on the unaffected side of the larynx is spared. A primitive tracheopharyngeal sphincter with the laryngeal "leftovers" and a mucosal flap from the pharynx are techniques used to allow for a prosthesis-free method of speech and to prevent aspiration.

Nerve-muscle pedicle graft to the larynx. A technique for reinnervating a paralyzed larynx using the ansa of the hypoglossal nerve and the omohyoid muscle as a nerve-muscle pedicle.

Palatoplasty. Surgical repair of the palate, as in cleft palate surgeries.

Parotidectomy. Resection of the parotid gland.

Partial laryngectomy. Subtotal removal of the larynx.

Periapical tissue biopsy. Biopsy of tissue from the roots of the teeth to examine for a malignant process.

Pharyngectomy. Removal of pharyngeal tissue.

Phonosurgeries. Surgeries done for the purpose of improving phonation; include **thyroplasties**, **recurrent nerve resection**, **laser therapy** for *plica ventricularis*, and **injection of bulking substances** into the vocal folds (Teflon injection, lipoprotein [fat] injections, collagen injections).

Radical neck dissection (RND). Surgical removal of the lymph nodes of the neck on the side of a malignant tumor that contain, or potentially contain, cancerous cells.

Septectomy. Surgical correction of a deviated nasal septum.

Sialadenectomy. Removal of a salivary gland.

Sialolithotomy. Removal of a salivary stone.

Stoma revisions, Z-plasties of the stoma. Plastic surgical technique to reduce stoma scar tissue stenosis by releasing the circular tension on the stoma.

Stomatoplasty, stoma plasty. Plastic surgical repair of the mouth, or stoma.

Supraglottic laryngectomy. Removal of the endolaryngeal structures from the tip of the epiglottis down to the upper laryngeal structures without sacrificing the remaining larynx; **subtotal horizontal laryngectomy** is synonymous.

Thyroidectomy, partial thyroidectomy, hemithyroidectomy, parathyroidectomy, partial parathyroidectomy. Excision of all or part of the thyroid gland or parathyroid gland.

Thyroplasties, laryngeal framework surgeries. Referring to surgeries that involve creating a window in the ala of the thyroid between the inner and the outer perichondrium on the side of a weakened vocal fold and implanting a Silastic wedge to medialize the fold for improved phonation.

Tonsillectomy and adenoidectomy (T & A). Removal of hyperthrophic tonsillar and adenoid tissue in the pharynx to prevent recurrent infections, sleep disturbances, dysphagia, and airway obstructions. Tonsillar hyperthrophy is graded as follows: 1+ (tissue obstructs 0–25% to midline); 2+ (25–50%); 3+ (50–75%); and 4+ (75–100%).

Tracheoesophageal puncture (TEP) voice restoration. Creation of a fistula from the tracheal wall of the tracheostoma after laryngectomy into the esophagus for the purpose of fitting a TEP prosthesis for alaryngeal speech. This surgery may be performed as a part of the **primary procedure** (at the time of the laryngectomy) or may be a **secondary procedure** (performed sometime following the total laryngectomy).

Tracheostomy. Opening into the trachea (Figure 13–2).

Tracheotomy. Incision into the trachea.

Tympanoplasty. Repair of large perforations of the tympanic membrane with grafting.

Uvulopalatopharyngoplasty (UP). Either a laser-assisted (LAUP) or cold steel (scalpel) procedure to remove wedges of the uvular tissue bilaterally to improve or eliminate snoring.

Vocal fold fusion. Surgical technique that closes the glottis to prevent severe aspiration. Patients require a tracheostomy following this surgery and an alaryngeal method for speech.

Voice restoration techniques. Surgeries designed to provide a phonation alternative following removal of all or most of the larynx. These surgeries may involve anatomical reconstructions without the use of mechanical aids or other prostheses or reconstructions performed to accommodate either implanted or removable prostheses. Reconstructive surgeries include construction of a neoglottis (such as the **Staffieri technique**), creating a mucoarytenoid shunt of the airway into the esophagus, creating a pharyngoesophageal mucosal flap, creating a reed-fistula from the trachea to the hypopharynx, and creating a tracheoesophageal fistula to insert a valved prosthesis (see *tracheoesophageal puncture* voice restoration).

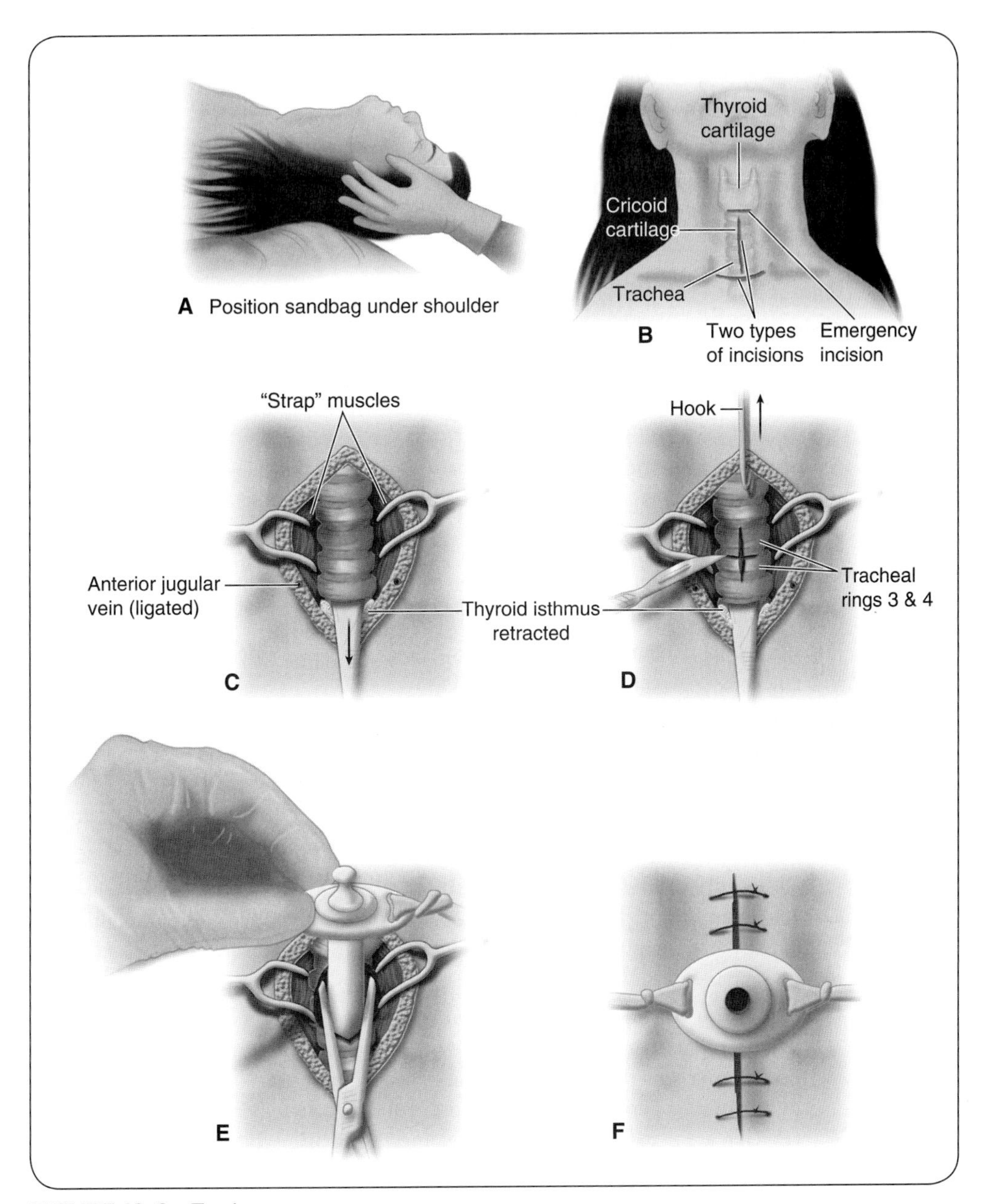

FIGURE 13–2 Tracheostomy. Source: Delmar/Cengage Learning

B. Gastrointestinal and Other Abdominal Surgeries and Procedures

Adrenalectomy. Removal of all or part of the adrenal gland(s).

Antrectomy. Removal of the gastrin-producing pyloric gland of the stomach.

Appendectomy. Removal of the appendix.

Brunschwig's operation. Removal of all of the pelvic organs in order to stop massive spread of cancer.

Celiotomy. Any surgery that opens the abdomen.

Cholecystectomy. Removal of the gallbladder.

Cholecystogastronomy. Surgically joining of the gallbladder to the stomach.

Choledocholithotomy. Removal of stones from the common bile duct leading from the gallbladder.

Colectomy. Removal of a section of the colon.

Colostomy. Surgical creation of an abdominal output (stoma) from the colon, usually following a colectomy.

Diverticulectomy. Surgical correction of an outpouching, or diverticulum, of the esophagus (or intestines).

Esophageal myotomy. Surgical dissection of a portion of esophageal muscle.

Esophagectomy. Removal of all or part of the esophagus.

Esophagojejunostomy. Surgical joining of the esophagus and jejunum.

Fundic patch. Surgical repair of a ruptured esophagus or an acid-peptic stricture at the distal esophageal-stomach juncture.

Fundoplication. Surgical procedure to relieve severe gastroesophageal reflux and improve gastroesophageal competence (see Figure 5–5).

Gastric bypass surgery. Procedures, for example, the **Roux-en-Y gastric bypass (RGB)** and **biliopancreatic diversion,** performed for weight control with severely obese patients involving a surgical reduction of the size of the stomach and repositioning of the small intestine, bypassing the duodenum and part of the jejunum.

Gastric resection. Removal of the majority of the stomach and joining the resected stomach to the *duodenum* (Billroth I procedure) or to the *jejunum* (Billroth II procedure).

Gastric transposition (pull-up) operation. Method for reconstructing the gullet usually after esophageal cancer surgery by creating an end-to-end anastomosis of the hypopharynx and stomach.

Gastrostomy tube placement. Creation of an opening into the stomach for insertion of a permanent or temporary tube. **Operative gastrostomy (OG)** refers to procedures done under general anesthesia usually by a general surgeon (Figure 13–3). Gastrostomies performed by percutaneous methods, or **percutaneous endoscopic gastrostomies (PEGs),** are usually done under local anesthesia by a surgeon or a gastroenterologist. Complications associated with gastrostomies include wound infections, gastric wall hematoma, gastrocolic fistula, and benign **pneumoperitoneum** (air entering the lining of the body cavity). Figure 13–4 illustrates the pediatric gastrostomy tube in place.

Hemorrhoidectomy. Removal of hemorrhoids.

Hepatic lobectomy. Removal of a lobe of the liver.

Hiatus (hiatal) hernia repair. Surgical procedures to correct a defect that permitted the esophagus to pass through the diaphragm.

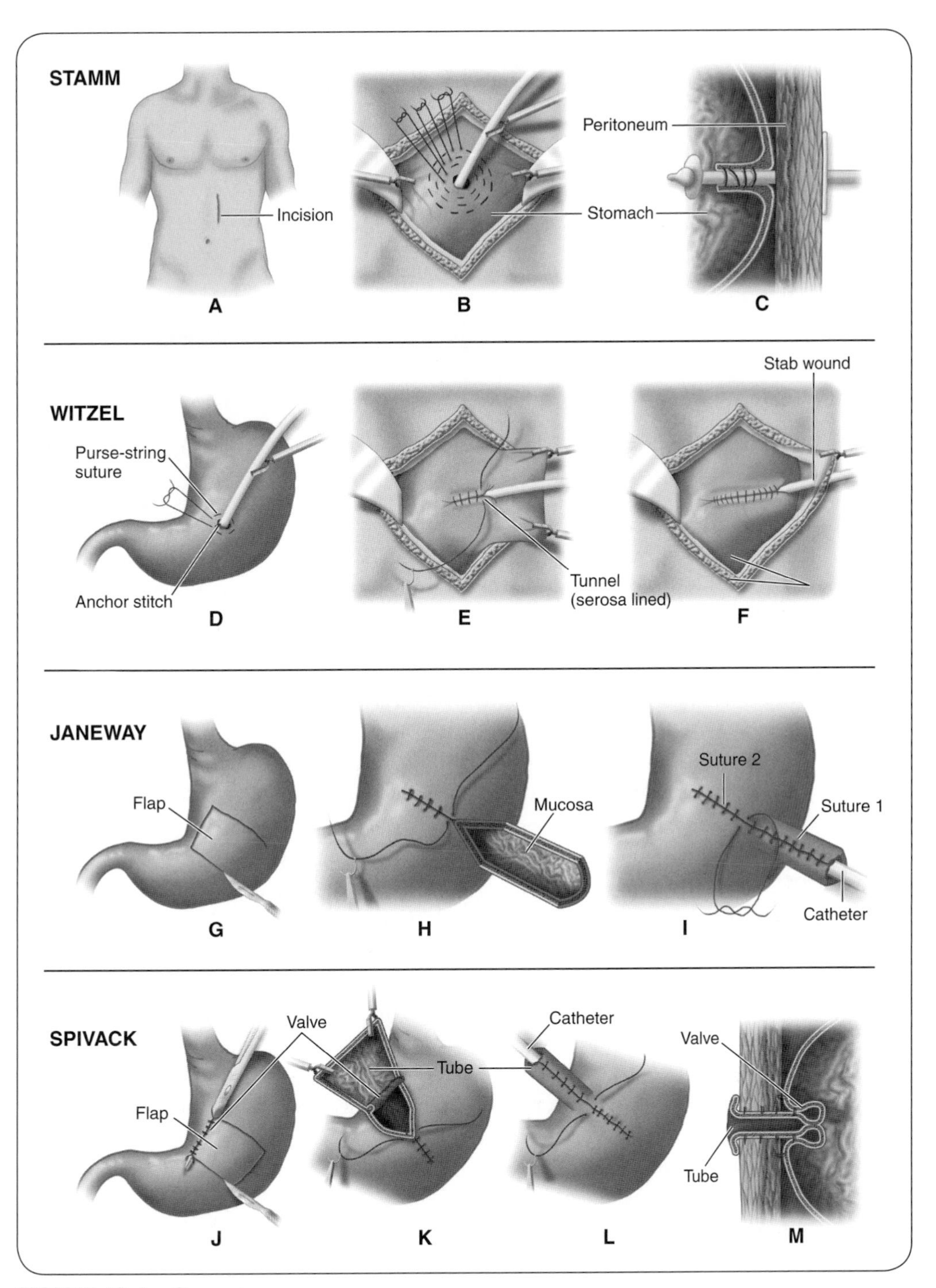

FIGURE 13–3 Gastrostomy. Source: Delmar/Cengage Learning

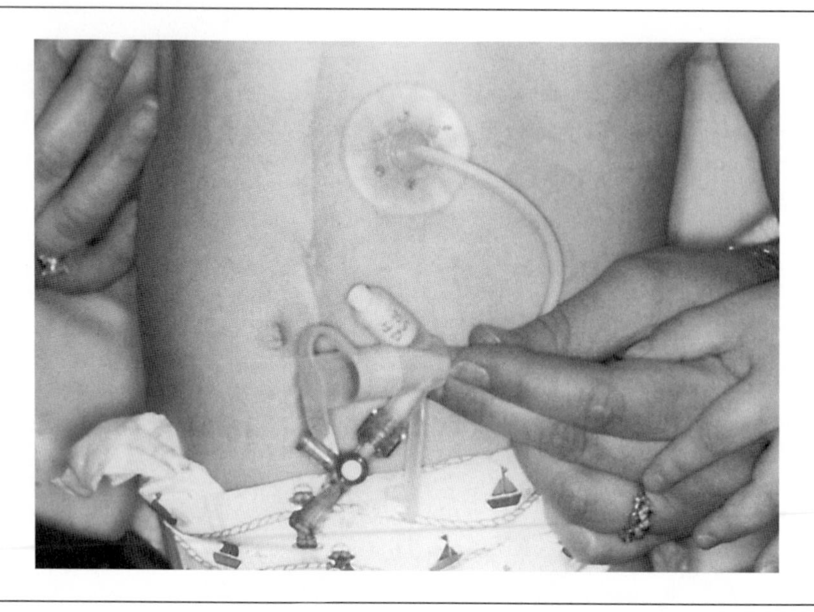

FIGURE 13–4 Pediatric patient with gastrostomy tube. Source: Arvedson, J. C., & Brodsky, L. (Eds.). (2002). *Pediatric swallowing and feeding: Assessment and management* (2nd ed.). Clifton Park, NY: Delmar Cengage Learning.

Ileostomy. Creating an opening into the ileum.

Imperforate anus repair. Surgical creation of an anal opening when one has failed to develop.

Inguinal hernia repair. Surgical correction of a tear or defect in the abdominal wall in the groin area of a male that had allowed abdominal contents to protrude (herniation).

Jejunostomy. Creating an opening into the jejunum.

Jejunostomy tube placement. Procedure for placing an enteral feeding tube into the jejunum. A percutaneous endoscopic jejunostomy placement is similar to a PEG (see earlier), except that a dual-lumen tube is used. The distal tip of the feeding tube is directed into the duodenum endoscopically with the proximal port left to decompress the stomach.

Lapband Procedure. A procedure performed for the purpose of weight reduction in severely obese individuals that involves the insertion of a fluid-filled band around the upper portion of the stomach by way of laparoscopy.

Pancreatectomy. Removal of part or all of the pancreas. The Whipple procedure, or *pancreaticojejunostomy*, refers to a large surgical resection of the pancreas as well as the duodenum, part of the stomach, and bile duct.

Percutaneous endoscopic gastrostomy (PEG). G-tube inserted through the abdominal wall under endoscopy.

Pharyngostomy and esophagostomy tube placement. Procedures performed under general or local anesthesia to place an enteral feeding tube in the pharynx or esophagus.

Proctoplasty. Removal and reconstruction of the rectum.

Resection of esophageal stricture. Removal of a narrowed portion of the esophagus followed by a colonic bypass anastomosis.

Thymectomy. Removal of all or part of the thymus gland(s).

Vagotomy. Denervation of the vagal nerve branch to the stomach to eliminate excessive stimulation of acid production to treat chronic gastric or duodenal ulcers.

C. Neurosurgeries and Procedures

Aneurysm repair. Surgical clipping or ligation of an artery to correct an aneurysm (ballooning out of a weakened vessel wall). In some cases, vascular bypass may be performed to prevent ischemia distal to the affected vessel.

Brain resections. Removal of brain tissue to treat intractable epilepsy or to remove all or a portion of brain tumors.

Cerebral artery bypass, enarterectomy, and anastomosis. Microvascular surgeries on the cerebral arteries to treat cerebrovascular disease.

Cervical fusion. Excision of one or more herniated cervical intervertebral disc(s) and placement of bone grafts to cause fusion of the discs.

Commissurotomy. Sectioning the anterior commissure or some part of the corpus callosum of the brain.

Cordotomy. Sectioning of the lateral pathways of the spinal cord to alleviate pain.

Cranioplasty. Replacement of an area of cranial bone with an autograft, metal prosthesis, or methylmethacrylate plate.

Craniotomy. Creating an opening into the skull to expose the brain or its coverings.

Evacuation of a hematoma (hemorrhage). Aspiration and drainage of a blood mass located in or causing pressure on the brain.

Laminectomy. Creating an opening into the lamina of the spinal cord usually to repair a herniated disc.

Lobectomy. Resection of a large portion of the brain.

Neurorrhaphy. Peripheral nerve repair with anastomosis of a severed nerve.

Rhizotomy. Sectioning a nerve root. **Neurectomy** refers to removing a nerve segment.

Shunts (cerebrospinal fluid). Diverting CSF away from the ventricles to another location to correct or prevent hydrocephalus, such as with **ventriculoatrial shunts** (in which a thin catheter with a valve to prevent reflux is tunneled under the scalp from a ventricle to an exit site through the common facial vein and reinserted percutaneously through the internal jugular vein to the superior vena cava) or **ventriculoperitoneal shunts** (in which the shunt tube is placed into the peritoneal cavity for drainage) (see Figure 11–1).

Sympathectomy. Sectioning of a sympathetic nerve.

Thalamotomy. Removal of a part of the thalamus.

D. Cardiothoracic and Pulmonary (Chest) Surgeries and Procedures

Also see Chapter 9, Cardiac, Pulmonary, and Hematologic Functions.

Atrial septal defect correction. Surgical closure of a congenital anomaly that had allowed blood from the left atrium to flow across into the right atrium.

Balloon catheterization. Placement of a catheter having a distal, inflatable (helium-filled) balloon into a blood vessel or heart chamber.

Cardiac catheterization. Passage of a long, thin catheter that is specially designed for passage through the blood vessels into the heart chambers for examination and to take special samples of blood, blood pressure, and cardiac output measures.

Cardiopulmonary bypass. Temporary diversion of the blood from the heart and lungs to be able to perform surgery on the heart or major vessels.

Closure of a patent ductus arteriosus. Surgical closure of an unnatural communication between the pulmonary artery and the thoracic aorta.

Coronary artery bypass grafts (CABG). Surgery to improve blood flow to the heart that involves taking an autogenous vein graft (vein from elsewhere in the patient's body), such as the saphenous vein from the lower leg, and *anastomosing* one end of the grafted vein to the ascending aorta and the other end to one or more of the arteries supplying the heart.

Correction of a coarctation of the thoracic aorta. Surgical correction of a congenital stenosis of the thoracic aorta.

Insertion of chest tubes. Surgical insertion of drainage tubes into the pleural cavity to remove blood or air that has accumulated after a thoracotomy.

Lobectomy. Removal of a lobe of the lung.

Lung biopsy. Excision of a small piece of lung tissue for microscopic analysis to establish a diagnosis of lung disease.

Pacemaker insertion. Suturing electrodes (with external batteries) to the heart to correct *bradycardia*, *heart block*, or *arrhythmias*.

Percutaneous transluminal coronary angioplasty (PTCA). Catheterization guided by radiologic imaging to examine and repair coronary artery disease.

Pneumonectomy. Removal of a lung.

Resection of an aneurysm of the ascending aorta. Surgical removal of an aneurysm section in the ascending aorta that typically has caused the aorta valve to become incompetent.

Resection of an aneurysm of the descending thoracic aorta. Surgical removal of an aneurysm section from the descending aorta.

Sternotomy. Cutting through the sternum to gain access to the heart.

Thoracotomy. Surgical opening into the thoracic region.

Valve replacements. Surgical implantation of prosthetic valves in place of irreversibly damaged heart valves (aortic valve, mitral valve, and tricuspid valve).

E. Orthopedic Surgeries, Devices, and Procedures

Amputation. Surgical removal of a limb, most often necessitated by diabetes-related peripheral vascular insufficiency or a malignancy.

AO/ASIF plates, screws, system. *AO* refers to "Arbeitsgemeinscraft fur Osteosynthesefragen," and in English-speaking countries it is known as the Association for the Study of Internal Fixation (ASIF). AO/ASIF devices or systems include any orthopedic apparatus designed based on the principles of the AO or ASIF.

Arthroplasty. Reconstructive surgery to a joint.

Arthroscopy. Direct visualization of a joint through a fiberoptic instrument.

Hand tendon surgeries. Surgical treatment of diseases affecting the hand tendons, such as tendon release surgery for *Dupuytren's contracture* (disease causing finger contractures) or surgery to release pressure on the median nerve of the wrist found with carpal tunnel syndrome.

Joint replacement surgeries. Surgical implantation of prosthetic joints (e.g., hip, knee, and shoulder joint replacement prostheses); includes **total hip arthroplasty (THA)** and **total knee arthroplasty (TKA).**

Knodt rod. A type of orthopedic fixation rod used in spinal reconstructive surgeries.

Knowles pin. An orthopedic fixation pin.

Kuntscher nail. An intramedullary nail used for fracture fixation.

Kurosaka screw. A type of headless orthopedic screw used to anchor grafts in the metaphysis of the femur and tibia.

Lane plate. A metal plate used for bone fixation following fractures.

Neufeld nail. A fixation device used for intertrochanteric femur fractures.

Neutralization plate. Device used in the shafts of long bones to provide stabilization of fragments.

Orion plate. A type of anterior fixation plate used in cervical fusions.

Osseointregration. Forming a chemical bond between bone and an implant.

Somi brace. A cervical spine brace.

Total hip arthroplasty, total hip replacement. Repair and reconstructive surgery to the hip with placement of a prosthetic hip joint.

Universal rod. A type of spinal fixation rod.

Wiltse system. A type of spinal fixation system using pedicle screws that are connected to a rod by clamps.

Yale brace. A type of cervical spine brace.

Zickle rod. A spinal fixation device using a unilateral plate attached laterally with screws into the vertebral spine.

F. Vascular and Lymph System Surgeries

Abdominal aortic aneurysm and aortic femoral bypass. The surgical removal of an abdominal aortic aneurysm and insertion of a bifurcated vessel prosthesis.

Carotid endarterectomy. Surgical removal of atherosclerotic plaque from an obstructed carotid artery.

Femoral-popliteal bypass. Surgical implantation of an artificial or autogenous (from elsewhere in the patient's body) vessel graft into the femoral and popliteal arteries.

Lymphadenectomy. Excision of lymph nodes.

Lymphadenotomy. Incision and drainage of a lymph gland.

Portacaval shunt. The surgical anastomosis of a portal vein of the liver to the vena cava to alleviate portal hypertension.

Portal shunt. Surgical method used to treat variceal hemorrhaging by diverting the blood of a hypertensive portal liver system into a normal systemic venous system.

Vein stripping. Surgical removal of the saphenous veins to alleviate severe varicose veins in the legs.

G. Urogenital Surgeries and Procedures

Adenectomy. Removal of all or part of a gland.

Circumcision. Removal of a part of the prepuce to expose the glans penis.

Cystectomy. Removal of part or all of the bladder.

Cystoplasty. Surgical repair of the bladder.

Hysterectomy. Removal of the uterus.

Kidney transplant (KTx). Organ donor transplantation surgery of a kidney.

Nephrectomy. Excision of one or both kidneys.

Nephrotomy. Incision into a kidney.

Orchiectomy. Removal of the testes.

Orchioplasty. Surgical repair of the testes.

Pyeloplasty. Surgical repair of the renal pelvis.

Renal transplantation. Removal of irreversibly diseased kidneys and replacement with a donor kidney from a tissue-matched living donor or cadaver organ donor.

Transurethral resection of the bladder (TURB). Endoscopic resection of the bladder to remove nonelastic tissues causing poor bladder control.

Transurethral resection of the prostate (TURP). Endoscopic resection of some portion of a hypertrophic prostate gland.

Tubal ligation. Sectioning and ligating the uteral tubes for birth control.

Ureteral resection. Excision of a ureteral lesion.

Ureterectomy. Removal of the ureter.

Vasectomy. Removal and ligation of the vas deferens.

H. Plastic, Aesthetic, Reconstructive, and Other Surgeries and Procedures

Augmentation mammoplasty. Surgery to enhance the size of breasts, usually with implants.

Blepharoplasty. Surgical repair of the eyelid, usually to remove redundant tissue.

Blephrectomy. Excision of an eyelid.

***Botulinum* toxin injection.** Needle injection of *botulinum* toxin (botulism), or **Botox**, a neurotoxin, into muscles usually under electromyographic guidance; botox is used in treatment for a wide variety of disorders, chiefly the treatment of dystonia in certain facial, neck, and laryngeal muscle groups, and as an aesthetic procedure to reduce facial wrinkles.

Cataract surgery. Removal of an opaque lens.

Chronal atresia repair. Surgical correction of a congenital condition occurring when the bucconasal membrane fails to separate, leading to a nasopharyngeal obstruction, respiratory distress, and nasal breathing.

Cleft lip repair. Cosmetic repair of a congenital cleft lip; the timing for surgery will generally follow what is referred to as the "rule of 10s" in which repair surgery will be performed when the infant is more than 10 weeks old, weighs more than 10 pounds, and has a hemoglobin (Hgb) greater than 10. Repair procedures can include a **lip adhesiolysis**, **rotation advancement** procedure, or **triangular flap** procedure.

Cleft palate repair. Various surgical techniques used to close the opening between the oral cavity and the nasal cavity to improve feeding, swallowing, and speech intelligibility. Procedures can include a **levator swing reconstruction,** in which surgery is performed at around 18 months of age to allow for better speech development (but also potentially hindering facial development); a **Furrows palatoplasty**; **V-Y push back technique**; **von Langenbeck's palatoplasty** (bipedicled mucoperiosteal flap); or the **Schweckendieck procedure** (primary veloplasty wtih closure of the velum at 4–12 months). Cleft lip and palate descriptive terms include: *complete cleft lip* (involves the entire lip and alveolar arch); *incomplete cleft lip* (involves a portion of the lip); *primary cleft palate* (involves the anterior to incisive foreman); *secondary cleft palate* (involves the posterior to incisive foreman); and *submucous cleft* (mucosa is intact but there is underdeveloped musculature, bifid uvula, or notching of the posterior hard palate).

Corneal surgery. Surgical repair of cornea defects. **Cornea transplant** surgery involves replacing a full-thickness cornea with a donor graft.

Dacryocystectomy. Removal of a lacrimal gland.

Ectropion repair. Plastic surgical repair of a sagging lower eyelid.

Enucleation. Removal of an eye.

Evisceration of the eye. Removal of the contents of an eye.

External ear malformation repairs. Surgeries to correct a variety of congenital malformations of the pinna, including *prominent ear*; *microtia* (graded from I, mild/nearly normal, to III, only a small lobule or skin tag is present; and *cup ear deformity* (the upper part of the ear is bent).

Functional endoscopic sinus surgery (FESS). Surgery using endoscopic instruments to correct nasal sinus abnormalities.

Labyrinthectomy. Destruction of the labyrinth of the inner ear to treat intractable vertigo.

Mammoplasty. Plastic surgery of the breast, usually to improve the appearance.

Mastoidectomy. Removal of diseased mastoid tissue.

Myringoplasty. Surgical repair of the tympanic membrane with a graft.

Myringotomy. Opening into the tympanic membrane, usually as a result of surgery.

Otoplasty. Surgical repair of a deformed pinna.

Ptosis correction. Plastic surgical correction of a drooping eyelid often caused by weakness of the levator palpebrae muscle.

Reduction mammoplasty. Plastic surgery to reduce the size of the breasts.

Rhinoplasty. Reconstruction of the nose.

Rhytidectomy. Plastic surgery to remove wrinkles.

Stapedectomy. Removal of the stapes, usually followed by prosthetic repairs (partial ossicular replacement prosthesis [PORP], or total ossicular replacement prosthesis [TORP])

Tarsorrhaphy. Surgical closure of an eyelid.

IV. SURGICAL INSTRUMENTS

A variety of instruments are used in head and neck surgery, neurosurgery, cardiothoracic and pulmonary, orthopedic, vascular and lymph systems, gastrointestinal and abdominal, urogenital, and plastic reconstructive surgeries. Figure 13–5 illustrates a few of the typical surgical setup tray and Figure 13–6 illustrates some of the commonly used surgical instruments.

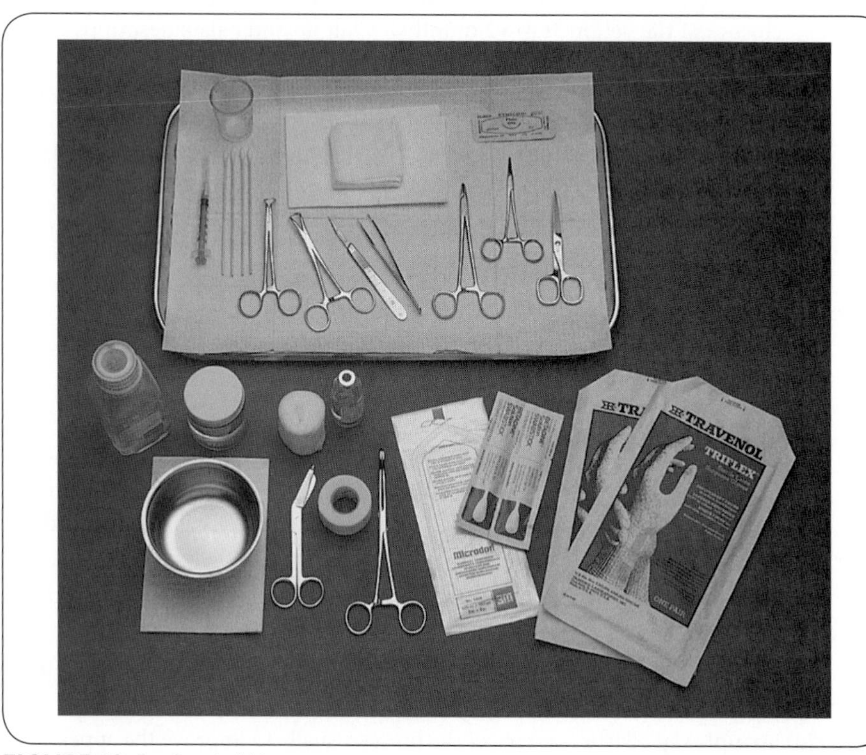

FIGURE 13–5 Surgical kit setup. Source: Delmar/Cengage Learning

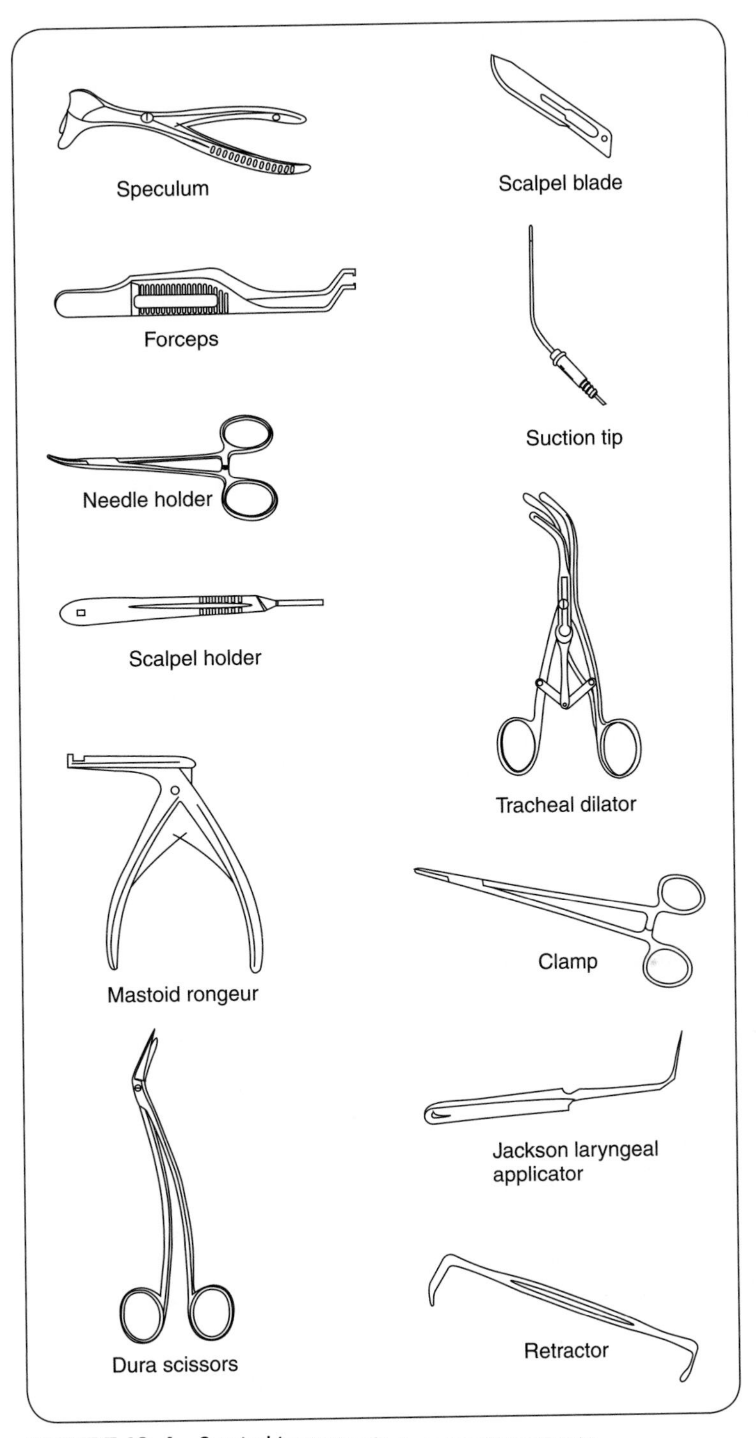

FIGURE 13–6 Surgical instruments. Source: Delmar/Cengage Learning

V. CLINICAL COMPETENCIES

The learner outcomes, skills, and competencies gained from information contained in this chapter include the ability to:

- Read, interpret, and use terminology and abbreviations related to surgeries and other procedures frequently performed by a surgeon.
- List and describe common eye, ear, oral, vocal, and laryngeal surgeries and procedures.
- List and describe common gastrointestinal, neurologic, cardiopulmonary, orthopedic, vascular, and urogenital surgeries and procedures.
- Identify common surgical instruments.

VI. REFERENCES AND RESOURCES CONSULTED

Anderson, D. (Ed.). (2003). *Dorland's illustrated medical dictionary* (30th ed.). Philadelphia: W. B. Saunders.

Arvedson, J. C., & Brodsky, L. (Eds.). (2002). *Pediatric swallowing and feeding: Assessment and management* (2nd ed.). San Diego, CA: Singular.

Bailey, B. J., & Biller, H. F. (1985). *Surgery of the larynx.* Philadelphia: W. B. Saunders.

Casper, J. K., & Colton, R. H. (1993). *Clinical manual for laryngectomy and head/neck cancer rehabilitation.* San Diego, CA: Singular.

Davies, J. J. (2008). *Essentials of medical terminology* (3rd ed.). Clifton Park, NY: Delmar Cengage Learning.

Dhillon, R. S., & East, C. A. (2006). *Ear, nose and throat and head and neck surgery: An illustrated colour text* (3rd ed.). Edinburgh: Churchill Livingstone Elsevier.

Flaherty, A. (2000). *The Massachusetts General Hospital handbook of neurology.* Philadelphia: Lippincott Williams & Wilkins.

Fogle, P. (2008). *Foundations of communication sciences & disorders.* Clifton Park, NY: Delmar Cengage Learning.

Friedman, M. (Ed.). (1986). Nonsquamous tumors of the head and neck: I. *The Otolaryngologic Clinics of North America.*

Fuller, J. R. (1981). *Surgical technology: Principles and practices.* Philadelphia: W. B. Saunders.

Hunter, T. B., & Taljanovic, M. S. (2003). Glossary of medical devices and procedures: Abbreviations, acronyms, and definitions. *Radiographics, 23,* 195–213.

Jablonski, S. (2005). *Dictionary of medical acronyms and abbreviations* (5th ed.). Philadelphia: Elsevier Saunders.

Johnson, A. F., & Jacobson, B. H. (Eds.). (2007). *Medical speech-language pathology: A practitioner's guide* (2nd ed.). New York: Thieme.

Keir, L., Wise, B., Krebs, C., & Kelley-Arney, C. (2008). *Medical assisting: Administrative and clinical competencies* (6th ed.). Clifton Park, NY: Delmar Cengage Learning.

Keith, R. L., & Darley, F. L. (Eds.). (1986). *Laryngectomee rehabilitation* (2nd ed.). San Diego, CA: College-Hill Press.

Layland, M. K. (Ed.). (2003). *Otolaryngology survival guide.* Philadelphia: Lippincott Williams & Wilkins.

Lucente, F. E., & Sobol, S. M. (1983). *Essentials of otolaryngology.* New York: Raven Press.

Schedd, D. P., & Weinberg, B. (Eds.). (1980). *Surgical and prosthetic approaches to speech rehabilitation.* Boston: G. K. Hall.

Shapshay, S. M., & Ossoff, R. H. (Eds.). (1985). Squamous cell cancer of the head and neck. *The Otolaryngologic Clinics of North America.*

Thorek, P. (1970). *Atlas of surgical techniques.* Philadelphia: J. B. Lippincott.

Wind, G. G., & Rich, N. M. (1987). *Principles of surgical technique* (2nd ed.). Silver Spring, MD: Urban & Swartzenberg.

CHAPTER 14

Rehabilitation Medicine and Geriatrics

Inpatient and outpatient rehabilitation services are often directed by a **Physical Medicine and Rehabilitation (PM & R)** physician (**physiatrist**). Medical care in nursing homes and in the geriatric "step down" or "recuperative care" units in hospitals are likely to be directed by **geriatricians**. Consequently, medical speech-language pathologists (SLPs) work particularly closely with geriatric and PM & R physicians and the nurse specialists associated with these disciplines. Practitioners in geriatrics and rehabilitation medicine are likely to use a **multidisciplinary approach** to patient care. Multidisciplinary treatment planning and implementation is generally viewed as optimal for patient care outcomes in geriatric and rehabilitation settings, and that is the care model generally mandated by rehabilitation accrediting bodies (The Joint Commission, The Commission on Accreditation of Rehabilitation Facilities [CARF]).

The medical disciplines of geriatric medicine and rehabilitation medicine have been leaders in preventive medicine and outcomes-oriented care in the United States. Rehabilitation medicine and geriatric medicine were among the earliest practitioners of **disease management**—an approach to patient care that emphasizes maintenance of health and psychosocial wellness despite chronic illnesses. These medical disciplines focus on maintaining functional independence and preventing additional debilitating disease by optimizing physical and mental activity. Because these two disciplines share many commonalities in their patient care philosophy, principles, and practices, they are discussed together in this chapter.

I. CHAPTER FOCUS

This chapter builds on the material reviewed in the preceding chapters by adding terminology, procedures, and descriptions specific to rehabilitation and geriatric practices and that have not yet been introduced. Many of the patients seen by SLPs will be under the care of practitioners in rehabilitation medicine and geriatrics, and SLP programs may receive medical direction from PM & R or geriatric medicine specialists; thus, familiarity with the language and practices of these professions is particularly important to medical SLPs. Also included in this chapter are discussions of two areas pertinent to rehabilitation and geriatric medicine and other areas of health care services regardless of the setting or the age groups treated, **biomedical ethics**, and **end-of-life** issues.

II. TERMINOLOGY

Geriatric medicine is a specialty within internal medicine. PM & R specialists may have had training or background in internal medicine, orthopedics, pediatrics, family practice, general surgery, or other medical disciplines. Thus, the medical terminology and abbreviation lists provided throughout this text, particularly in Chapter 3 (Vital Signs and the Physical Examination), Chapter 4 (Mental Status and the Neurologic Examination), and Chapter 10 (Neurologic and Psychiatric Disorders), in particular, pertain to the practices, procedures, and principles of rehabilitation and geriatric medicine. For the most part, the terminology that follows has not been provided elsewhere in this text and is commonly encountered in PM & R and geriatric services communication.

Abducted gait. Swinging the leg through a step in an abducted position.

Active. Motion performed with voluntary muscle action.

Active-assisted. Movements using voluntary muscles with gravity effects removed by assistance from another person, a device, or an unaffected limb.

Acupressure. The application of pressure to acupuncture sites.

Adaptive equipment. Devices that support or compensate for an impaired function.

Ambulation. Walking.

Amputation. Removal, usually by surgery, of a body extremity or protrusion.

Amputee chair. Wheelchair with rear wheels set back to compensate for a change in the user's center of gravity.

Ankylosing spondylitis. A group of nonspecific, chronic inflammatory spondyloarthropathies that include Reiter's syndrome, psoriatic arthritis, and other spondyloarthropathies. Patients with ankylosing spondylitis complain of stiff necks and back pain and have radiographic evidence of large cartilaginous and small synovial joints of the axial skeleton.

Antitips. A right-angled extension to the tipping lever on a wheelchair that prevents backward tipping of the chair.

Brain dead. No evidence of brain activity in an individual who is receiving life support.

Cardiac rehabilitation. Multistaged (Phase I, II, III, and IV) cardiac fitness programs usually prescribed for post myocardial infarction (MI) or post bypass graft surgery patients.

Cervical orthoses. Various types of cervical braces or collars used for the purpose of treating pain and instability after cervical injury or dysfunction. Types of cervical orthoses include *Halo vests, head-cervical thoracic orthoses* (HCTOs), *sternal-occipital-mandibular immobilizers* (SOMIs), and *skull cervical thoracic lumbar-pelvic orthoses* (SCTLOs).

Complex lymphedema massage therapy. Treatment for edematous swelling (usually after mastectomy or other surgery) using massage and pneumatic pumps.

Conditioning. Referring to exercises or activities that improve fitness.

Constraint Induced Therapy (CIT), Constraint Induced Movement Therapy (CIMT). A treatment approach for hemiplegia/hemiparesis that emphasizes mass practice of the affected limb by restricting the use of the unaffected limb during 90% of the patient's waking hours.

Constraint Induced Language Therapy (CILT), Constraint Induced Verbal Therapy (CIVT). A treatment approach for aphasia that applies the principles of CIT to word retrieval and naming tasks. In this treatment paradigm, the patient is "constrained" and required to use only the weakest modality (i.e., spoken expression) while the use of other modalities (drawing, writing, or gesturing) are effectively eliminated by a visual barrier screen placed between the patient and the SLP.

Cryokinetics. Referring to cold pack (iced) massage.

Decubitus ulcers. Pressure sores caused by a combination of several factors, including pressure on a body part, shearing (rubbing) forces, malnutrition, edema, sensory loss, weakness, sepsis, maceration, and inactivity.

Degenerative joint disease (DJD). A noninflammatory disease of the joints characterized by the degeneration of articular hyaline cartilage and secondary hypertrophy of a subchondral and marginal bone.

Diathermy. Therapeutic deep-heating modality of treatment using high-frequency electromagnetic radiation.

Dorsal column stimulator, spinal dorsal column stimulator. Electrical stimulator to reduce muscle spasticity or chronic pain.

Effleurage. Superficial or deep massaging motions.

Euthanasia. In medicine, an assisted, easy death.

Facilitation. In physical therapy, facilitation refers to stimulation to increase muscle tone to enhance muscle function. In the context of speech and language management, facilitation can refer either to underlying cognitive-linguistic mental processes or the application of therapy procedures that elicit or increase the likelihood of a particular motor speech or language response. For example, slips of the tongue in normal speakers are "facilitated" (more likely to occur) when words share phonologic or semantic similarities, and naming accuracy in aphasic individuals is "facilitated" by the clinician's use of priming with the initial sound of the word.

Footboards and foot blocks. Special supports at the foot of the bed used to keep the feet in proper alignment to prevent outward rotation and also serve to keep blanket pressures off the toes.

Footdrop. Foot posturing lacking dorsiflexion.

Footplate. Metal support for the foot attached to a wheelchair.

Footrest. Part on a wheelchair that supports only the feet without calf support.

Forward stabilizers. An attachment to the front of a wheelchair that prevents forward tipping.

Frailty. Referring to multiple physical and mental factors (such as cerebrovascular disease and other chronic and disabling illnesses, confusion, falls, polypharmacy, depression, sensory impairments) that contribute to an individual's inability to maintain functional independence, place the individual at risk for additional medical complications or declines, and require services from medical professionals. A commonly used scale for frailty in the elderly is the **Winograd Scale** (Winograd et al., 1991), in which these and other factors are weighted and scored to arrive at a degree of frailty score.

Friction. Deep circular massaging motions.

Genu recurvatum. Hyperextension of the knee on the weight-bearing, or stance, leg.

Geriatrics. A specialty area of medical practice (analogous to *pediatrics*).

Gerontology. A field of study that crosses disciplines (medicine, sociology, psychology, and other disciplines) and encompasses the psychosocial, emotional, economic, and physical aspects of aging.

Gluteus maximus gait. Backward lurching of the trunk, producing lordosis and shortened step.

Grip strength. Measurement in weight (pounds or kilograms) of the patient's grasp strength; grip strength is measured by a *goniometer.*

Halo vest. Cervical immobilization apparatus with a metallic ring fixed to the skull with screws and attached by rods to a padded thoracic vest.

Hospice. In the United States, hospice care is based on Medicare benefits. Hospice benefits cover all medications, durable medical equipment (DME), physician services, visiting nurse services, transportation, short-term hospital stays, respite care, bereavement support, pastoral care, and home assistants. To be eligible for Medicare-supported hospice services, two physicians must certify that the individual has no more than 6 months to live and that treatments will be aimed at palliation (described later). Hospice care can be provided in the home or nursing home or on a special bed service in a hospital. Patients or their representatives are *not* required to sign a "do not resuscitate" (DNR) agreement to obtain this benefit.

Hubbard tank. Tank with a mechanical lift and whirlpool used as a form of hydrotherapy to treat open wounds (such as burns), pressure sores, rheumatoid arthritis, tendon surgery and joint replacement surgeries, and fractures.

Inhibition. Stimulation to reduce muscle tone.

Jobst stocking. Type of compression stocking worn to reduce leg edema.

Local cooling. Cold packs or immersion therapy to reduce spasticity.

Lower extremity orthoses. Brace or splint supports to parts of the lower extremity, including *above the knee orthoses* (AKOs), *ankle-foot orthoses* (AFOs), *knee-ankle-foot orthoses* (KAFOs), and *hip-KAFOs.*

Milwaukee brace. An external device used with skeletally immature patients to stabilize or correct their spinal deformity.

Mobilization. Referring to the use of passive movements to regain fluidity and range of movement between joint parts.

Neurogenic bladder or bowel. Inhibition of the reflex for urinary or fecal voiding due to a disturbance in neurologic control of the bladder or bowel. The forms of neurogenic bladder and bowel disorders include *uninhibited neurogenic, sensory paralytic, motor paralytic, reflex neurogenic,* and *autonomous neurogenic.*

One-arm drive. A wheelchair with both hand rails on the same side of a chair, each controlling a different wheel; used with patients who have only one functional upper extremity.

Orthoses. Braces or splints; devices that support dysfunctional body parts.

Palliative care. A multidisciplinary approach to care of patients with end-stage disease that is aimed at enhancing quality of life and comfort.

Paraffin bath. Tub of very warm (melted) paraffin used for emersion of the hands for relief of painful joints and to improve joint mobility.

Passive. Referring to movements assisted by another person or with assistance from the functional extremity.

Passive euthanasia. In medicine, applying techniques to relieve pain at the end of life and while not taking active measures to prevent a natural death.

Percussion. Repeated tapping motions.

Petrissage. Compression or kneading massage motions.

Phantom pain. A sensation of pain coming from a missing part following an amputation.

Philadelphia collar. A cervical stabilization collar made from plastic that is molded to support the back of the head and the chin.

Plinth. Padded table, or platform, on which the patient performs therapeutic exercises.

Pneumatic lymphedema device. Pump "sleeves" or "stockings" that apply pressure on extremities that are *lymphedematous.*

Polypharmacy. Referring to the administration or use of multiple medications, which when taken in combination, contribute to adverse side effects such as gastrointestinal disorders or decreased cognitive status. Polypharmacy is a particular concern in geriatric medicine and with individuals who have central nervous system (CNS) damage and require medications for other medical problems (e.g., combining medications for blood pressure, diabetes, thyroid dysfunction, and pain control).

Postmortem care. Care of the body after death.

Prone cart. Self-propelled stretcher.

Prosthesis. An artificial body part.

PULSES. Acronym for a profile for evaluating independence in self-care and mobility, where *P* refers to physical condition; *U* refers to upper limb functions (such as dressing, grooming, etc.); *L* refers to lower extremity functions (walking, transferring, etc.); *S* refers to sensory components (speech, hearing, and vision); *E* refers to excretory functions; and *S* refers to support from the caregivers (intellectual, emotional, and financial).

Seattle Foot. A prosthesis designed at the University of Washington, in Seattle, for unilateral, lower limb amputees. It has a patented monolithic keel spring that allows for dynamic response from the prosthesis and greater functionality than other types of lower extremity prostheses.

Short opponens orthosis. Hand-wrist brace that maintains the thumb in opposition with the index and middle finger.

Sjögren's syndrome. A syndrome most often found in postmenopausal women thought to be a form of a collagen disease, characterized by rheumatoid arthritis, xerostomia, and keratoconjunctivitis sicca.

Spinal orthoses. Spinal support braces, including *trochanteric belts, sacroiliac orthoses* (SIOs), *thoracic lumbosacral orthoses* (TLSOs), and *lumbosacral orthoses* (LSOs).

Stance phase, Trendelenburg sign. Abnormal angle or drop of the pelvis contralateral to the affected limb that is noted by observing the gluteal fold. When standing on the affected limb, the gluteal fold of the unaffected side falls instead of rises when the unaffected leg swings forward through a step. A positive Trendelenburg sign is seen in poliomyelitis, fractures of the femoral neck, and congenital dislocations.

Syme's amputation. Removal of the foot, sparing the heel.

Tapotement. Clapping-type percussion motions made with a cupped hand.

Thanatologist. Individual who studies death and dying.

Transportation. Moving from one place to another.

Trochanter rolls. Rolled bath blankets or towels that are placed on both sides of the patient while in bed, near the trochanters (the bony ridges at the head of the femur near the hips), to prevent outward rotation of the legs.

Vibratory. Referring to the use of a vibratory mechanical device in massage or to promote bronchial drainage.

Walking belts. Wide fabric belts, with handles for the person assisting the patient on the sides and back, that are fitted snuggly around the patient's waist and used to provide support during ambulation.

Yale brace. A type of cervical spine brace.

III. ABBREVIATIONS

Abd. Abduction

Add. Adduction

ADLs. Activities of daily living

AFO. Ankle foot orthosis

AKO. Above the knee orthosis

AROM. Assisted range of motion

B & B. Bowel and bladder

BFO. Balanced-frame orthosis

BKWP. Below the knee walking plaster

BoS. Base of support

CoG. Center of gravity

CTS. Carpal tunnel syndrome

ETT. Exercise tolerance test

F. Fair

FES. Functional electrical stimulation

FIM. Functional Index Measure

G. Good

GIP care. General inpatient care (hospital stays as a part of hospice benefits)

KD. Knee disarticulation

LE. Lower extremity

Left hemi. Left hemiparesis/plegia

MHB. Maximal hospital benefits

N. Normal

NDT. Neurodevelopmental therapy

P. Poor

PNF. Proprioceptive neuromuscular facilitation

PREs. Progressive resistive exercises

PROM. Passive range of motion

PULSES. Physical, upper extremity, lower extremity, sensory, excretory, support

Right hemi. Right hemiparesis/plegia

ROM. Range of motion

ROM (p). Range of motion (passive)

St. c. Standard cane

T. Trace

TENS. Transcutaneous electrical nerve stimulation

THA, THR. Total hip arthroscopy, total hip replacement

TSR. Total shoulder replacement

UE. Upper extremity

WFL. Within functional limits

WNL. Within normal limits

WO. Wrist orthosis

IV. FUNDAMENTAL PRINCIPLES

A. Rehabilitation Medicine

Rehabilitation medicine has been a recognized medical specialty since the mid-1930s. The preferred professional titles for these physician practitioners in the United States are either *physiatrist* or *Physical Medicine and Rehabilitation* (PM & R) physician/specialist. Rehabilitation medicine seeks to enhance the functional abilities of children and adults who have a disabling impairment due to a congenital condition, trauma, injury, acute illness, chronic medical disease, or transient medical episode that has limited their ability to live independently (Landrum, Schmidt, & McLean, 1995). Medical rehabilitation is directed toward improved function through the combination of medical therapies and rehabilitation therapies. This emphasis on *improved functional status* of the patient is a fundamental principle of both rehabilitation and geriatric medicine. Geriatric and rehabilitation medicine place a strong emphasis on improving functional status and *quality of life* through multidisciplinary and, in some settings, interdisciplinary management. The management plans in rehabilitation and geriatric medicine nearly always incorporate and place the goals and wishes of the patient and the family or caregivers ahead of the goals of the care team. One of the key differences between PM & R and geriatrics compared to most other medical specialties, with the exception of disciplines such as Behavioral Neurology and Psychiatry, is the use of functional, quality of life, and behavioral measurement scales to evaluate the status of the patient and the treatment outcomes. Some of the instruments and screening tests one finds frequently in rehabilitation and geriatric services are discussed in Chapter 4, in Section III, Mental Status Examination. Additional examples of rating scale instruments are provided later in this chapter.

B. Neurologic Rehabilitation

One of the most exciting advances in rehabilitation today is the science and practice of **neurologic rehabilitation**. Neurologic rehabilitation applies research from an array of neurosciences concerned with the recovery of function following injury to the nervous system. This research examines the plasticity of normal and damaged tissues in the CNS, mechanisms of neuronal death, axonal regeneration, stem cell biology, and other physiologic factors in neurologic recovery. The results of these investigations are challenging long-held notions that damage to the nervous system is irreversible. Neurologic rehabilitation research has been applied to a host of neurologically based disorders, including pain control, movement disorders, dysphagia, aphasia, apraxia, neglect, cognitive deficits with traumatic brain injury (TBI), muscular dystrophy, multiple sclerosis, spinal cord injury, dementia, and executive functions (Selzer, Clark, Cohen, Duncan, & Gage, 2006). This exciting work will provide guidance for designing effective, physiologically based rehabilitation protocols for individuals with neurologic injuries and diseases.

C. Geriatric Medicine

Most hope to live to old age as "healthy elders" with fairly well-intact mental faculties and physical abilities. However, mentally and physically *healthy* elders are not likely to make up the majority of a geriatrician's practice. Geriatricians are usually internists who, like pediatricians, specialize in the medical management of a particular age group. The age at which one reaches the status of a "geriatric" patient is probably best discussed as a combination of chronologic age (sometime after the sixth decade of life) and physical status. Geriatricians manage the range and types of medical problems that other internists manage but within the context of the physical, cognitive, and other factors associated with advanced chronologic age (Palmer & Hunter, 2007). Medical management in geriatric medicine requires considering the psychosocial well-being of the patient along with the physiologic, cognitive, and functional disabilities that could account for or contribute to increased **frailty** (Winograd et al., 1991). The H & P examination in geriatric medicine, more than any other age group, includes a close scrutiny of all of the medications, both prescription medications and over-the-counter drugs, taken by the patient and any alcohol or other recreational drug use. It is essential for the physician to determine if multiple drug interactions are present, a condition referred to earlier as *polypharmacy,* because the effects may contribute to the medical, cognitive, or functional disability of the patient.

Nutrition status is also a key feature of the physical examination and therapy with the elderly. Issues in the management of nutrition in the elderly are discussed in detail in Chapter 5. Sensory, cognitive, and mobility status are also of special concern with the elderly. Hearing and visual losses, for example, can affect the patient's ability to follow verbal and written directions. Hearing and visual sensory losses may diminish socialization, potentially leading to isolation of the elder. Decreased pain sensation places the elderly person at risk for injury and infection. Decreased taste sensation places the elderly person at risk for decreased nutrition. Poor cognitive status may indicate the onset of a neurologic disease (e.g., dementing diseases) or depression. Cognitive impairment may be the result of correctable conditions, including polypharmacy or unintended medication effects, malnutrition, inadequate hydration, sensory losses, and depression. Muscle strength, balance, and mobility are highly correlated with other areas of functioning, including independence in activities of daily living (ADLs), nutrition and hydration (having independent access to food and water), bowel and bladder control, and socialization. Maintaining mobility and muscle strength is important in the prevention of difficult-to-manage complications, for example, **decubitus ulcers** and **deep vein thromboses (DVTs)**, and for maintaining good bone density to prevent fractures.

A frequent complaint in elders relates to **balance disorders**. Distinguishing between light-headedness, vertigo, disequilibrium, and gait disturbances is essential to defining the treatment course. **Balance function testing** by an audiologist can identify vestibular dysfunction and risk for falls. Along with the increased risk for having more than one serious, chronic medical disease (such as heart disease, hypertension, arthritis, diabetes, or cancer), aging brings special medical risks, some of which are correctable or controllable. The fundamental goals of the geriatrician, beyond the medical management of the patient's chronic diseases, is improving the patient's sensory, cognitive, and mobility status to increase independent functioning and delay or prevent the onset of frailty in the elderly. Thus, audiology and speech-language pathology services, along with rehabilitation therapies, are often a part of the management plans.

D. Functional Ratings in Rehabilitation and Geriatric Medicine

Although rehabilitation and geriatric medicine require the use of objective laboratory and impairment measurement data (e.g., blood chemistries, goniometric measurements of grip strength), these specialties also measure quality of life, functional independence, self-perceptions of health, and patient and family satisfaction. Functional status of mobility, ADLs, speech, transportation, and so forth are typically rated with qualifiers such as *independent* (no assistance from others is required), *with supervision* (stating how much and in what manner), *with assistance* (stating what manner), and *dependent.* One copyrighted system for formal ratings of functional status that is commonly used in rehabilitation programs is the ***Functional Independence Measure (FIM)*** (SUNY Research Foundation, 1993). This assessment methodology was developed by the State University of New York's Department of Rehabilitation Medicine as a method for rating functional outcomes in rehabilitation. The FIM data are submitted to a national database called the "Uniform Data Set for Medical Rehabilitation." Eighteen functional status variables are rated by seven qualifiers from "complete independence" (7) to "total assistance" (1) (SUNY Research Foundation, 1993). Another rating measure that is an adaptation of the FIM for head-injured patients adds ratings for parameters related to cognitive, behavioral, communication, and community functioning and is called the ***Functional Assessment Measure (FAM)*** (Hall, Hamilton, Gordon, & Zasler, 1993; Hawley, Taylor, Hellawell, & Pentland, 1999). The pediatric rehabilitation version of the FIM is the ***Wee FIM*** (Msall et al., 1994; SUNY Research Foundation, 1991). In addition to the Wee FIM, pediatric rehabilitation programs may use a rating scale called the ***Pediatric Evaluation of Disability Inventory (PEDI)*** (Haley, Coster, Ludlow, Haltiwanter, & Andrellos, 1992), which rates self-care, mobility, and social functions. That instrument was designed for children aged 6 months through 7.5 years.

A popular rating scale in rehabilitation and geriatric medicine is the **SF-36** (Ware & Sherbourne, 1992), which assesses physical status, role limitations due to physical and emotional problems, social functioning, general mental health, pain level, energy and fatigue, and general health perceptions. This 36-item scale has good interrater reliability and is frequently encountered in medical rehabilitation and geriatric inpatient programs (Frattali, 1998). Also widely used in rehabilitation facilities is the ***Level of Rehabilitation Scale – III (LORS III)*** (Parkside Associates, 1996), which rates ADLs, mobility, communication, and cognitive abilities.

V. BIOMEDICAL ETHICS

At some point in their careers, medical SLPs are highly likely to encounter ethical decisions and dilemmas. One of the sources for guidance in biomedical ethics related specifically to SLP practices is found in a chapter by Strand, Yorkston, and Miller (2007). Strand and colleagues review the basic principles of ethics that can guide the practitioner's behavior, including **autonomy** (the right to self-determination), **beneficence** and **nonmaleficence** (doing what is kind and merciful along with doing no harm), **justice** (doing what is fair), **veracity** (telling the truth), **confidentiality** (protecting confidences), and **fidelity** (keeping promises and agreements). Dilemmas arise when one ethical principle or proscription is inconsistent with another. For example, a dilemma may result from the desire to allow the patient his or her autonomy if that is different from what the team feels is more likely to be of benefit. Ethical care questions and dilemmas arise in clinical practices across the age span, but they are particularly present and salient in nursing home settings, where patients may have cognitive or communicative impairments and cannot express their preferences. Such dilemmas occur whenever health care providers are caught between the facility's policies and procedures, the families' wishes, the patients' wishes, or their profession's "best practices." There also may be conflicting family, religious, or cultural values that contribute to ethical dilemmas.

Chapter 2 discusses *living wills* and *advance medical directives*, which are now commonly required to be a part of the medical record at or prior to admissions to health care facilities. These legal documents are the best indicators of the patient's wishes about care decisions, and the implementation of advance medical directives respects the ethical principle of autonomy.

Health care organizations will have established policies and protections to guide staff members, including ethical review committees, or **Biomedical Ethics Boards**. These committees are intended to provide support for the patient's autonomy and the staff in their decisions. Facilities typically have policies that allow employees to decline to be involved in any procedure or practice that is not consistent with their cultural, religious, or personal values (e.g., refusal to participate in abortions).

In research studies, **Institutional Review Boards (IRBs)** oversee research activities to ensure compliance with ethical principles and practices such as autonomy and informed consent. In the United States, the ethical principles and decision-making guidelines and practices regarding the conduct of research with human subjects evolved from a document published in the late 1970s, known as **"The Belmont Report"** (The Belmont Report, 1979). Research subjects and patients undergoing both experimental and tested medical/surgical procedures are given the opportunity to express their wishes, to acknowledge that they understand the risks and benefits of procedures, and to decline a procedure or to participate in an investigation. These "patient rights and responsibilities" support an important role for SLPs, who can help ensure that communicatively impaired patients understand the risks and benefits of a procedure, that they can express their preferences, and that they are able to give informed consent.

VI. END OF LIFE

Medical therapies and technology are largely directed toward saving lives and seeking a cure for diseases. The consequences of that technology are seen throughout the age spectrum—increased survivability of very low birth weight neonates and survival of adults who have suffered devastating injuries or diseases (such as TBIs, strokes, cardiac arrest, or cancer). Individuals are living longer than would have been possible in years past, and a greater number of geriatric patients are surviving to reach *frailty* within their 9th and 10th decades of life. Despite advances in medical technologies, death can be the consequence of many of the diseases and disorders that bring an SLP in contact with a patient and his or her family. SLPs, like other health care providers, must be prepared to face the impending end of life or sudden death of one of their patients. The impending or ultimate death of a patient can bring an emotional burden to every member of the health care team, particularly those who have grown close to the patient or the family. Clinicians who work in neonatal intensive care units, trauma wards, cancer services, burn units, amyotrophic lateral sclerosis (ALS) teams, or nursing homes are likely to have experienced times when they have grieved the loss of a patient, and they often will have grieved along with family members and other members of the care team. One cannot enter a profession that requires us to communicate empathy and not feel sad when a patient, regardless of the age, dies.

Health care providers may be aided in these situations by having considered their own feelings about death and dying. One way to clarify and objectify personal feelings about death is to prepare a living will or advance medical directives for oneself. The preparation of these documents requires asking questions such as: "Would I want to know if I had a terminal condition? What events would I want to control? In what, if any, circumstances would I want to have life-supportive technologies used? Who do I want to make decisions for me? Where would I prefer to die? What fears do I have?" (Lewis & Trimby, 1988).

In terminally ill patients, the plan of care is directed less toward "life sustaining" and more toward providing palliation by providing physical and psychological pain relief, providing comfort, and allowing the patient to die on his or her own terms. During end stages of terminal diseases, the SLP may have a special role with those individuals who have speech or language impairment by helping patients express their preferences to their family, physicians, and others. The ability to question the need for uncomfortable medical tests or routines (taking vital signs every 4 hours) and to refuse chemotherapy, tubes, or blood tests is an essential right for the terminally ill patient. All patients deserve the right to question or refuse care. Checking vital signs and other routine hospital procedures and exposing a patient to the risks and complications of a percutaneous endoscopic gastrostomy (PEG) or other forms of enteral feeding may be unwanted and unwarranted with the terminally ill individual. SLPs are able to provide guidance on feeding dysphagic patients with end-stage disease so they can enjoy the social and sensory satisfaction of eating and avoid the discomforts and complications of tubes in their last weeks and days of life. In the last days of life patients typically have little appetite and may refuse food and drink orally or via tubes. Families can become frustrated when they can no longer get their terminally ill family member to take nutrition, and they may worry that if they do not intervene (with tube feeding) they will be complicit in starving their loved one. SLPs and other members of the care team can provide reassurance that when individuals come to the end of their lives disinterest in food and a refusal to eat is not "starvation" but rather a normal part of the "shutting down" process.

The SLP who is working with the patient, family, medical team, and, ideally, a palliative medicine consultant can help sort out the patient's questions, concerns, and preferences and help the team meet its ethical obligations in ensuring that the patient's rights to autonomy, self-determination, and dignity have been respected.

VII. CLINICAL COMPETENCIES

The learner outcomes, skills, and competencies gained from information contained in this chapter include the ability to:

- Read, interpret, and use terminology and abbreviations encountered in rehabilitation and geriatric medicine.
- Describe the fundamental principles and practices that are shared by rehabilitation and geriatric medicine.
- List commonly encountered functional rating scales that are used in rehabilitation and geriatric medicine.
- Identify the ethical principle that applies to all health care documentation and other communications.
- Describe the role of the SLP when ensuring that the ethical principle of autonomy and self-determination is respected with the patient who is communicatively impaired.

VIII. REFERENCES AND RESOURCES CONSULTED

Anderson, D. (Ed.). (2003). *Dorland's illustrated medical dictionary* (30th ed.). Philadelphia: W. B. Saunders.

Andreoli, T. A., Carpenter, C., & Grigg, R. C. (Eds.). (2007). *Cecil essentials of medicine* (7th ed.). Philadelphia: W. B. Saunders.

(The) Belmont Report. (1979, April). Retrieved July 2008, from http://www.hhs.gov/ohrp/humansubjects/guidance/belmont.htm

Frattali, C. M. (1998). *Measuring outcomes in speech-language pathology.* New York: Thieme.

Haley, S. M., Coster, W. J., Ludlow, L. W., Haltiwanter, J. T., & Andrellos, P. J. (1992). *Pediatric evaluation of disability inventory, version 1.0.* Boston: New England Medical Center Hospitals, Inc.

Hall, K. M., Hamilton, B. B., Gordon, W. A., & Zasler, N. D. (1993). Characteristics and comparisons of functional assessment indices: Disability rating scale, functional independence measure, and functional assessment measure. *Journal of Head Trauma Rehabilitation, 8,* 60–74.

Hawley, C., Taylor, R., Hellawell, D. J., & Pentland, B. (1999). Use of the functional assessment measure (FIM+FAM) in head injury rehabilitation: A psychometric analysis. *Journal of Neurology, Neurosurgery, & Psychiatry, 67,* 749–754.

Hunter, T. B., & Taljanovic, M. S. (2003). Glossary of medical devices and procedures: Abbreviations, acronyms, and definitions. *Radiographics, 23,* 195–213.

Jablonski, S. (2005). *Dictionary of medical acronyms and abbreviations* (5th ed.). Philadelphia: Elsevier Saunders.

Landrum, P. K., Schmidt, N. D., & McLean, A. (1995). *Outcome-oriented rehabilitation: Principles, strategies, and tools for effective program management.* Gaithersburg, MD: Aspen.

Lewis, L. W., & Trimby, B. K. (1988). *Fundamental skills and concepts in patient care* (4th ed.). Philadelphia: J. B. Lippincott.

Msall, M. E., DiGaudio, K., Rogers, B. T., LaForest, S., Catanzaro, N. L., Cambell, J., et al. (1994). Functional independence measure for children (Wee-FIM). Conceptual basis and pilot use in children with developmental disabilities. *Clinical Pediatrics, 33,* 421–430.

Palmer, T. R., & Hunter, M. B. (2007). Issues in geriatric medicine. In A. F. Johnson & B. H. Jacobson (Eds.), *Medical speech-language pathology: A practitioner's guide* (2nd ed.). New York: Thieme.

Parkside Associates. (1996). *Level of rehabilitation scale – III.* Park Ridge, IL: Author.

Salter, R. B. (1999). *Textbook of disorders and injuries of the musculoskeletal system: An introduction to orthopaedics, fractures, and joint injuries, rheumatology, metabolic bone disease and rehabilitation* (3rd ed.). Baltimore: Williams & Wilkins.

Selzer, M. E., Clark, S., Cohen, L. G., Duncan, P. W., & Gage, F. (Eds.). (2006). *Textbook of neurologic repair and rehabilitation, vol. II: Medical neurorehabilitation.* Cambridge: Cambridge University Press.

Singer, P. (1994). *Ethics.* Oxford: Oxford University Press.

State University of New York (SUNY) at Buffalo, Research Foundation. (1991). *Functional independence measure for children (Wee FIM), version 1.5.* Buffalo: Author.

State University of New York (SUNY) at Buffalo, Research Foundation. (1993). *Guide for the use of the Uniform data set for medical rehabilitation: Functional independence measure.* Buffalo: Author.

Strand, E. A., Yorkston, K. M., & Miller, R. M. (2007). Medical ethics and the speech-language pathologist. In A. F. Johnson & B. H. Jacobson (Eds.), *Medical speech-language pathology: A practitioner's guide* (2nd ed.). New York: Thieme.

Ware, J., & Sherbourne, C. (1992). The MOS 36-item short form health survey (SF-36). *Medical Care, 30,* 473–483.

Winograd, C. H., Gerety, M. B., Chung, M., Goldstein, M. K., Dominguez, F., & Vallone, R. (1991). Screening for frailty criteria and predictors of outcomes. *Journal of the American Geriatrics Society, 39,* 778–784.

APPENDIX A

Selected Normal Laboratory Values and Ranges

The values in this appendix are adapted from Gomella (1989, 1993), Hendricks and Duggan (2005); Kenner (1992); Rothstein, Roy, and Wolf (1991); and Thomas (2001).

I. NORMAL VALUES

Ranges for "normal" laboratory values will vary slightly between laboratories, and for some values the expected levels for normal will differ between men and women and children and adults. Other factors also affect the acceptable ranges for normal values, including diet, nutrition and hydration status, medications, activity level, and medical status. Some of the ranges for normal values that are likely to appear in the medical records of adults, children, and neonates are provided in this appendix for illustration. Laboratory values are often referenced in units from the *Système International d'Unités* (SI). The SI units for reporting laboratory values are generally preferred but there are some differences in conventions between the U.S. system and the SI system. Electronic medical records now reference the range of normal values in laboratory data and will highlight findings outside of normal. Most medical dictionaries contain a complete list of laboratory norms with equivalent units for both conventional and SI values and conversion formulas. These references will contain laboratory parameters that are not included in this list. In the tables that follow, a **gram** (g) is the common measure of weight, with *pg* referring to **picograms**, *mg* referring to **milligrams**, and *mcg* or *μ g* referring to **micrograms**. These units will be expressed per *liter* (mg/l or L) or *decaliter* (mg/dL). A "gram molecular weight" is based on the atomic weight of the substance. In the SI system, results are expressed in moles per liter. In the United States, these units may be expressed in grams per liter, or *millimoles* (mmol), *micromoles* (μm), *nanomoles* (nmol), or *picomoles* (pmol). The **micrometer** (μm) is the common unit for length in reporting laboratory values; for example, *mean corpuscular volume* is expressed in micrometers.

II. NORMAL LABORATORY VALUES FOR ADULTS AND CHILDREN

Normal values for some parameters may vary in children depending on their age and weight, and those for older adults may vary depending on a variety of factors (medications or health and activity status). Always refer to the normal ranges for the reporting lab.

A. Blood Counts and Chemistry

Albumin (Alb). 3.2–5 g/dL (protein)
Alkaline phosphatase (Alk. Pho). 50–136 units/L (enzyme)
Amylase. 44–128 units/L (enzyme)
Bicarbonate (HCO_3). 24–30 mmol/L (electrolyte)
Calcium (Ca). 8.5–10.5 mg/dL (electrolyte)
Chloride (Cl). 100–106 mmol/L (electrolyte)
Creatine kinase (CK). 60–400 units/L; **or creatine (phospho)kinase (CPK).** 3–350 units/L (a measurement of muscle, including cardiac, enzyme)
Creatinine. 0.6–1.5 mg/dL (electrolyte)
Glucose (fasting). 70–110 mg/dL (electrolyte)
Iron (Fe). 18–250 ng/mL (electrolyte)
Lactate dehydrogenase (LDH). 60–170 units/L (enzyme)
Lipase. 40–210 units/L (enzyme)
Lipids (total). Cholesterol less than 200 mg/dL; HDL 35–50 mg/dL; LDL less than 159 mg/dL; triglycerides 35–200 mg/dL
Phosphate (PO_4). 2–4 mg/dL (mineral)
Potassium (K). 3.4–5.3 mmol/L (electrolyte)
Prealbumin (PAB). 17–42 mg/dL
Protein (total). 6.0–8.4 g/dL
Magnesium (Mg). 1.4–2.4 mg/dL (electrolyte)
Sodium (Na). 135–145 mmol/L (electrolyte)
Transaminase (AST, SGOT). 0–50 units/L (enzyme)
(Blood) Urea nitrogen (BUN). 5–25 mg/dL (hydration, kidney function)

B. Blood Gases

HCO_3. –23 to –25 mmol/L
Oxygen saturation (arterial) (O_2 sat.). 90–100%
Partial pressure of arterial carbon dioxide ($PaCO_2$, pCO_2). 35–45 mmHg
Partial pressure of arterial oxygen (PaO_2, pO_2). 75–100 mmHg when breathing room air (dependent on age)
pH. 7.35–7.45 (arterial), 7.32–7.42 (venous)

C. Urinalysis

Bacteria. None; negative
Bilirubin. None; negative
Calcium (Ca). 100–250 mg/24 h

Chloride (Cl). 110–250 mmol/24 h
Creatinine. 15–25 mg/kg of body weight/24 h
Creatinine clearance. 140–180 L/24 h
Glucose. None; negative
Potassium (K). 40–80 mmol/24 h
Protein. Less than 150 mg/24 h
Sodium (Na). 130–200 mmol/24 h

D. Hematologic Values

Differential cells. Segmenteds 41–71%; eosinophils 1–3%; basophils 0–1%; lymphocytes 24–44%; monocytes 3–7%; and stab neutrophils 5–10%
Erythrocytes (RBC). 4.2–5.9 × $10^6/\mu L^3$
Mean corpuscular hemoglobin (MCH): 27–32 pg
Mean corpuscular volume (MCV): 80–94 μm^3
Mean corpuscular hemoglobin concentration (MCHC): 33–37 g/dL
Erythrocyte sedimentation rate (sed rate). Males: 1–20 mm/h; Females: 1–30 mm/h
Hematocrit (HCT). 45–52% (males); 37–48% (females)
Hemoglobin (HgB). 13–19 g/dL (males); 12–16 g/dL (females)
Leukocytes (WBC). 16–46%
Platelets. 1.5–3.5 $10^3/mm^3$
Thrombocytes. 130–400 × $10^3\mu L$

E. Cerebrospinal Fluid Analysis

Bacteria. None; negative
Cell count. 0–5 mononuclear cells (lymphs)
Glucose. 45–100 mg/dL
Pressure (initial). 70–180 mm of water
Protein. 15–45 mg/dL

III. NORMAL LABORATORY VALUES FOR NEONATES

A. Blood Chemistries

Bicarbonate (HCO_3). 18–23 mmol/L
Bilirubin tot/dir. Less than 0.6 mg/dL
Calcium (Ca). 7–10 mg/dL
Carbon dioxide (CO_2). 15–25 mmol/L
Chloride (Cl). 90–114 mmol/L
Cholesterol HDL. Greater than 60 mg/dL
Cholesterol LDL. Less than 150 mg/dL
Creatinine. 0.3–1 mg/dL
Glucose. 40–80 mg/dL
Iron. 100–250 mcg/dL
Potassium (K). 4–6 mmol/L

Protein. 4–7 g/dL
PTT. 35–65 sec
SGOT (AST). Less than 75 units/L
SGPT (ALT). Less than 35 units/L
Sodium (Na). 135–148 mmol/L
Triglycerides. 32–106 mg/dL
Urea (BUN). 3–25 mg/dL
Uric acid. 2.4–614 mg/dL

B. Hematologic Values and Blood Gases

Differential cells. Segmenteds 9400/mm^3 (52%); eosinophils 400/mm^3 (2.2%); basophils 100/mm^3 (0.6%); lymphocytes 5500/mm^3 (31%); monocytes 1500/mm^3 (5.8%); and stab neutrophils 1600/mm^3 (9%)
HCO_3. 18.6–22.6 mEq/L
Hematocrit (HCT). 51–56%
Hemoglobin (HgB). 16.5 g/dL (cord blood)
O_2 saturation. Greater than 95%
pCO_2. 29.4–60.6 mmHg
pH. 7.20–7.41
Platelets. 1.5–4.0 10^3/mm^3)
pO_2. 70–100 mmHg
White cells total. 18,000/mm

IV. REFERENCES AND RESOURCES CONSULTED

Gomella, L. G. (Ed.). (1993). *Clinicians pocket reference* (7th ed.). Norwalk, CT: Appelton & Lange.

Hendricks, I. M. & Duggan, C. (Eds.). (2005). *Manual of pediatric nutrition* (4th ed.). Hamilton, Ontario: BC Decker.

Kenner, C. A. (1992). *Nurses' clinical guide: Neonatal Care.* Springhouse, PA: Springhouse.

Rothstein, J. M., Roy, S. H., & Wolf, S. L. (1991). *The rehabilitation specialist's handbook.* Philadelphia: F. A. Davis.

Thomas, C. L. (Ed.). (2001). *Tabers' cyclopedic medical dictionary* (15th ed.). Philadelphia: F. A. Davis.

APPENDIX B

Anatomical Figures

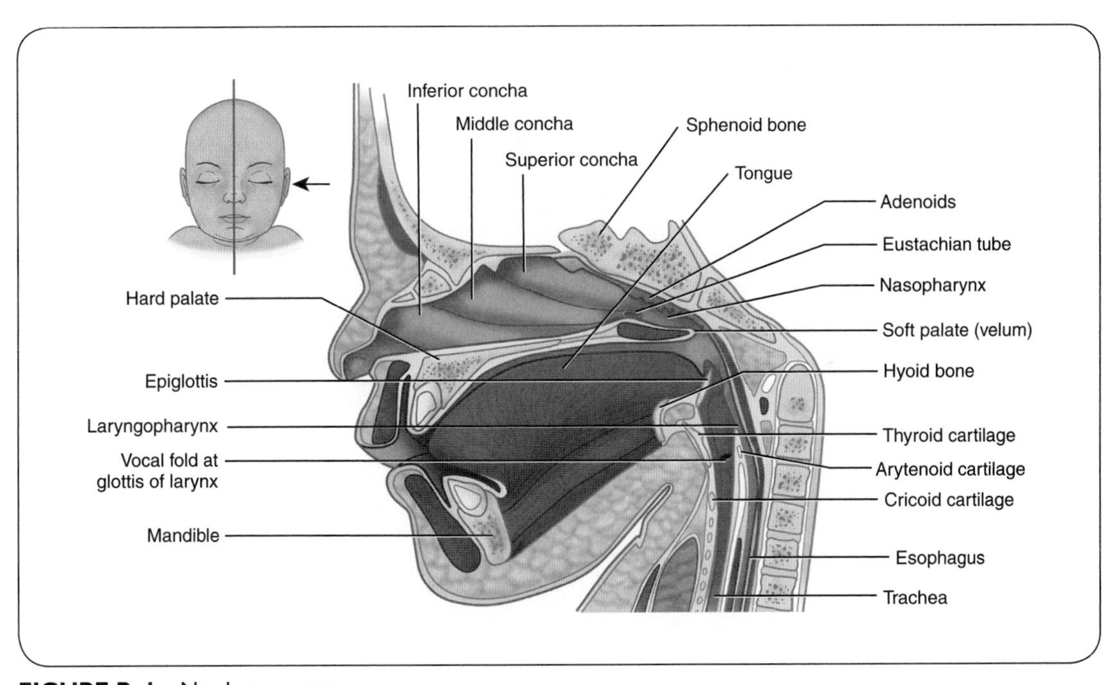

FIGURE B–1 Newborn anatomy. Source: Delmar/Cengage Learning

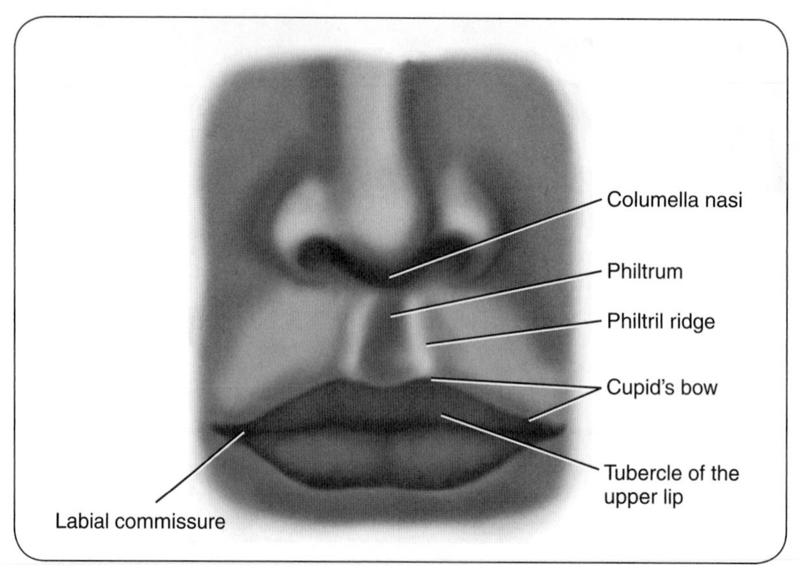

FIGURE B–2 Anatomy of the external mouth. Source: Delmar/Cengage Learning

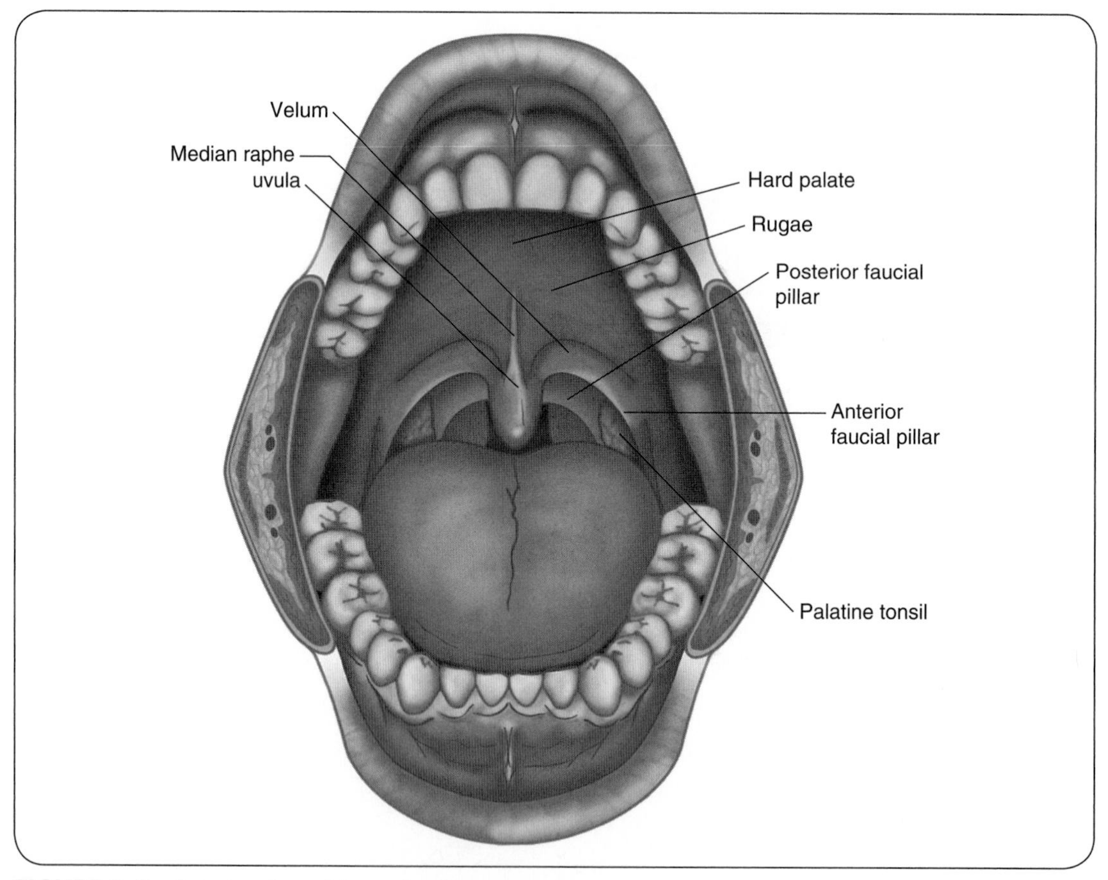

FIGURE B–3 Anterior view of the oral cavity. Source: Delmar/Cengage Learning

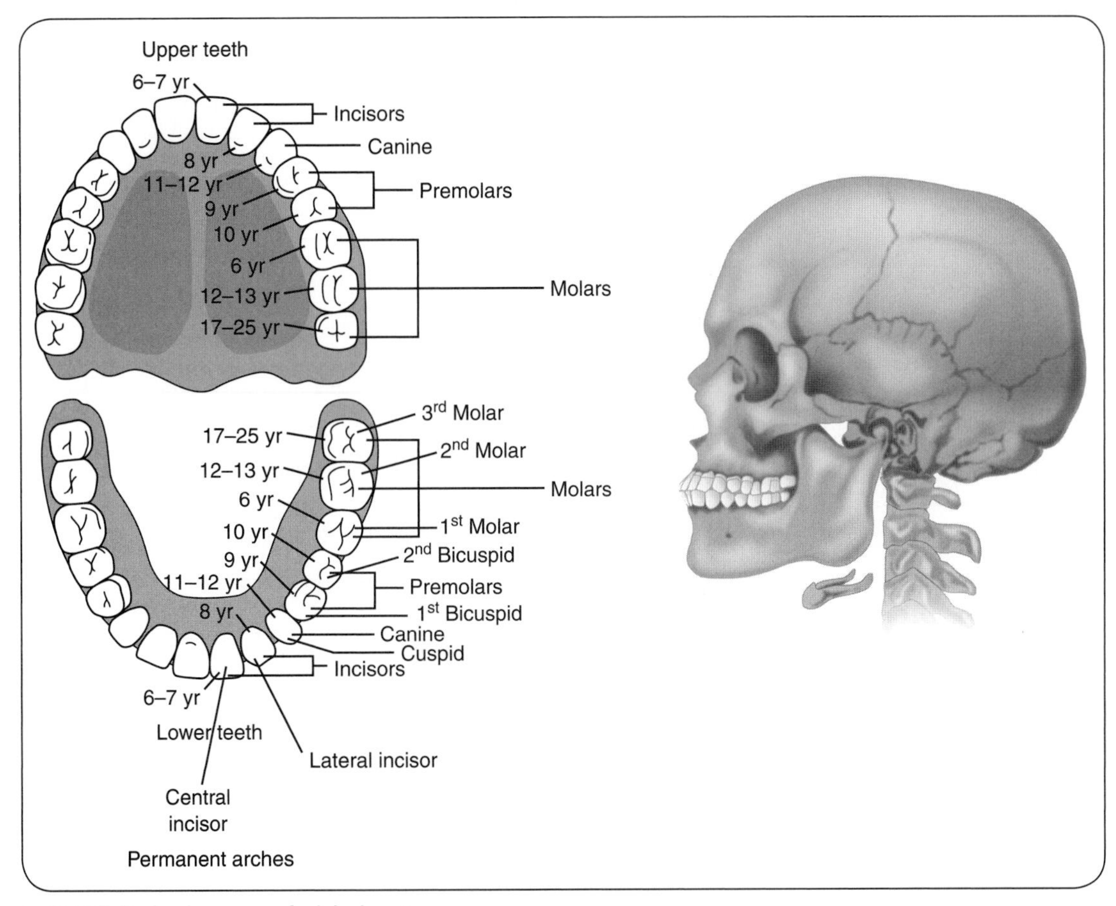

FIGURE B–4 Anatomy of adult dentition. Source: Delmar/Cengage Learning

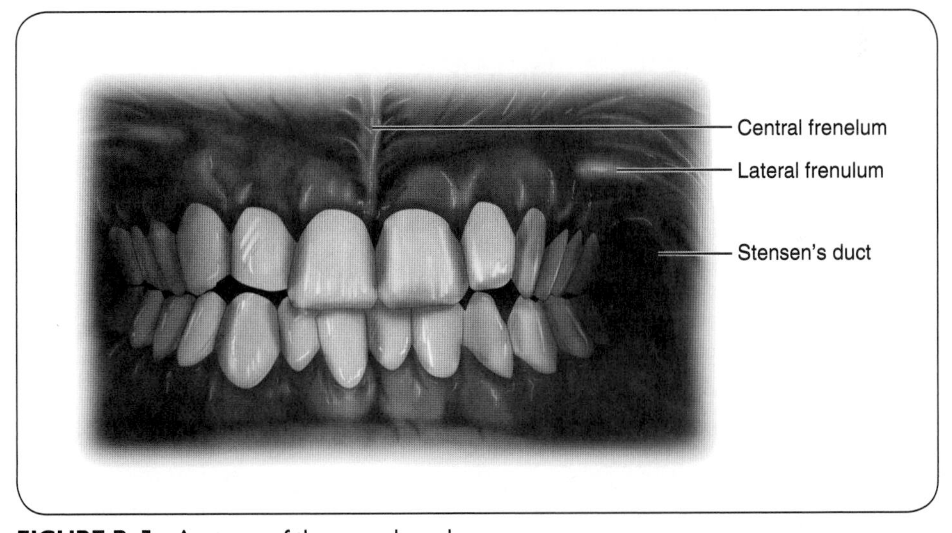

FIGURE B–5 Anatomy of the upper buccal space. Source: Delmar/Cengage Learning

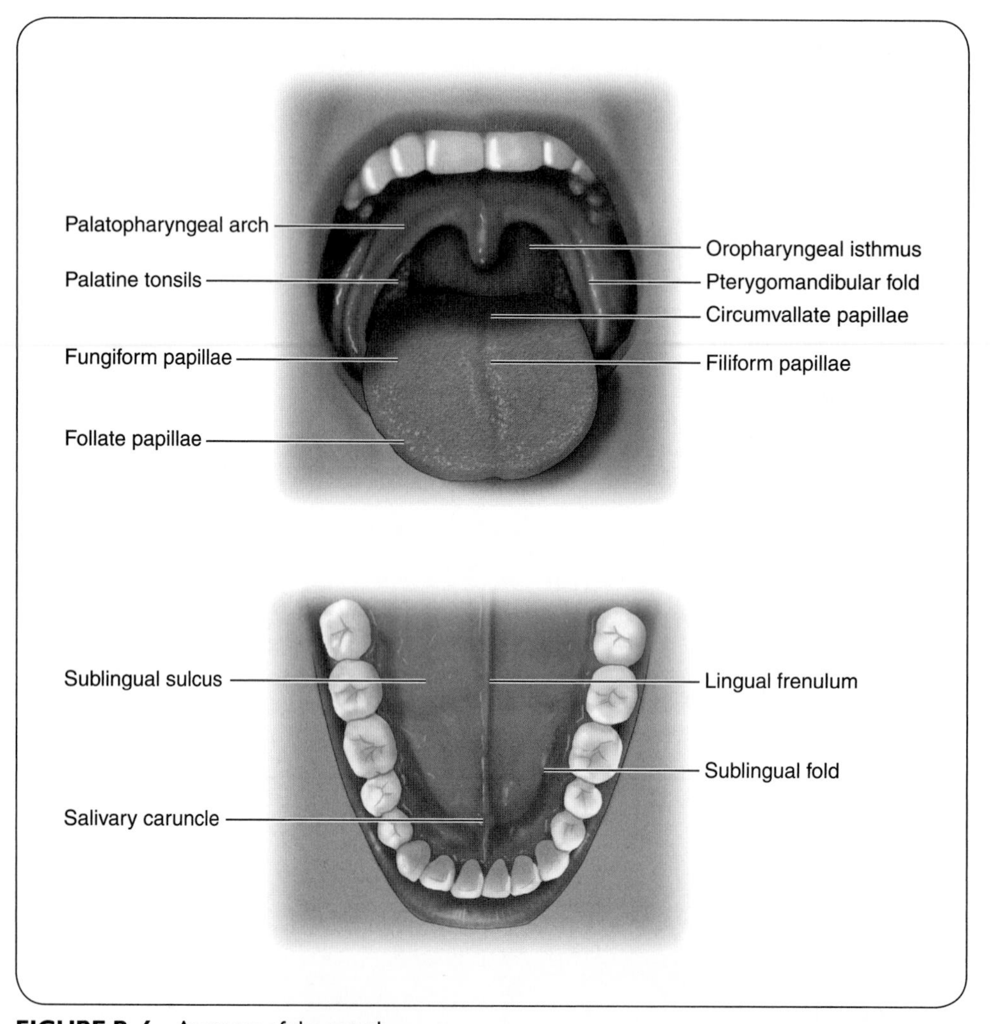

FIGURE B–6 Anatomy of the mouth. Source: Delmar/Cengage Learning

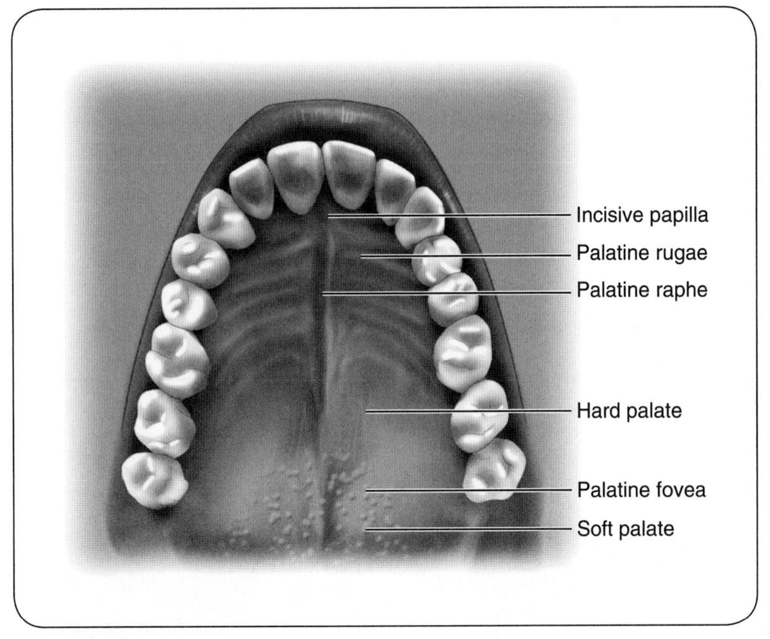

FIGURE B–7 Anatomy of the palate. Source: Delmar/Cengage Learning

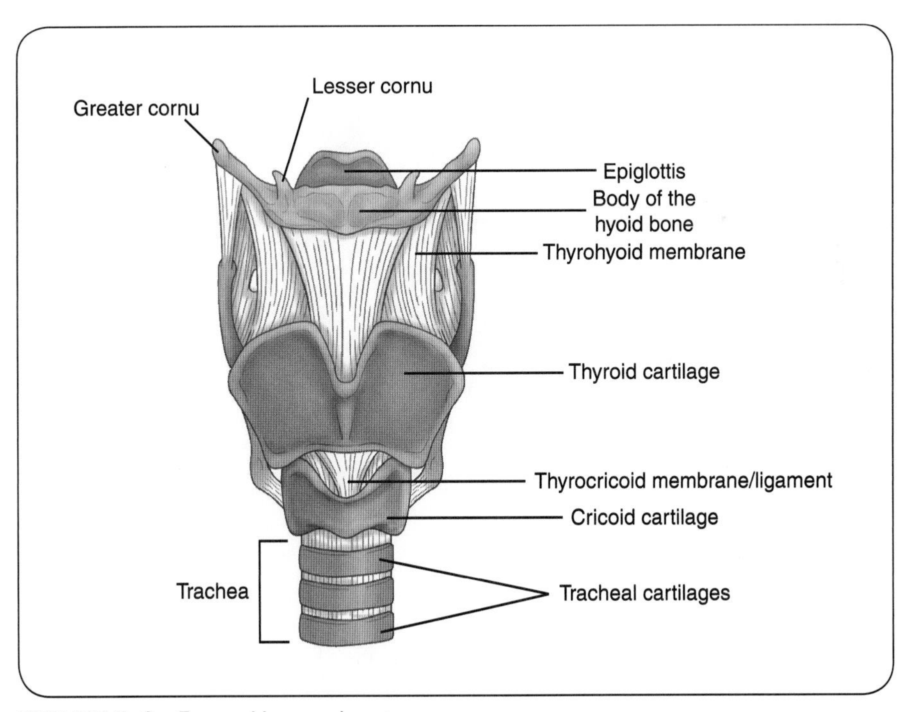

FIGURE B–8 External laryngeal anatomy. Source: Delmar/Cengage Learning

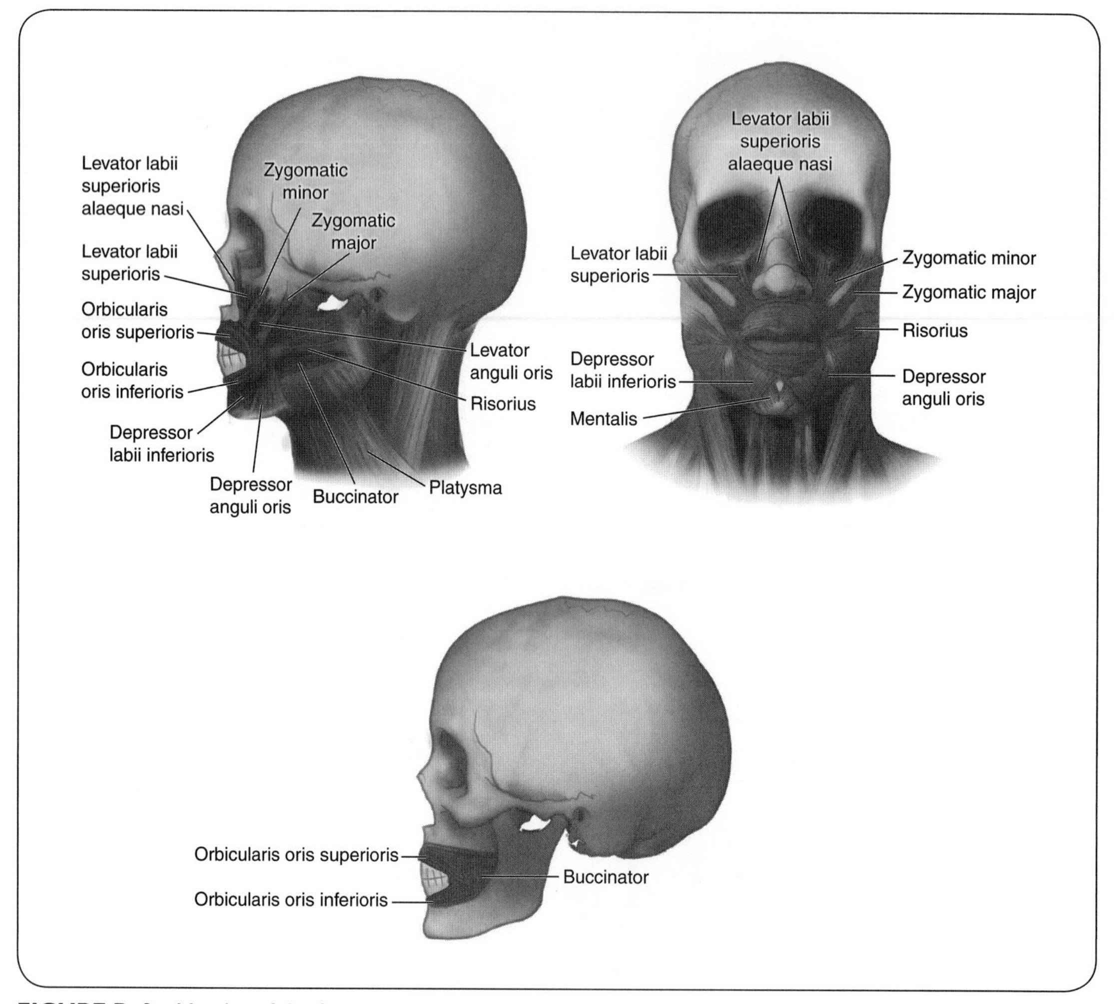

FIGURE B–9 Muscles of the face. Source: Delmar/Cengage Learning

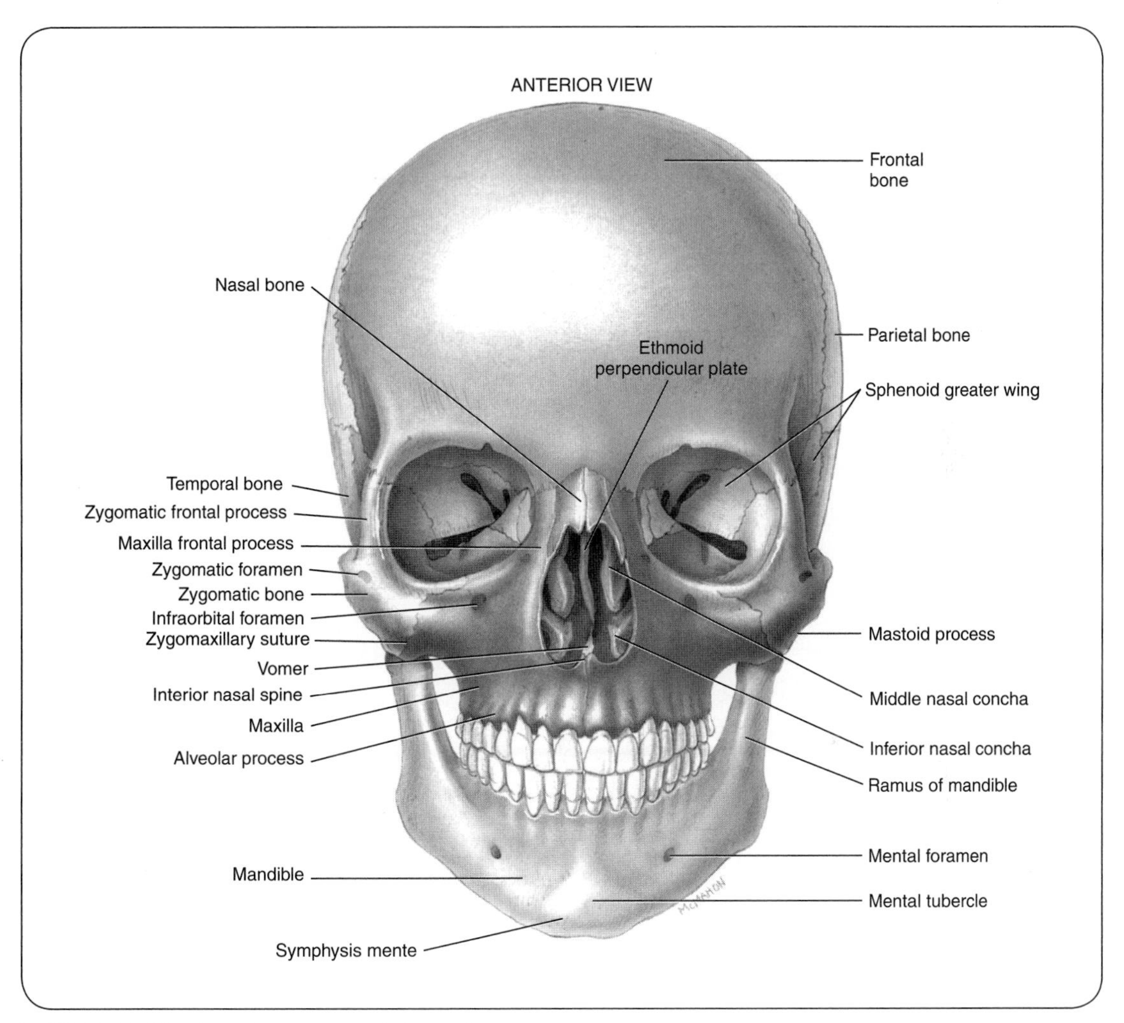

FIGURE B–10 Anterior anatomy of the skull. Source: Delmar/Cengage Learning

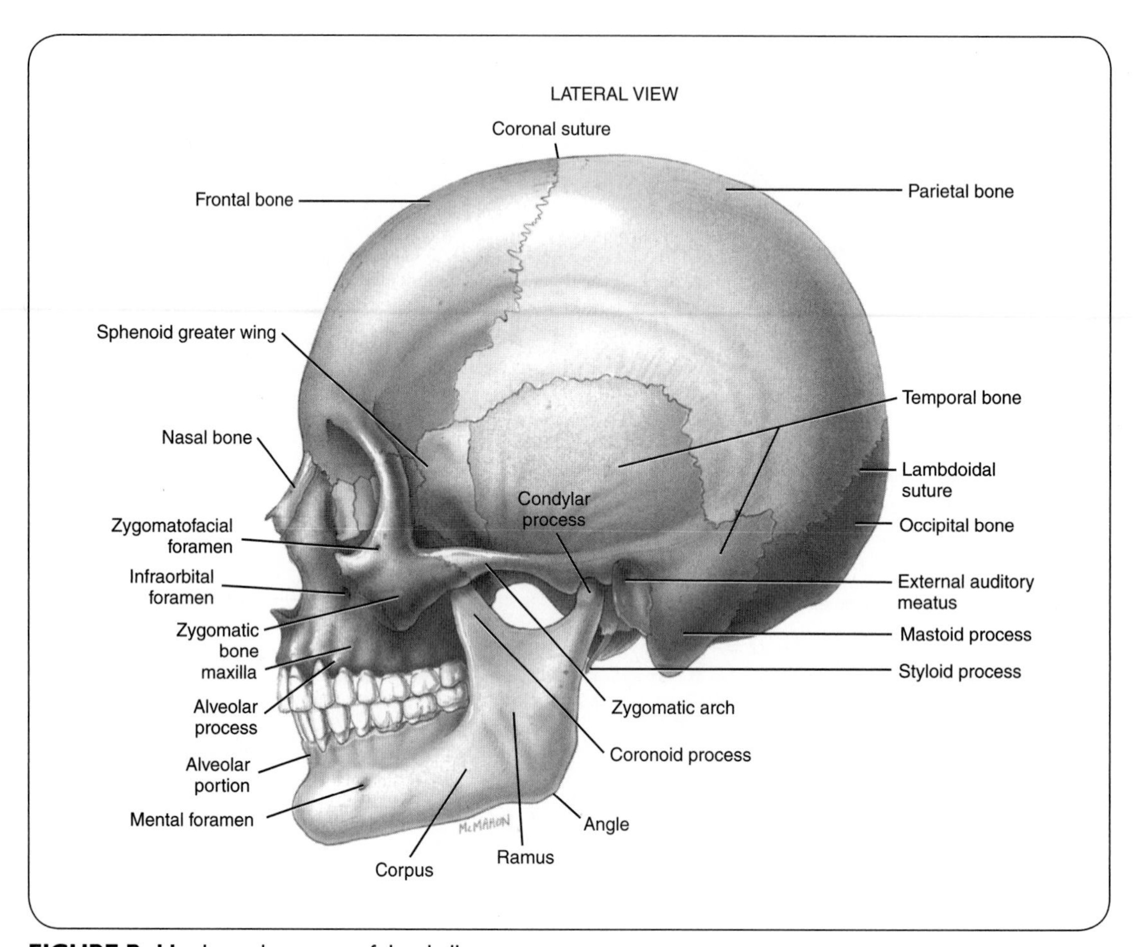

FIGURE B–11 Lateral anatomy of the skull. Source: Delmar/Cengage Learning

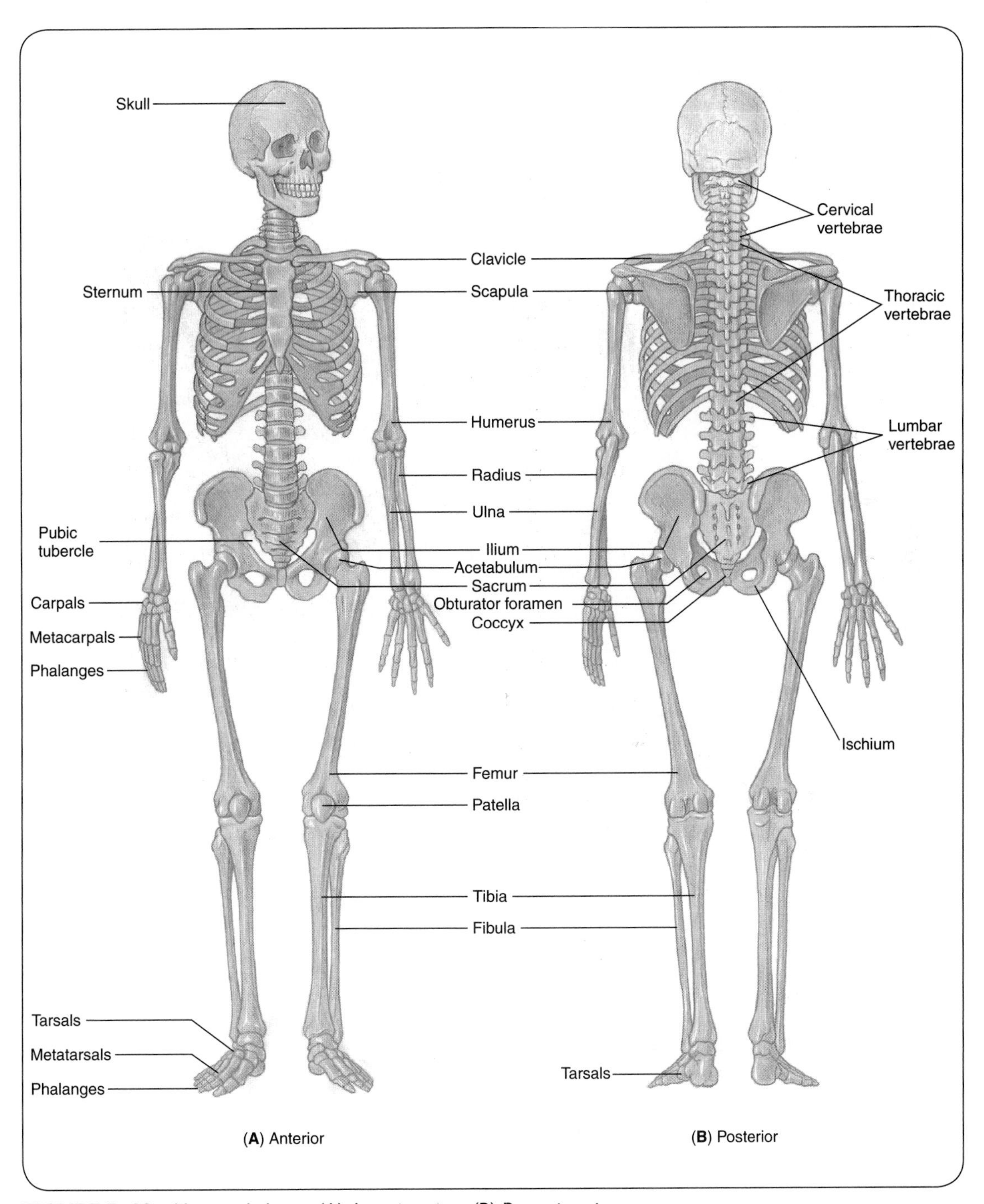

FIGURE B–12 Human skeleton: (A) Anterior view. (B) Posterior view. Source: Delmar/Cengage Learning

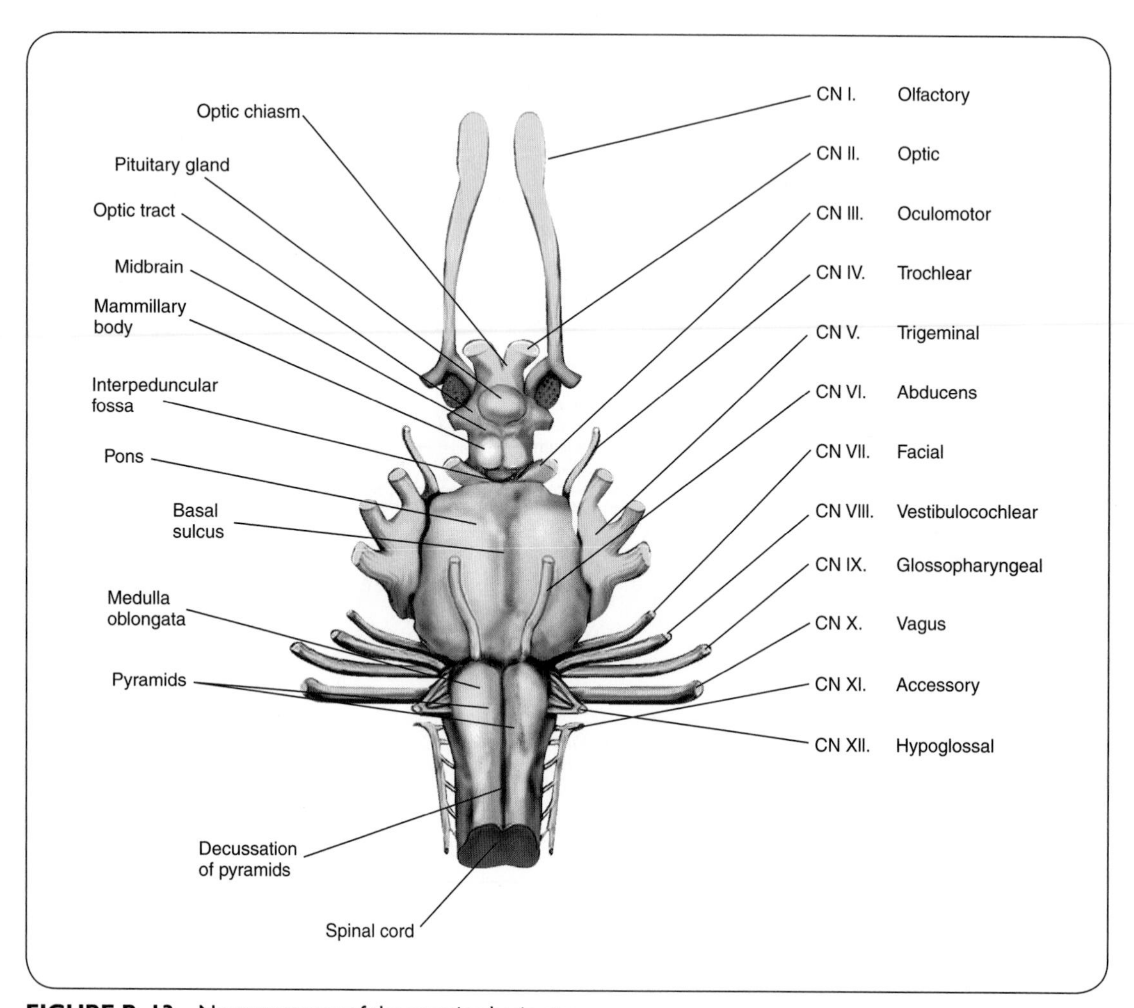

FIGURE B–13 Neuroanatomy of the anterior brain stem. Source: Delmar/Cengage Learning

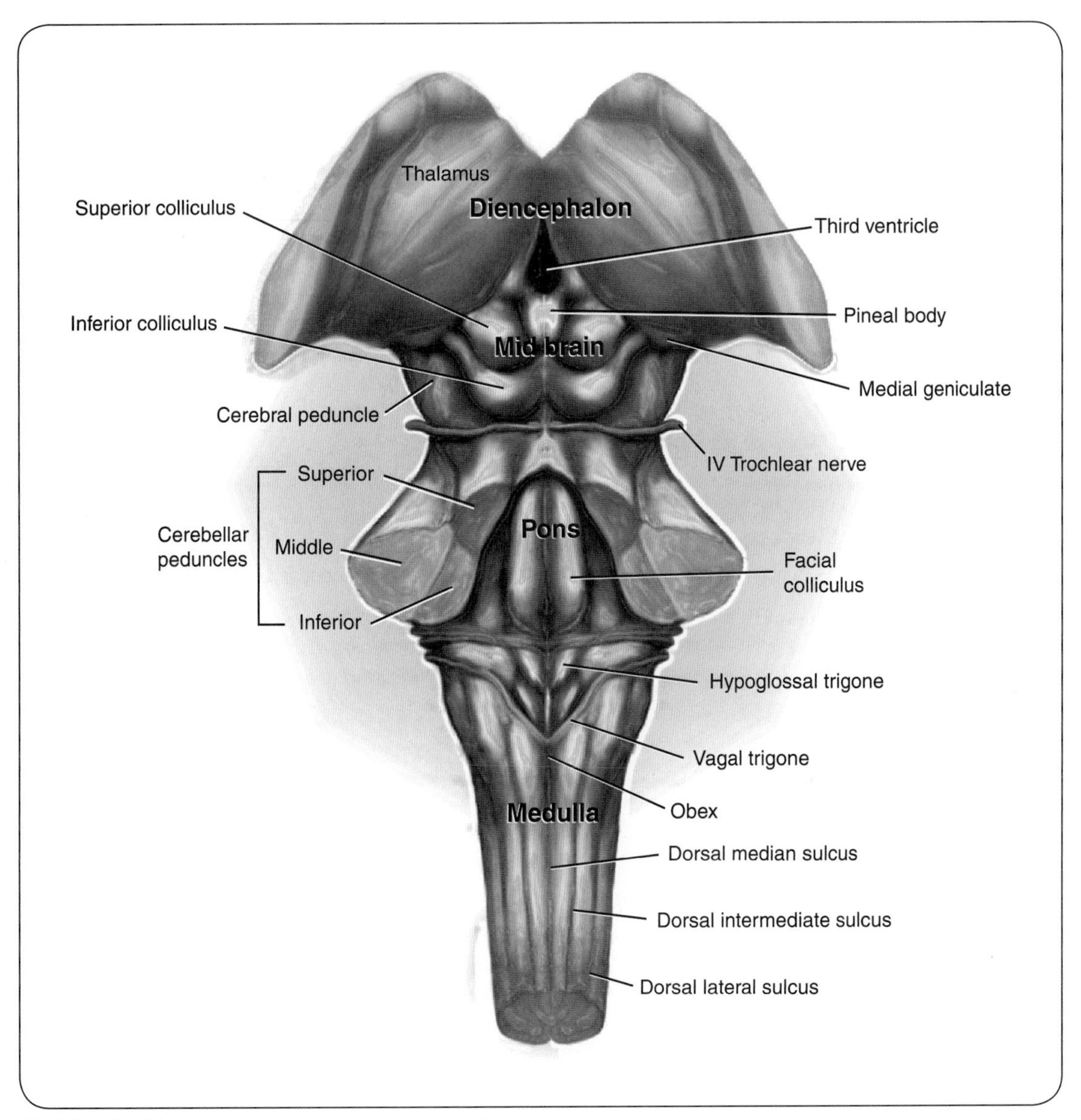

FIGURE B–14 Neuroanatomy of the posterior brain stem. Source: Delmar/Cengage Learning

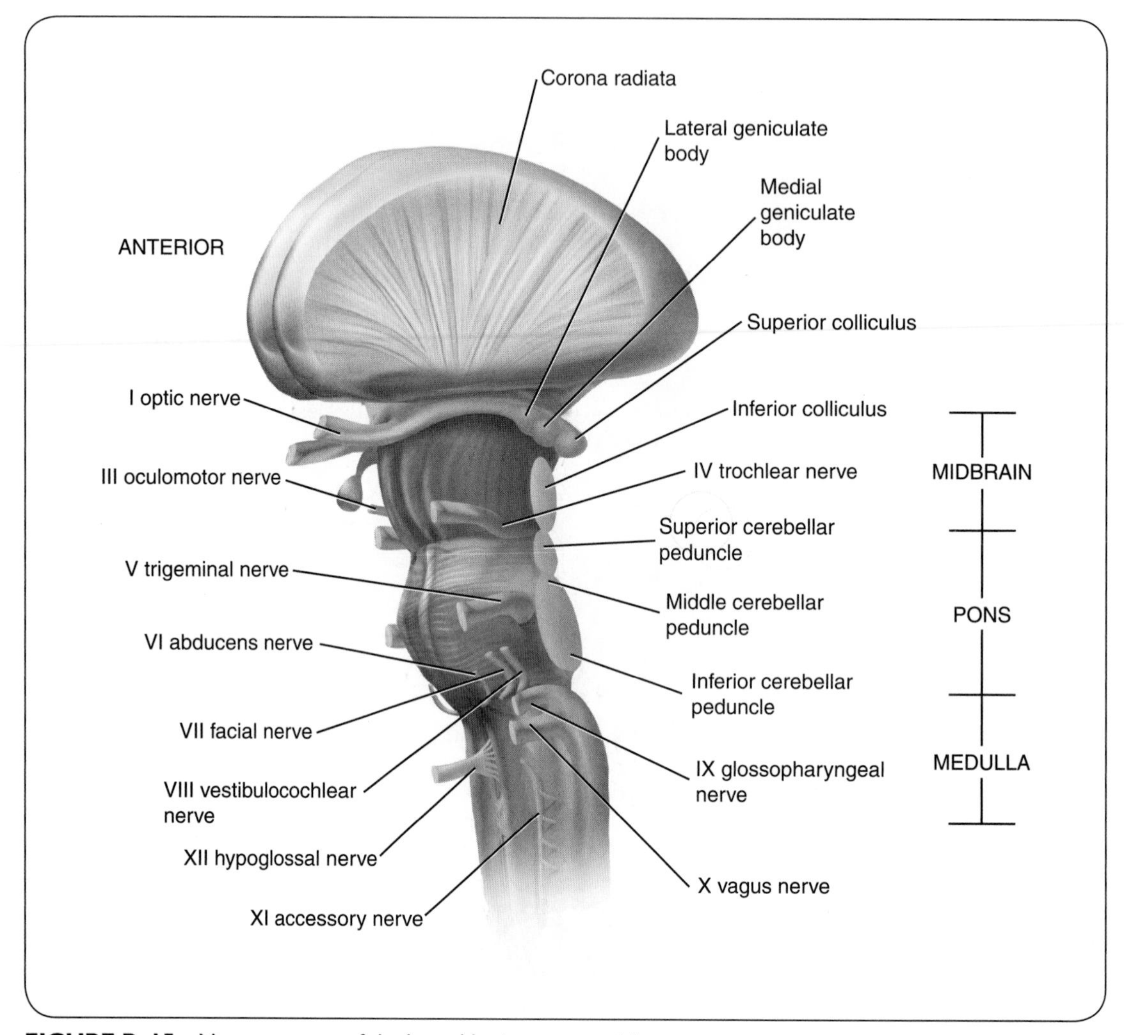

FIGURE B–15 Neuroanatomy of the lateral brain stem cranial nerves. Source: Delmar/Cengage Learning

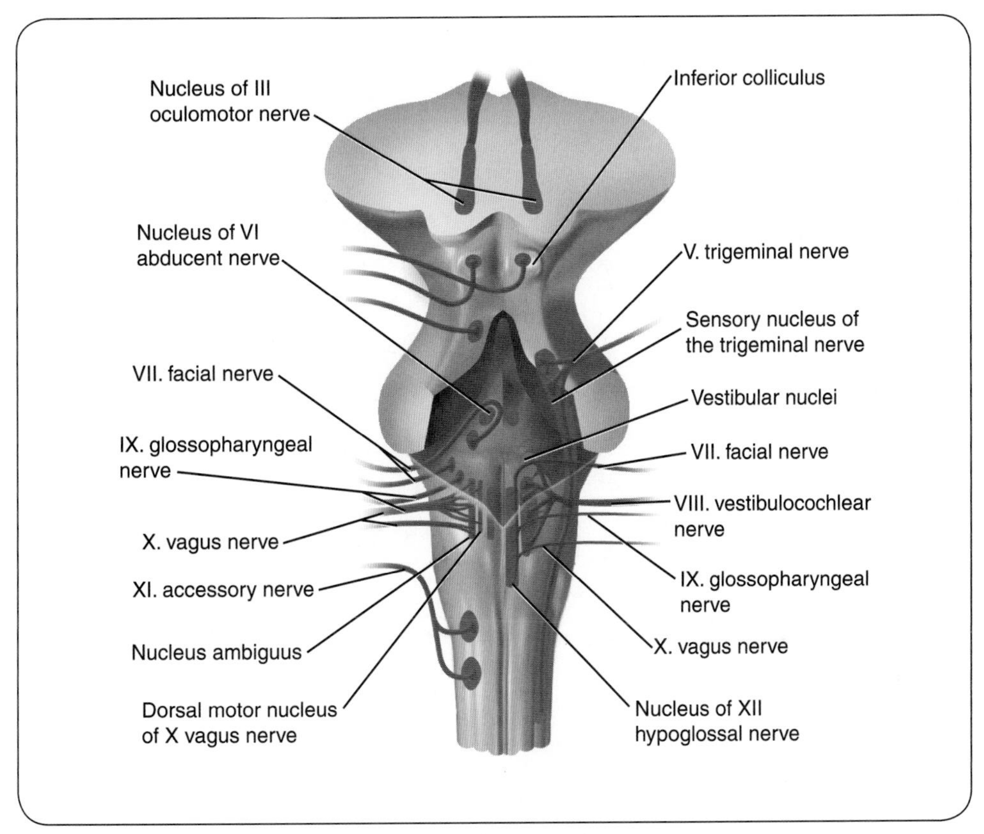

FIGURE B–16 Neuroanatomy of the nuclei of the cranial nerves. Source: Delmar/Cengage Learning

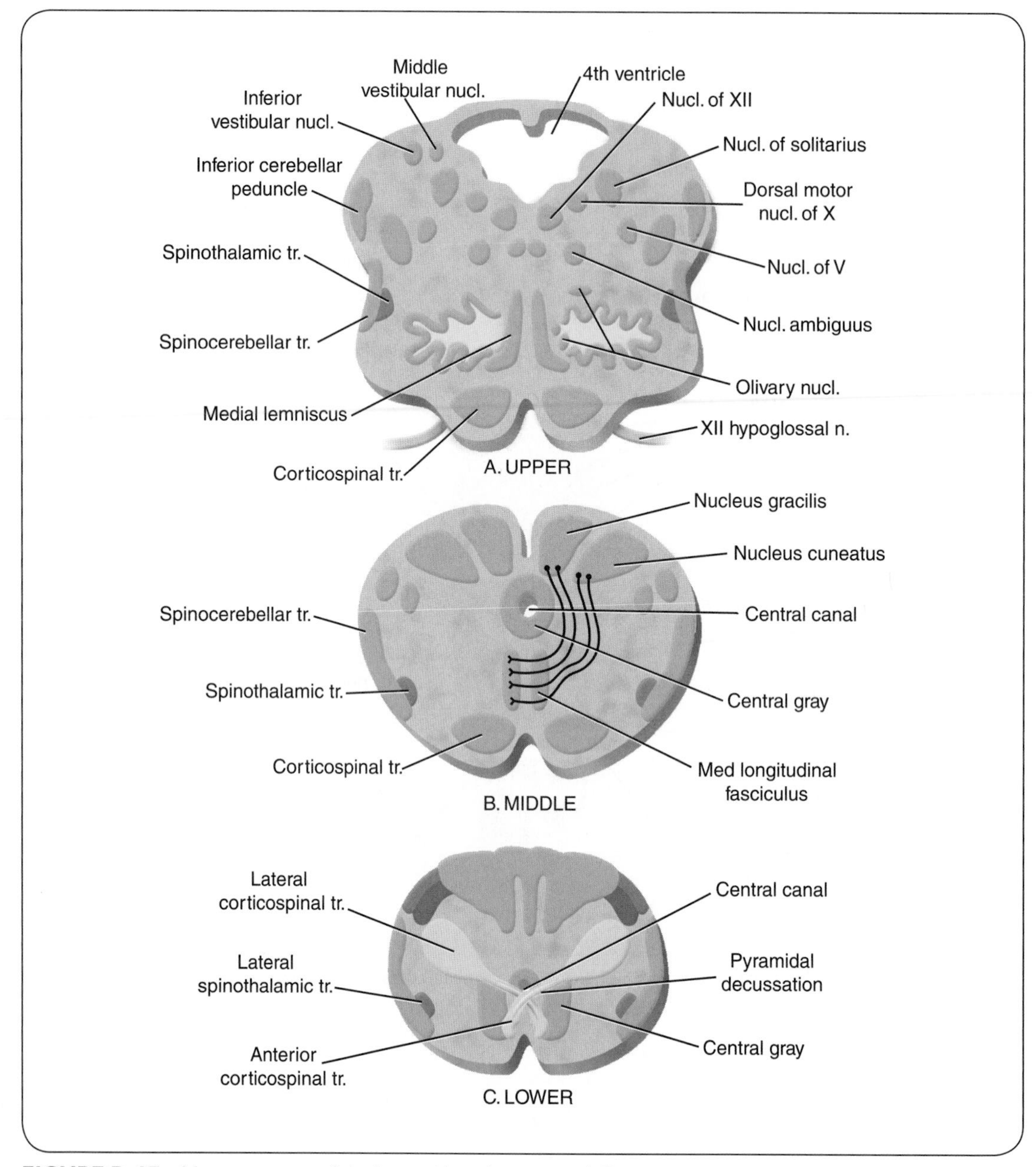

FIGURE B–17 Neuroanatomy of the low, mid, and upper medulla in transverse sections. Source: Delmar/Cengage Learning

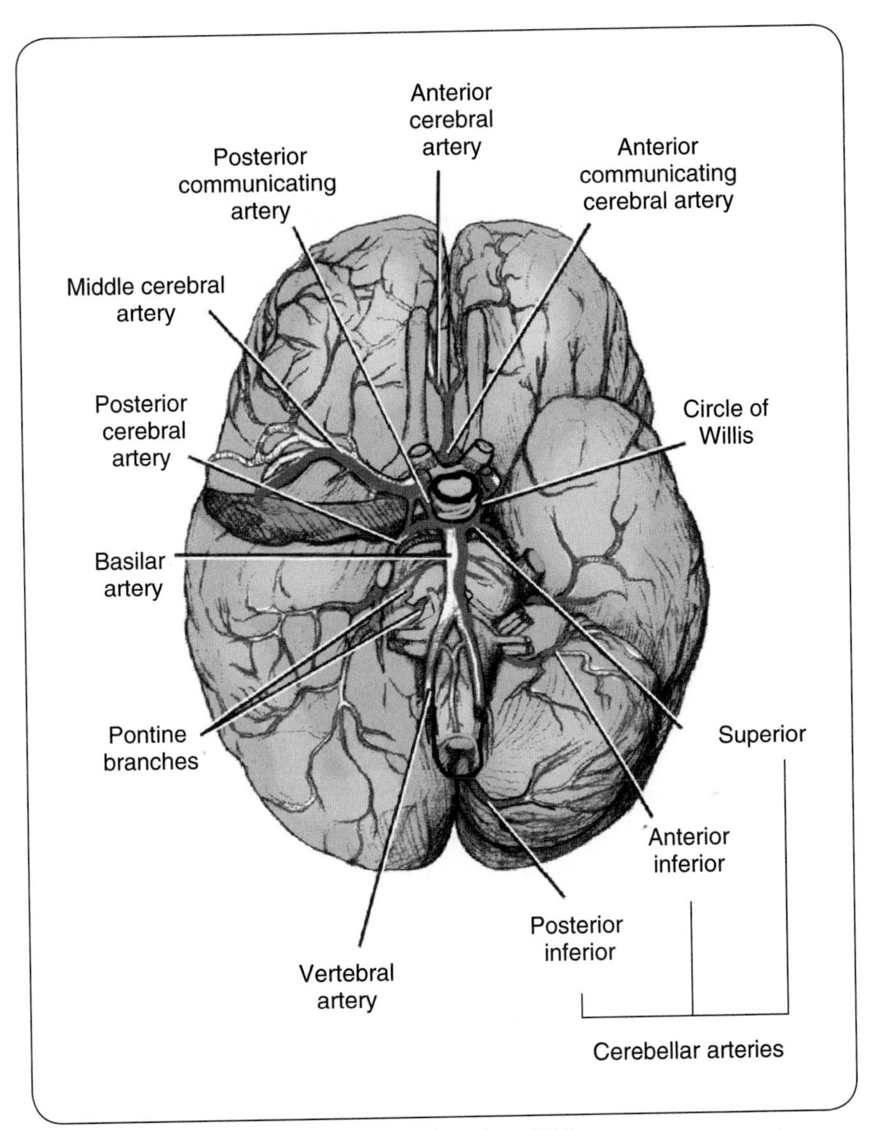

FIGURE B–18 Arteries of the brain and Circle of Willis. Source: Delmar/Cengage Learning

INDEX

A

B

C

D

E

F

G

H

I

K

L

M

N

O

P

R

S

T

U

V

W

X